Lecture Notes of the Institute for Computer Sciences, Social-Informatics and Telecommunications Engineering 16

Rashid Mehmood   Eduardo Cerqueira
Radoslaw Piesiewicz   Imrich Chlamtac (Eds.)

Communications Infrastructure

Systems and Applications in Europe

First International ICST Conference,
EuropeComm 2009
London, UK, August 11-13, 2009
Revised Selected Papers

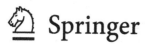 Springer

Volume Editors

Rashid Mehmood
Swansea University, School of Engineering
Swansea SA2 8PP, United Kingdom
E-mail: r.mehmood@swansea.ac.uk

Eduardo Cerqueira
University of Coimbra
Department of Informatics Engineering
3030-290 Coimbra, Portugal
E-mail: ecoelho@dei.uc.pt

Radoslaw Piesiewicz
Wroclaw Research Centre, R&D: ICT Development
54-066 Wroclaw, Poland
E-mail: radoslaw.piesiewicz@eitplus.pl

Imrich Chlamtac
University of Trento
CreateNet Research Consortium
Trento 38100, Italy
E-mail: chlamtac@create-net.org

Library of Congress Control Number: 2009941787

CR Subject Classification (1998): C.2, D.4.4, J.3, K.4.1, I.2.9, C.1.3, C.2.5

ISSN   1867-8211
ISBN-10   3-642-11283-8 Springer Berlin Heidelberg New York
ISBN-13   978-3-642-11283-6 Springer Berlin Heidelberg New York

springer.com

© ICST Institute for Computer Science, Social Informatics and Telecommunications Engineering 2009
Printed in Germany

Typesetting: Camera-ready by author, data conversion by Scientific Publishing Services, Chennai, India
Printed on acid-free paper   SPIN: 12827985   06/3180   5 4 3 2 1 0

Preface

The First International ICST Conference on Communications Infrastructure, Systems and Applications in Europe (EuropeComm 2009) was held August 11–13, 2009, in London. EuropeComm 2009 brought together decision makers from the EU commission, top researchers and industry executives to discuss the directions of communications research and development in Europe. The event also attracted academia and industry representatives, as well as government officials to discuss the current developments and future trends in technology, applications and services in the communications field.

Organizing this conference was motivated by the fact that the development and deployment of future services will require a common global-scale infrastructure, and therefore it is important that designers and stakeholders from all the systems stacks come together to discuss these developments. Rapidly decreasing costs of computational power, storage capacity, and communication bandwidth have led to the development of a multitude of applications carrying an increasingly huge amount of traffic on the global networking infrastructure. What we have seen is an evolution: an infrastructure looking for networked applications has evolved into an infrastructure struggling to meet the social, technological and business challenges posed by the plethora of bandwidth-hungry emerging applications.

Developments in optical communication technologies have shown the potential to meet the technological challenges for bandwidth demands. Various solutions have been proposed so far for the discrete parts of the optical network infrastructure; however, the most fundamental challenge at this point of the optical networking evolution, apart from enhancing these solutions and inventing novel ones, is to combine these parts under a unified control and management framework. Although wireless technologies have undergone massive improvements, wireless is far from meeting mobility, bandwidth and other QoS challenges posed by the current and future applications and services. With an increasing number of collocated personal, local and cellular wireless communication systems, the questions of optimum coexistence and internetworking are being raised.

While bandwidth, mobility and QoS requirements for many existing applications are on the rise, new applications and services are emerging, such as in the healthcare and transportation sectors. These emerging services are making the design space for infrastructure developers even more challenging. Privacy, security and trust are increasingly critical and are adding significantly to the challenges posed to the development of global networking infrastructures and services. The search for appropriate business models and innovation platforms to kick-start the process has begun globally.

We organized this conference on communications encompassing mobile, optical and converged technologies as well as services and applications. We focussed on two key application themes of these technologies for the discussions during the event: intelligent transportation systems and healthcare services. We also foresaw Future Internet Infrastructure and Services, Open Models and Innovation Processes as the key cross-cutting subjects for the conference. Our vision is to establish, in the next few years, the EuropeComm event as *the* meeting place for European telecommunication infrastructure and services, an annual event where stakeholders meet from different communities and where business can be done.

Future Internet infrastructure: Progress in the field of Future Internet infrastructure is crucial to support new bandwidth-hungry applications and hence sustain the growth of the European knowledge-based society. We envision ubiquitous data access to end-users with bandwidth and connectivity adapting to specific application requirements and dynamically changing network and context conditions. The key challenges along the way that we have identified are (a) coexistence and cooperation of different access technologies, (b) self-organization and reconfigurability of communication networks, (c) converged optical-wireless systems and (d) control and management of service-oriented plug and play next-generation optical networks. The aim is to develop innovative solutions for cooperating wireless and optical communication systems in order to provide ubiquitous broadband access to end-users offering them seamless and adaptive connectivity in a cost-effective manner. Specifically, solutions toward flexible self-x network infrastructure for the Future Internet are sought. In our view, cognitive and reconfigurable paradigms are enablers toward true heterogeneous cooperating and coexisting communication systems, that eventually will merge the properties of short-range with wide-area, mobile with fixed, wireless with optical into one underlying network infrastructure with only services and applications visible to the end-user.

Intelligent Transportation Systems: We have seen the convergence of telephony and the Internet. ICT is converging rapidly into our lives, and transportation at the moment seems to be the prime target of this convergence, i.e., intelligent transportation systems (ITS). Conventional inductive loops are increasingly being used alongside mobile phones and GPS to devise efficient mobility solutions, and what we see now is the convergence of mobile telephony, Internet and transport infrastructure. Many factors are driving the growth of the ITS industry: congestion costs, energy usage, environment, deaths, injuries and other health effects, mobility, safety and security are the major ITS drivers. Cooperative vehicle infrastructure systems are high on government agendas. FCC has approved 75MHz of licensed bandwidth in the 5.9 GHz band for vehicle-to-vehicle and vehicle-to-infrastructure communications. A number of projects are underway and hopefully the ITS vision of vehicles talking to each other for reduced congestion and improved safety will soon be a reality. However, the ITS community has to address several challenges: aggregation and analysis of traffic data produced by the vehicles in real time, network design for high-speed nodes with rapidly changing topology, security, user privacy and business models are among the prime challenges.

Healthcare is perhaps the biggest service sector in many economies of the planet. However, the healthcare industry has been relatively static compared to the rapid developments in ICT and peoples' changing, highly demanding, behaviours. The developments in science, engineering and computational biology have opened many new opportunities for customized and preventative healthcare, but the healthcare delivery systems and channels have been unable to exploit these opportunities. ICT developments have led to people having higher demands for quality, value and customization. Ageing populations have created another imbalance in the demand and supply equation for the healthcare sector. Several well-known inefficiencies in the healthcare systems, such as multiple reactive treatments rather than preventative, have further exacerbated the situation. Healthcare is a service industry, it will increasingly be traded and offered on the Internet as we have seen with many other services (marketplace, shopping) utilizing the Internet. Many of the problems in health systems will be resolved by augmenting the healthcare industry with a global Internet. Furthermore, the Internet has increasingly become an accessible and influential medium between the marketplace and consumers, and so it will lead to public adaptability and will resolve some of the social and operational challenges. However, as the next-generation healthcare systems go live on the global Internet, many new social and technical challenges such as privacy, trust, security, safety, and reliability will emerge.

Open Models and Innovation Processes: This is a cross-cutting theme overarching all sessions including Internet Infrastructure, ITS, Healthcare and Digital Divide. Much of the innovation in networked distributed systems, such as the Internet, came from their decentralized and open development models. Many open source projects, directly and indirectly, opened the gates to the developments and innovations in science and engineering research. However, we have not really tried to understand and to capture the opportunities offered by open models. With recession looming, it is becoming increasingly important that we give serious thought to our methods and ideals of doing business and developing the economy. In yesterday's slowly evolving business environment, innovation rendered a reward. Today, innovation is the only way to attain competitive advantage. Tomorrow, perhaps only those businesses will survive that infuse innovation into their fiber and are able to understand and innovate in an increasingly dynamic and complex environment.

The call for papers attracted 52 submissions from several countries around the world. After a peer-review process, 15 full papers and 6 work in progress and short papers were accepted by the Technical Programme Committee (TPC) in order to assure a high-quality programme. We also invited carefully selected experts in their fields to submit papers, and received an additional seven papers, which further improved the quality and diversity of the conference proceedings. The TPC comprised researchers from industry and academia working in wide-ranging disciplines including engineering, computing science, telecommunications, life sciences, sociology and business. It is our sincere hope that the proceedings of EuropeComm 2009 will serve as a valuable reference for researchers and developers. The conference programme also included a one-day business track with invited presentations on the conference themes from leading industry experts.

We would like to thank all authors who submitted their papers for consideration and our congratulations to all those who had their papers accepted after a rigorous peer-review selection process. We express our gratitude to the TPC members and additional reviewers who all worked hard in reviewing the submitted papers. We thank Beatrix Ransburg, Edit Marosi and the ICST team for their invaluable support. We would also like to thank Paulo T. de Sousa, John G. Williams, John Hand and

John Polak for kindly agreeing to give keynote speeches at the conference. Our thanks also go to the invited speakers of the EuropeComm'09 Business Track; Jerry Fishenden, Jeremy Evans, Richard Harris, Bryan Manning, Christopher Reed, Janne Sillanspa, Len Starnes, and Dirk Trossen.

August 2009

Rashid Mehmood
Eduardo Cerqueira
Radoslaw Piesiewicz
Imrich Chlamtac

Organization

Steering Committee

Imrich Chlamtac	CREATE-NET, Italy
Rashid Mehmood	Swansea University, UK
Radoslaw Piesiewicz	Wroclaw Research Center EIT+, Poland

Conference General Chair

Rashid Mehmood	Swansea University, UK

Conference General Vice-Chair

Eduardo Cerqueira	Federal University of Para, Brazil, & University of Coimbra, Portugal

Conference Coordinator

Beatrix Ransburg	ICST

Industry Liaison

Edit Marosi	ICST

Technical Programme Committee Members and Session Chairs

Antônio Jorge Abelém	Federal University of Para (UFPA), Brazil
Sajid Ahmed	School of Engineering, University of Edinburgh, UK
Omar Alani	School of Electronic and Electrical Engineering, University of Leeds, UK
David Al-Dabass	Nottingham Trent University, UK
Hamada Alshaer	School of Electronic and Electrical Engineering, University of Leeds, UK
Mohamed Aziz	Department of Electronic and Electrical Engineering, University of Bath, UK
Eduard Babulak	Fairleigh Dickinson University, Canada
Abdur Rahim Biswas	CREATE-NET, Italy
Behzad Bordbar	School of Computer Science, University of Birmingham, UK
Mohamed Boucadair	France Telecom, France
Iain Buchan	University of Manchester, UK

Vasa Curcin   Imperial College London, UK
Mario Dantas   Universidade Federal de Santa Catarina (UFSC),
                             Brazil
John Darlington   Imperial College London, UK
Martin De Heaver   Capital Project Consultancy Ltd, UK
Kelvin Dias   Federal University of Para, Brazil
Christos Efstratiou   Computing Department, Lancaster University, UK
Brian Fuchs   Imperial College London, UK
Alex Galis   University College London, UK
Z Ghassemlooy   University of Northumbria, UK
Gary Graham   Manchester Business School, University of
                             Manchester, UK
Oubay Hassan   MBE, Swansea University, UK
Benjamin Heydecker   Head of Centre for Transport Studies, University
                             College London, UK
Finola Kerrigan   King's College London, UK
Shahzad Khan   DISTIL Interactive Ltd., Ottawa, Canada
Mikolaj Leszczuk   AGH University of Science and Technology, Poland
Ronan Lyons   Professor of Public Health, Co-Director of the Health
                             Information Research Unit (HIRU), Swansea
                             University, UK
Azeem Majeed   Imperial College London, UK
Andy Miah   School of Media, Language and Music, University of
                             the West of Scotland, UK
Keith Mitchell   Department of Computing and Information System
                             Services, Lancaster University, UK
Anil Namdeo   Newcastle University, UK
Maziar Nekovee   BT Research and University College London, UK
Augusto Neto   Institute of Telecommunications, Universidade de
                             Aveiro, Portugal
P. Nithiarasu   Civil and Computational Engineering Centre,
                             Swansea University, UK
Salah Obayya   Faculty of Advanced Technology, University of
                             Glamorgan, UK
Patrick Olivier   Newcastle University, UK
Antonio Orlando   Civil and Computational Engineering Centre,
                             Swansea University, UK
John Polak   Head of CTS, Imperial College London, UK
Mustafizur Rahman   University of Oxford, UK
Soren Riis   Queen Mary, University of London, UK
Thomas C. Schmidt   HAW Hamburg, Germany
Huseyin Seker   De Montfort University, UK
Kandeepan
   Sithamparanathan   CREATE-NET, Italy
Mike Smith   University of York, UK
Tony Solomonides   University of the West of England, UK
Peter Stoker   General Motors Europe Engineering

Table of Contents

Emerging Infrastructure and Technologies I

Emerging Infrastructure and Technologies II

Intelligent Transportation Systems (ITS)

Intelligent Healthcare Systems (IHS)

Work-in-Progress and Short Papers

Emerging Infrastructure
and Technologies I

Building Digital Economy – The Research Councils Programme and the Vision

John Hand

Head of Research Councils UK Digital Economy Programme, UK

Abstract. We at the Research Councils believe that there are many aspects of society and business that could be transformed by the innovative design and use of digital technologies. This has led to the Digital Economy Programme. The Digital Economy is an RCUK Cross-Research Council Programme, led by the EPSRC, but working closely with ESRC, MRC, AHRC and TSB. What is Digital Economy? Digital Economy is the novel design or use of information and communication technology to help transform the lives of individuals, society or business. All Digital Economy research involves the user community. This can include industry, government, society, charities or other groups as applicable. The research will understand the technologies and also why change is needed, what the impacts will be and who will benefit. Research in this cross-research council area can be driven by economic, social or technical need. The early involvement of the user community is vital if new technologies are to be integrated successfully into business opportunities, technical solutions or commercial products and processes. Challenges in the Digital Economy will require multi-disciplinary academic input, including, but not limited to, the arts and humanities, economic and social sciences and medical sciences, in addition to engineering and physical sciences.

R. Mehmood et al. (Eds.): EuropeComm 2009, LNICST 16, p. 3, 2009.
© Institute for Computer Science, Social-Informatics and Telecommunications Engineering 2009

Why the Internet Is So 'Small'?

Shi Zhou

Department of Computer Science, University College London
Malet Place, London, WC1E 6BT, United Kingdom
s.zhou@cs.ucl.ac.uk

Abstract. During the last three decades the Internet has experienced fascinating evolution, both exponential growth in traffic and rapid expansion in topology. The size of the Internet becomes enormous, yet the network is very 'small' in the sense that it is extremely efficient to route data packets across the global Internet. This paper provides a brief review on three fundamental properties of the Internet topology at the autonomous systems (AS) level. Firstly the Internet has a power-law degree distribution, which means the majority of nodes on the Internet AS graph have small numbers of links, whereas a few nodes have very large numbers of links. Secondly the Internet exhibits a property called disassortative mixing, which means poorly-connected nodes tend to link with well-connected nodes, and vice versa. Thirdly the best-connected nodes, or the rich nodes, are tightly interconnected with each other forming a rich-club. We explain that it is these structural properties that make the global Internet so 'small'.

Keywords: Internet, network, topology, autonomous systems, BGP, shortest path, power-law, scale-free, assortative mixing, rich-club.

1 Introduction

The Internet is a network of autonomous systems (AS) which are collections of IP networks and routers under the control of one entity, typically an Internet service provider. The Border Gateway Protocol (BGP) is a critical component of the Internet's infrastructure as it serves to connect these ASes together [1]. Performance of the BGP depends strongly on properties of the topological connectivity between these ASes. Surprisingly, it was only in 1999 that researchers reported that the Internet AS graph is a 'scale-free' network [2]. This discovery effectively invalidated all previous Internet models based on random graphs.

Since then researchers have reported many other topological properties of the Internet [3,4]. In this paper we review three of them, namely the power-law degree distribution [5], the disassortative mixing [6,7] and the rich-club phenomenon [8]. We explain that it is these structural properties that make the global Internet so 'small' in the sense that it is extremely efficient to route data packets across the global Internet.

So far much of the research on Internet topology occurs in the communities of physics, mathematics and complexity science. Interdisciplinary communication

R. Mehmood et al. (Eds.): EuropeComm 2009, LNICST 16, pp. 4–12, 2009.

with other communities is much needed [9]. This paper is an effort towards this direction. The network under study is the Internet, but the statistical methods and the topological properties introduced here can be applied to any other network in nature and society.

2   Internet Topology at AS Level

The Internet is a capital example of complex networks. It is unlike any previous human invention in both scale and effect, and is now a global resource important to all of the people in the world. The Internet provides a low-level communication infrastructure upon which other communication mechanisms can be built, e.g. the ubiquitous email and Web protocols. Internet service providers (ISP) offer billions of users access to the Internet via telephone line, cable and wireless connections. Data packets generated by users are forwarded across the Internet toward their destinations by routers through a process known as routing.

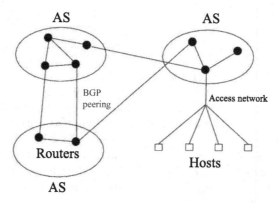

Fig. 1. Nodes of the Internet topology. (1) Hosts, that are the computers of users; (2) routers, that arrange data traffic across the Internet; and (3) autonomous systems (AS) that are subnetworks in the Internet.

The Internet contains millions of routers, which are grouped into thousands of subnetworks, called autonomous systems (AS) (see Fig. 1). The global Internet structure is characterised at the AS-level because the delivery of data traffic through the Internet depends on the complex interactions between ASes that exchange routing information using the Border Gateway Protocol (BGP). On the Internet AS-level topology, a node is an AS, which is usually controlled by an ISP; and a link represents a BGP peering relation between two ASes, which a commercial agreement between two ISPs on forwarding data traffic.

Measurement data of the Internet AS-level topology became available in late 1990's. Since then there have been a number of projects to collect the topology data of the Internet [4]. These measurements have greatly improved our understanding of the structure and evolution of the Internet [3]. The Internet macroscopic structure has become relatively stable in recent years. This suggests that the Internet has entered a fairly mature stage in terms of network evolution. Today the Internet AS graph is very large. It contains about twenty thousand AS nodes and fifty thousands of links. It is important to realise that the Internet is actually very much sparsely connected. The actual number of links present in the Internet is only about 0.04% of all possible links that the network can have. This is relevant because the fewer links the Internet has the cheaper and easier to invest, manage and maintain the network.

A remarkable property of the Internet is that it is extremely efficient in routing data packets across the global network. On the AS graph the average of shortest path between any two nodes is around 3 hops. The length of routing path observed on real BGP data is around 4 hops. This is in spite of the fact that the Internet contains tens of thousands of nodes and the network is very sparsely connected. Why is the Internet so 'small'? The key lies in the topological structure of the Internet.

3   Node Connectivity

In graph theory, degree k is defined as the number of links or immediate neighbours a node has. The average node degree is $\langle k \rangle = \frac{1}{N} \sum_i k_i = 2L/N$, where k_i is the degree of node i, N is the number of nodes and L is the number of links. The average node degree in the Internet is around 6. The principal statistical property to describe and discriminate between different networks is to measure the degree distribution $P(k)$, i.e. the fraction of nodes in the network with degree k.

It had been assumed that the Internet topology resembles a random graph where nodes are connected with each other randomly (with a uniform probability). A random network features a Poisson degree distribution where most node degrees are close to the average degree and only a few nodes have very large or very small degrees. It is known from graph theory that a random graph is small in the sense that one node is never too far away from other nodes. Is this the reason that the Internet is so small?

The answer is no, because in 1999 it was discovered that the internet topology at the AS level (and at the router level) exhibits a power law degree distribution $P(k) \sim Ck^\gamma$ [5], where $C > 0$ is a constant and the exponent $\gamma \simeq -2.2 \pm 0.1$ (see Fig. 2). This means a few nodes have very large numbers of connections, whereas the vast majority of nodes have only a few links. The power law property is an evidence that the Internet AS-level topology has evolved into a very heterogeneous structure, which is completely different from the random graph model. A power-law network is called a 'scale-free' network [2] because it is not the average degree, but the exponent of power-law distribution that fundamentally characterises the network's connectivity and the value of the exponent is not related to the size (scale) of the network.

Recently the small-world theory [10] has attracted a lot of attention. A small-world network resembles a typical social network which is highly clustered where one's friends are likely to be friends to each other. At the same time a small-world

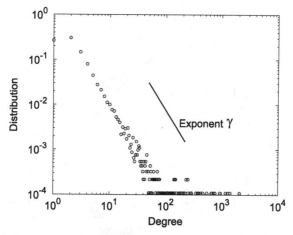

Fig. 2. Internet power-law degree distribution on log-log scale

contains random connections which serve as shortcuts and make the network small. Most scale-free networks can be regarded as small-world networks in the sense that the average shortest paths of scale-free networks are always small. But some scale-free networks are smaller than others. For example the average shortest path of many social networks is around 6 (which is comparable to that of random graphs); whereas the Internet's average shortest path is 3 which is actually substantially smaller than predicted by the random graph and small-world theories.

In the last few years many studies have shown [4,11] that the degree distribution alone does not uniquely characterise a network topology. Networks having exactly identical degree distribution can exhibit vastly different other topological properties. The fact that a network is scale-free only tells us limited information. In order to obtain a full picture of a network's structure, we need to look beyond the question of 'how many links does a node have?' and ask 'To whom the node is connected to?'

4   Who Connects with Whom?

4.1   Disassortative Mixing

Recently a number of studies have shown that the degree correlation plays a significant role in defining a network's structure [4,7,12,13]. The degree correlation defines the mixing pattern in a network. Social networks are assortative mixing where nodes tend to attach to alike nodes, i.e. high-degree nodes to high-degree nodes and low-degree nodes to low-degree nodes. On contrast technological and biological networks, including the Internet, are disassortative mixing where high-degree nodes tend to connect with low-degree nodes, and visa versa. We can not use a network's degree distribution to predict its mixing pattern. Networks with the same degree distribution can have completely opposite mixing patterns [11].

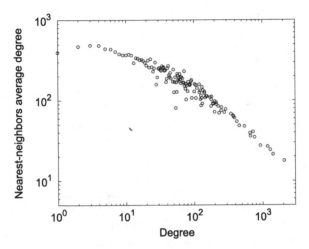

Fig. 3. Nearest-neighbours average degree of k-degree nodes

A network's mixing pattern can be inferred by the correlation between a node's degree k and its nearest-neighbours average degree k_{nn} [6]. Fig. 3 shows the Internet exhibits a negative correlation between the two quantities suggesting the network is disassortative mixing. For example for a node with degree 1000, the average degree of its 1000 neighbours is around 20; whereas for a node with degree 2, the average degree of its two neighbours is around 500.

The mixing pattern can also be inferred by computing the so-called assortative coefficient [7], $-1 < \alpha < 1$, which is defined as

$$\alpha = \frac{L^{-1}\sum_m j_m k_m - [L^{-1}\sum_m \frac{1}{2}(j_m + k_m)]^2}{L^{-1}\sum_m \frac{1}{2}(j_m^2 + k_m^2) - [L^{-1}\sum_m \frac{1}{2}(j_m + k_m)]^2},$$

where L is the number of links a network has, and j_m, k_m are the degrees of the nodes at the ends of the mth link, with $m = 1, ..., L$. If $0 < \alpha < 1$, a network is assortative mixing; and if $-1 < \alpha < 0$, a network is disassortative mixing, e.g. $\alpha = -0.19 \sim -0.24$ for the Internet.

The disassortative mixing property of the Internet is relevant because it means the peripheral, low-degree nodes are almost always connect directly with some high-degree nodes. On the other hand the chance of finding a chain of low-degree nodes is low. Then, how about the high-degree nodes themselves? Are they interconnected with each other? Does the disassortative mixing property mean that the high-degree nodes only connect with low-degree nodes?

4.2   Rich-Club Phenomenon

We call nodes with large numbers of links the 'rich' nodes. Fig. 4 shows that in the Internet the richest nodes are tightly interconnected with each other forming the core of the network. This is called the rich-club phenomenon [8]. This phenomenon does not conflict with the Internet's disassortative mixing property.

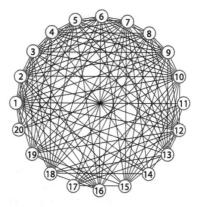

Fig. 4. Internet connections among the top 20 richest nodes themselves. Other connections to the nodes are omitted for clarity.

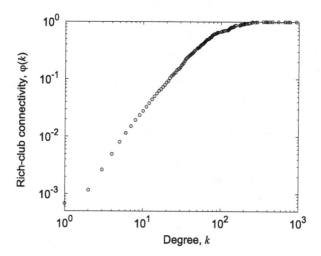

Fig. 5. Rich-club coefficient as a function of node degree

Each rich node shown in the figure has a large number of links. The majority the links are connect to poorly connected nodes (disassortative mixing) whereas only a few of them are enough to provide the interconnectivity with other rich nodes, whose number is anyway small.

The rich-club phenomenon can be quantitatively assessed by measuring the rich-club coefficient,

$$\phi(k) = \frac{2E_{\geqslant k}}{N_{\geqslant k}(N_{\geqslant k} - 1)}, \tag{1}$$

where $N_{\geqslant k}$ is the number of nodes with degrees greater or equal to k and $E_{\geqslant k}$ is the number of links among the $N_{\geqslant k}$ nodes themselves. The rich-club coefficient measures the ratio of the actual number of links to the maximum possible number of links among nodes with degrees no less than k. Fig. 5 shows the rich-club efficient as a function of node degree k. It shows that the rich nodes are becoming more tightly interconnected when the degree increases, in other words, when the club becomes more 'exclusive'. A small number of nodes with degrees larger than 300 have $\varphi = 1$ which means they are fully interconnected.

5   Discussion

The internet is ultra small because it exhibits both disassortative mixing and rich-club phenomenon. These two structural properties together contribute to the routing efficiency of the network. The rich club consists of a small number of highly connected nodes. The club members are tightly interconnected between each other. If two club members do not have a direct connection, they are very likely to share a neighbouring club member. Thus the hop distance between the members is very small(either 1 or 2 hops). The rich-club functions as a 'super' traffic hub of the Internet by providing a large selection of shortcuts for routing. The disassortative mixing property ensures that the majority of network nodes, which are peripheral low-degree nodes, are always near the rich-club. Thus a typical shortest path between two peripheral nodes consists of three hops, the first hop is from the source node to a member of the rich club, the second hop is between two rich-club members, and the final hop is to the destination node.

As we know a fully connected graph is the most efficient topology because the shortest path is 1 between any two nodes. Whereas for sparsely connected networks, the star-like topology is very efficient because the average shortest path is less than 2. If we abstract the rich-club as a single node then the Internet topology will look like a star topology, where all nodes connects with the centre of the star. A star topology has a big problem that the centre of the star is very easy to be congested and becomes the single-point-of-failure. The Internet 'solves' these problems by replacing the centre with a club of rich nodes. The rich-club contains plenty of redundant links. The network's performance and integrity will not be affected if some of the links between the club members are removed. In addition, incoming traffic to the 'centre' is handled in a distributed manner by a handful of rich-club members such that the chance of getting congested is reduced. In case a few club member are congested (or removed), the peripheral nodes served by these rich nodes may suffer, but the rest of the network can still work as normal. Of course if the rich-club core is broken by removing too many rich nodes or inter-rich links, the network will fall apart.

6   Summary

In a way the Internet has an ideal structure. It is very large in size and very sparse in connectivity. Yet the Internet has a sophisticated structure which makes the network very 'small' in terms of routing. At the same time the Internet is quite robust because the function of the network's core is shared by a group of rich nodes which are tightly interconnected with each other and therefore have plenty of redundant links. It is remarkable that such a structure is the consequence of the Internet evolution process which is driven by distributed, local decisions without any central plan. In fact until ten years ago there was not even any map of the global Internet.

In the last decade there is a increasing recognition that effective engineering of the Internet is predicated on a detailed understanding of issues such as the large-scale structure of its underlying physical topology, the manner in which it evolves over time, and the way in which its constituent components contribute to its overall function [14].

In recent years there have been a lot of research activities on characterising and modelling the Internet topology. Various metrics and models are proposed [15,16]. Researchers are interested in understanding not only the Internet's structure but also the dynamics and the evolution [17]. One important goal is to provide better models for more realistic simulations which differentiates the different natures of links between AS nodes and incorporates suitable traffic model as well as other relevant factors such as capacity and demo-geographic distributions of network elements.

Acknowledgments. S. Zhou is supported by The Royal Academy of Engineering/EPSRC Research Fellowship under grant no. 10216/70.

References

1. Quoitin, B., Pelsser, C., Swinnen, L.: Interdomain traffic engineering with BGP. IEEE Communications Magazine 41, 122–128 (2003)
2. Barabási, A., Albert, R.: Emergence of scaling in random networks. Science 286, 509 (1999)
3. Pastor-Satorras, R., Vespignani, A.: Evolution and Structure of the Internet - A Statistical Physics Approach. Cambridge University Press, Cambridge (2004)
4. Mahadevan, P., Krioukov, D., Fomenkov, M., Huffaker, B., Dimitropoulos, X., Claffy, K., Vahdat, A.: The internet AS-level topology: Three data sources and one definitive metric. Computer Comm. Rev. 36, 17–26 (2006)
5. Faloutsos, M., Faloutsos, P., Faloutsos, C.: On power–law relationships of the Internet topology. Computer Comm. Rev. 29, 251–262 (1999)
6. Pastor-Satorras, R., Vázquez, A., Vespignani, A.: Dynamical and correlation properties of the internet. Phys. Rev. Lett. 87 (2001)
7. Newman, M.E.J.: Mixing patterns in networks. Phys. Rev. E 67, 026126 (2003)
8. Zhou, S., Mondragón, R.J.: The rich-club phenomenon in the Internet topology. IEEE Comm. Lett. 8, 180–182 (2004)
9. Krioukov, D., Chung, F., Claffy, K., Fomenkov, M., Vespignani, A., Willinger, W.: The workshop on internet topology (WIT) report. Computer Comm. Rev. 37, 69–73 (2007)
10. Watts, D.J., Strogatz, S.H.: Collective dynamics of 'small-world' networks. Nature 393, 440 (1998)
11. Zhou, S., Mondragón, R.: Structural constraints in complex networks. New Journal of Physics 9, 1–11 (2007)
12. Vázquez, A., Boguñá, M., Moreno, Y., Pastor-Satorras, R., Vespignani, A.: Topology and correlations in structured scale-free networks. Phys. Rev. E 67 (2003)

13. Maslov, S., Sneppenb, K., Zaliznyaka, A.: Detection of topological patterns in complex networks: correlation profile of the internet. Physica A 333, 529–540 (2004)
14. Floyd, S., Kohler, E.: Internet research needs better models. Computer Comm. Rev. 33, 29–34 (2003)
15. Tangmunarunkit, H., Govindan, R., Jamin, S., Shenker, S., Willinger, W.: Network topology generators: Degree-based vs. structural. In: Proc. ACM SIGCOMM, pp. 147–159 (2002)
16. Zhou, S., Mondragón, R.J.: Accurately modelling the Internet topology. Phys. Rev. E 70, 066108 (2004)
17. Dorogovtsev, S.N., Mendes, J.F.F.: Evolution of Networks - From Biological Nets to the Internet and WWW. Oxford University Press, Oxford (2003)

Reactive Management of Quality of Service in Multimedia OBS Networks Based on GMPLS

Fernando N.N. Farias[1], Rafael P. Esteves[1], Waldir A. Moreira[2],
Antonio J.G. Abelém[1], and Michael A. Stanton[3]

[1] Research Group on Computer Networks and Multimedia Communications,
Federal University of Pará, Belém, Pará, Brazil
[2] Institute for System and Computer Engineering of Porto, Porto, Portugal
[3] Computing Institute, Federal Fluminense University, Niterói, Rio de Janeiro, Brazil
{fernnf,esteves,abelem}@ufpa.br, wjunior@inescporto.pt, michael@ic.uff.br

Abstract. This paper presents a proposal for dynamic control of Quality of Service (QoS) in optical networks based on optical burst switching (OBS) using a GMPLS control plane. In this proposal, monitoring agents are used to verify the QoS experienced by the burst classes and to deploy reactive mechanisms in order to guarantee absolute performance levels. Using GMPLS traffic engineering, these agents also offer idle resources to traffic flows whose service level is not being achieved. Simulation results show that the proposal can minimize the blocking probability when there are violations of burst flow parameters.

Keywords: Quality of Service, Optical Burst Switching, Generalized Multiprotocol Label Switching, Traffic Engineering.

1 Introduction

The consolidation of optical networking and wavelength division multiplexing (WDM) provides optical links with transmission capacity of tens of gigabits per second. However, with the aim of extending the benefits of optical communication and minimizing the disadvantages of electronic switching, all-optical switching was proposed. Basically, there are three approaches to all-optical switching: optical circuit switching (OCS) [1], optical packet switching (OPS) [2], and optical burst switching (OBS) [3].

Of these paradigms, OBS is notable since it is a hybrid proposal between OCS and OPS, capable of solving problems encountered in these two paradigms, such as lack of scalability, or the need for optical buffers or for sending control information along with the data.

The extension of the MultiProtocol Label Switching (MPLS)the control plane the Generalized MultiProtocol Label Switching (GMPLS) [4] has provided the best way for integrating the IP protocol with WDM, because with generalized labels an end-to-end label-switched path (LSP) can be established regardless of the multiplexing technology used, whether it be by wavelength, cell/packet

R. Mehmood et al. (Eds.): EuropeComm 2009, LNICST 16, pp. 13–22, 2009.

or time division, thus providing a simpler architecture, with intelligence and guarantees.

Quality of service (QoS) is important in all-optical networks and multimedia applications because of the increasing performance requirements of network applications, and also of the existing restrictions on optical technologies for temporary information storage. In [3], there are two basic models of QoS in OBS networks multimedia application: absolute QoS and relative QoS. In absolute QoS, quantitive performance limits are of great importance, such as in requirements of guarantees of maximum delay, minimum blocking, or minimum bandwidth. In relative QoS, the QoS parameters are not defined in absolute terms, but based on criteria that allow, for example, a high priority burst class to have a lower blocking probability than that of a low priority class, but there is no imposition on how small this probability must be.

However, in scenarios with a very high traffic load, the traditional QoS mechanisms cannot guarantee the desired performance, even if there are available resources in other routes of the network. GMPLS traffic engineering can be used for offering quality of service for OBS networks with a dynamic decision-making scheme to help in the choice of alternative routes. Reactive QoS management could monitor blocking probability levels of burst classes and offer idle network resources to these bursts, in order to reduce blocking in all classes.

The goal of this paper is to propose an architecture for dynamic control of QoS in OBS networks which uses the GMPLS control plane. Each class has its QoS context, which are metric values (e.g., delay, jitter or blocking probability) defined for a given class of service that must be satisfied. Dynamic QoS-control agents located at nodes in the OBS core monitor QoS measurements for each burst flow and, in the case of a parameter violation, they generate alarms and adjust the flow dynamically, using GMPLS traffic engineering, diverting affected flows to alternative routes that have idle resources. To validate this proposal, extensions were built for the Network Simulator 2, such as modules for QoS management and for OBS networks with GMPLS control plane and monitoring agents.

This paper is organized as follows. In Section 2, we describe related work. In Section 3, we provide an overview of OBS network architecture and of the detailed functioning of dynamic control agents. In Section 4, the proposal is analyzed in order to evaluate its impact on QoS in the OBS network. Finally, Section 5 concludes the paper and lists intended future works.

2   Related Work

In [5], a proposal for dynamic QoS is presented, using admission control at each OBS network node. A new model of admission protocol for bursts is proposed, using an OBS network architecture where each node is composed of a switching unit, a wait unit formed by fiber delay lines, a switching control unit (responsible for resource reservation and contention resolution), and entry and exit processing units. When it needs to send a burst, the entry edge node sends a burst control packet (BCP) with QoS information and delay statistics. Intermediate nodes receive the BCP, check the QoS values and estimate delay and blocking metrics. In the case of blocking, the control unit routes the incoming burst to a fiber delay line (FDL). If no FDL is available, the burst is discarded. On exit of the burst from the FDL, if blocking is still taking place, the burst is discarded. If the delay estimate exceeds the value defined in the QoS metric, the burst is also discarded.

In [6], it is proposed to use the differentiated services (Diffserv) architecture to offer QoS in OBS networks. Burst control packets are electronically processed to provide differentiated treatment to the corresponding bursts through different per hop behaviors (PHBs) for the services supported: Expedited Forwarding (EF), Assured Forwarding (AF) and Best Effort (BE). The definition of these PHBs has an impact on the process of burst assembly that varies according with the service class.

Both static and dynamic burst admission control mechanisms are proposed in [7]. The two mechanisms are similar, reserving a certain number of wavelengths in a link for each service class. Both are based on link usage for admitting bursts of each service class and, in this way, to differentiate the blocking probabilities experienced by different classes. The two mechanisms use the JET protocol and are used at those OBS network nodes where each burst occupies an entire wavelength during transmission and the node has complete capability for wavelength conversion.

The main problem of these previous approaches is that, in high traffic scenarios, none of them takes into account the availability of alternative network resources that could be used, even when the proposed techniques are incapable of guaranteeing the fulfillment of absolute restrictions on performance. The intention of this paper is to get around the limitations identified in the work mentioned here, through dynamic adaptations in the paths used by the burst flows, so that their QoS parameters are satisfied in an absolute way.

3   Dynamic Control of QoS in OBS Networks

3.1   Dynamic QoS Management Architecture (DQM)

In order to provide QoS in OBS networks, we propose an architecture for dynamic QoS management (DQM) that offers tools to provide improved control and monitoring of the service classes supported by the OBS network. In Figure 1, we present a general view of the DQM architecture.

In the proposed architecture, aspects related to the metrics, policies, decision making and agent are highlighted. The metrics are QoS measurements collected by the agent in the node where it is present. For this paper, we just observed the blocking probability.

The policies are restrictions on the QoS context that should be obeyed for the service classes of the OBS network. The context of each class contains thresholds with the maximum or minimum values of metrics that should be guaranteed.

Decision making defines the actions that are to be carried out as a result of possible policy violations (QoS context violation), and these actions can include the sending of an alarm to the network edge or the rerouting of flows using GM-PLS traffic engineering. The agents are responsible for monitoring the network and to carry out QoS management actions.

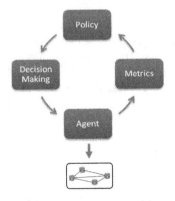

Fig. 1. View of the DQM architecture

3.2 DQM Agent

A Dynamic QoS Management Agent (DQMA) is incorporated into each node of the OBS network, as shown in Figure 2. A DQMA can be classified as a core DQMA or an edge DQMA.

A core DQMA has as function updating the metric tables while traffic goes through the node, and of sending an alarm to the edge DQMA in the case of a QoS context violation for a given service class. The metric stored in this table is the blocking probability that is calculated for each burst flow which is classified in one of the classes.

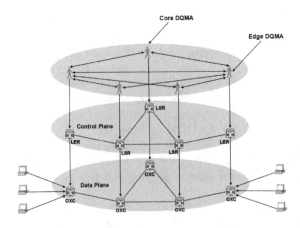

Fig. 2. DQM Agents

A core DQMA receives the context of each class, containing information on QoS measurements (for example: maximum value of blocking probability supported by the class) that should be obeyed in an absolute way. This information is stored in a policy table such as: High Class has 10% of blocking; Average Class has 20% of blocking; and Low Class has 30% of blocking. During network operation, comparisons are made between the metric values and the defined limits in the policy table. In case of detection of a QoS context violation, the core DQMA sends an alarm to the edge DQMA reporting which classes suffered as a result of policy violations, and which flows of those classes were the most affected.

An edge DQMA has the same functions as a core DQMA, with the difference of being capable of receiving and processing alarm signals sent by core agents and interacting with the GMPLS control plane to divert flows that are experiencing QoS context violations. An edge DQMA stores alternative routes that can be used in case of a QoS context violation. The number of alternative routes varies for each class, and is also in accordance with the available resources in the network. A high priority class will have a larger amount of additional routes to their flows. Figures 3a and 3b illustrate the agents' operation.

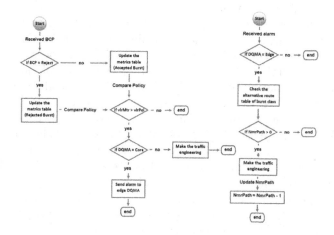

Fig. 3. DQMA operation for receiving: BCP (a) and alarm (b)

When a network node receives a BCP, the availability of wavelengths is verified for its outgoing link. If resources are available for the burst corresponding to the BCP being processed, the accepted burst counter for the DQMA of the node is updated. If there is no wavelength available for the burst at the moment of the request, the blocked burst counter is updated. In both cases, a comparison is made between the value of the blocking probability metric based on the collecte/stored values in the DQMA and the limits established in the policy table (if vlrMtr > vlrPol). In the case of a QoS context violation, the core DQMA sends an alarm to the ingress edge DQMA that makes a traffic engineering decision based on the existence of alternative routes for the service class (if NmrPath > 0). If an alternative route is available for the flow, then the flow is rerouted. An edge DQMA does not send an alarm to itself; in this case, traffic engineering is carried out automatically.

In order to incorporate DQMA into OBS networks, modifications to OBS signaling were needed to minimize the amount of control information exchanged by DQMAs and to take advantage of the OBS signaling, represented by BCP, to store the QoS context of each burst. This allows a burst class to change its context characteristics dynamically, as well as to offer the possibility of an individual flow altering its service class in a way that is transparent to the OBS network.

Three fields are added to the BCP structure: the flow identification (ID Flow), the identification of the class to which the burst belongs (ID Class) and the maximum blocking probability allowed for the class.

4   Analysis of the Proposal

This section evaluates the impact of the use of QoS monitoring and of a managing architecture based on the blocking probability of the burst classes in an OBS network using the GMPLS control plane. To this end, simulations were carried out using the NS-2 platform [8].

Several extensions to the simulator were developed to make it possible to analyze this proposal. Among the main contributions, we can enumerate: a component to simulate an edge OBS node that is capable of gathering packets into bursts and implementing JET signaling, a DQMA responsible for monitoring the burst flows, calculating the statistics of each flow and sending alarms to the network edge in the case of a QoS context violation.

The chosen topology for the simulations is based on a hypothetical extension to the backbone of the Brazilian National Research and Education Network (RNP) [9], with the addition of nodes and links that allowed the creation of alternative routes for the bursts. These links have a capacity of 10 Gb/s and a propagation delay of 1 millisecond. Each link has eight wavelengths and the high priority class (gold) can use up to four, the intermediate priority class (silver) has three reserved channels and the low priority class (bronze) can use up to two wavelengths. Figure 4 shows the network topology.

Fifteen traffic generators are used and are distributed according to four scenarios that differ in the amount of traffic attributed to each of the three service classes. In the first traffic scenario, the load was split in one third of the amount of burst traffic for each of the considered classes, namely class, silver, bronze. For the second traffic scenario, the load was divided in 46% for gold class, 27% for silver class and 27% for bronze class. As for the third traffic scenario, the distribution was of 27% for gold class, 46% for silver class and 27% for bronze class. Finally, in the fourth traffic scenario, the amount remained the same but with 27% for gold class, 27% for silver class and 46% for bronze class. Individual packets have size of 500 bytes [10]. The process of burst assembly is based on the fixed size, in other words, it will only be sent when it reaches a given size.

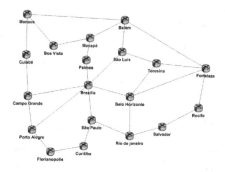

Fig. 4. Topology used in the simulations

In this paper, bursts are of 125KB on average [6]. The arrival of bursts follows a Poisson distribution.

The source of the flows of the gold class is the Brasília node and the destination is the Belém node. For the silver class, the source is the Recife node and the destination is the São Paulo node. Finally, the bronze class flows are sent from the Porto Alegre node to the Manaus node.

The alternative routes are known by the edge DQMAs and were defined according with the burst service class. There is a set of alternative routes for the bursts of a class. It was determined that the gold class bursts have three options of alternative routes, the silver class has two alternatives and the bronze class has only an additional route. Below, we have the original routes of each class and their respective alternative routes:

- *Gold:*
  Real route: São Luis, Brasília, Belém
  Alternative Route 1: Brasília,Palmas, Macapá, Belém
  Alternative Route 2: Brasília, Campo Grande, Cuibá, Belém
  Alternative Route 3: Brasília, Belo Horizonte, Fortaleza, Belém
- *Silver:*
  Real route: Recife, Salvador, Rio de Janeiro, São Paulo
  Alternative Route 1: Recife, Fortaleza, Belo Horizonte, Rio de Janeiro, São Paulo
  Alternative Route 2: Recife, Fortaleza, Teresina, São Luís,Brasília, São Paulo
- *Bronze:*
  Real route: Porto Alegre, Campo Grande, Cuiabá, Manaus.
  Alternative Route 1: Porto Alegre, Brasília, São Luís, Belém, Macapá, Boa Vista, Manaus.

A specific context was defined for each of the service classes. The maximum blocking probability allowed is of 5%, 15%, and 25% for the gold, silver and bronze classes, respectively.

Results regarding DQMA usage in the proposed scenarios are presented below. The goal is to analyze the impact of using agents for dynamic QoS control in an OBS network.

Each of the traffic generators produces a load that varies from 0.1 to 0.5 erlangs, and in the high load scenario the information generated in the network arrives at about 2000 bursts per second ($\simeq$ 2 Gbps). Fifty simulations were run for each point, with a confidence interval of 95% regarding the average of the samples.

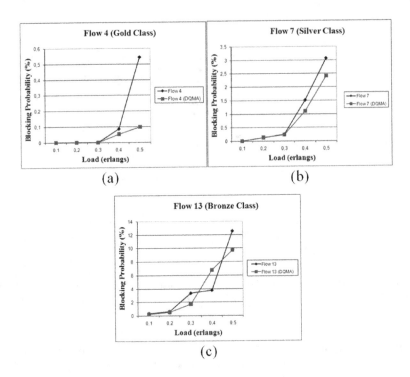

Fig. 5. Blocking probability in flow class: gold (a), silver (b) and bronze (c)

The blocking probability of each flow is calculated based on the average of the blocking probability registered in each node of the determined route. The blocking probability of each class is determined by the average of the blocking probabilities of each flow belonging to the class.

Figures 5a, 5b, and 5c show the blocking probability as a function of the load for a flow of each of the three service classes. Figures 6a, 6b, 6c, and 6d show the blocking probability for the whole class as a function of the defined traffic scenarios.

Figures 5a, 5b, and 5c show that there is a decrease of the blocking probability in the flows of all of the classes when DQMAs are used to perform dynamic QoS management. It is worth pointing out that not all of the flows will be served using explicit routing, since the number of alternative routes for each class is finite. A problem that can occur is when a given route explicitly shares links and wavelengths with other flows. In this case, the contention level can increase instead of decreasing, as can be seen in Fig. 5c for the load of 0.4 erlangs.

It can be observed from Figure 6 that there was a reduction in blocking probability for all of the classes with the use of DQMAs. It can be noticed that with an increase in the amount of traffic in each class, dynamic QoS control becomes even more necessary, so that absolute levels of performance for the bursts can be offered.

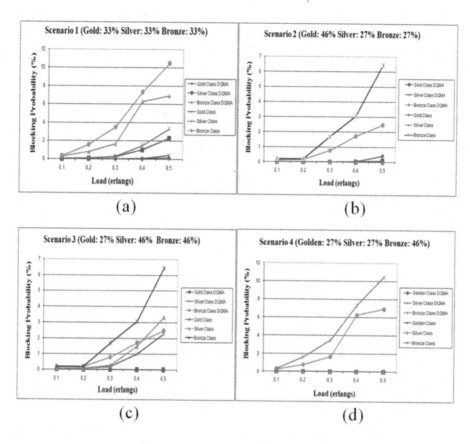

Fig. 6. Blocking probability for load class, In: Scenario 1 (a), Scenario 2 (b), Scenario 3 (c) and Scenario 4 (d)

5   Final Considerations and Future Work

This paper proposes an architecture for dynamic QoS control in OBS networks, based on traffic monitoring and automatic rerouting of bursts belonging to flows that suffer from high levels of blocking, according to the restrictions defined for each class. Thus, it is possible to define absolute levels of QoS for the applications that have strict performance requirements.

The proposal improved the performance of the service classes in a general way, besides guaranteeing the fulfillment of the given requirements. The results also show that, depending on the amount of traffic originating from each class, the demand for additional resources can really increase. For that reason, the main limiting factor of this proposal is the availability of additional network resources to meet the demands of the service classes. In case these are unavailable, there are no warranties that the proposal will provide the desired performance.

Another important aspect is related to the definition of the alternative routes that will be used. If these routes conflict with other existing ones, the level of contention experienced by the diverted bursts can be influenced by the existence of other flows.

In future studies, we intend to investigate the possibility of using a mechanism of automatic resource discovery to determine alternative routes for the bursts. In addition to performance requirements, resource discovery should also take into account the level of usage of candidate routes. Some means of admission control is also needed, as a more efficient means of avoiding disturbance of high priority flows by those of low priority. In addition, the metrics evaluated should include, besides the blocking probability, the delay and jitter relative to the thresholds defined in the QoS context, taking into account the synchronization between the agents.

References

1. Chlamtac, I., Ganz, A., Karmi, G.: Ligthpaths Communications: An Approach to High Bandwidth Optical WANs. IEEE Transactions on Communications 40(7), 1171–1182 (1992)
2. O' Mahony, M.J., et al.: The Application of Optical Packet Switching in Future Communication networks. IEEE Communications Magazine 39(3), 128–135 (2001)
3. Jue, J.P., Vokkaranne, V.M.: Optical Burst Switched Networks. Optical Networks Series, pp. 1–3. Springer, Heidelberg (2005)
4. Mannie, E.: Generalized Multi-Protocol Label Switching (GMPLS) Architecture, RFC 3945 (October 2004)
5. Lazzez, A., El Fatmi, S.G., Boudriga, N., Obiadat, M.S.A.: Dynamic QoS-based Scheme for Admission Control in OBS Network. In: IEEE Communication Society, ICC 2007, vol. 1, pp. 449–454 (2007)
6. Long, K., Tucker, R., Wang, C.: A New Framework and Burst Assembly for IP Diffserv over Optical Burst Switching Networks. In: IEEE Global Telecommunications Conference, GLOBECOM 2003, vol. 22(1), pp. 3159–3164 (2003)
7. Zhang, Q., Vokkarane, V.M., Jue, J.P., Chen, B.: Absolute QoS Differentiation in Optical Burst-Switched Networks. IEEE Journal on Selected Areas in Communications 22, 2062–2071 (2004)
8. VINT Project (2007, jul 07), The Virtual InterNetwork Testbed, http://www.isi.edu/nsnam/vint/index.html
9. RNP (2007, jul 07). Rede Nacional de Ensino e Pesquisa, http://www.rnp.br/backbone
10. Zhang, F., Macnicol, J., Pickering, M.R., Frater, M.R., Arnold, J.F.: Efficient Streaming Packet Video Over Differentiated Services Networks. IEEE Transactions on Multimedia 8(5), 1005–1010 (2006)

Enhancing Java RMI with Asynchrony through Reflection

Orhan Akın and Nadia Erdoğan

Istanbul Technical University, Computer Sciences, Informatics Institute,
Maslak-34469, Istanbul, Turkey
orhan@engineer.com, nerdogan@itu.edu.tr

Abstract. Java RMI's synchronous invocation model may cause scalability challenges when long duration invocations are targeted. One way of overcoming this difficulty is adopting an *asynchronous* mode of operation. An asynchronous invocation allows the client to continue with its computation after dispatching a call, thus eliminating the need to wait idle while its request is being processed by a remote server. This paper describes an execution framework which extends Java RMI functionality with asynchrony. It is implemented on top of RMI calls, using the thread pooling capability and the reflection mechanism of Java. It differs from previous work as it does not require any external tool, preprocessor, or compiler and it may be integrated with previously developed software as no modification of target remote objects is necessary.

Keywords: Asynchronous Communication, Asynchronous RMI, RMI, Reflection, parallel programming, distributed programming.

1 Introduction

Communication is a fundamental issue in distributed computing. Middleware systems offer a high level of abstraction that simplifies communication between distributed object components. Java's Remote Method Invocation (RMI) [1] mechanism is such an abstraction that supports an object-based communication framework. It extends the semantics of local method calls to remote objects, by allowing client components to invoke methods of objects that are possibly located on remote servers. In RMI, method invocation is synchronous, that is, the operation is blocking for the client if it needs the result of the operation or an acknowledgement. This approach generally works fine in LANs where communication between two machines is generally fast and reliable [2]. However, in a wide-area system, as communication latency grows with orders of magnitude, synchronous invocation may become a handicap. In addition, RMI's synchronous invocation model may cause scalability challenges when long duration invocations are targeted. One way of overcoming these restrictions is adopting an asynchronous mode of operation. This type of invocation provides the client with the option of doing some useful work while its call request is being processed, instead of being blocked until the results arrive. Asynchronous invocations have the following advantages:

R. Mehmood et al. (Eds.): EuropeComm 2009, LNICST 16, pp. 23–34, 2009.
© Institute for Computer Science, Social-Informatics and Telecommunications Engineering 2009

- to overlap local computation with remote computation and communication in order to tolerate high communication latencies in wide-area distributed systems,
- to anticipate the scheduling and the execution of activities that do not completely depend on the result of an invocation,
- to easily support interactions for long-running transactions
- to enforce loose coupling between clients and remote servers.

We propose an execution framework which extends RMI functionality with asynchrony. Clients are equipped with an interface through which they can make asynchronous invocations on remote objects and continue execution without the need to wait for the result of the call. They can later on stop to query the result of the call if it is required for the computation to proceed, or they may completely ignore it, as some invocations may not even produce a result.

Our framework focuses on the four most commonly used techniques, namely fire and forget, sync with server, polling, and result callback for providing client-side asynchrony. The design of the framework is based on a set of asynchrony patterns for these techniques described in detail in [3]; actually implementing the asynchrony patterns on top of synchronous RMI calls.

This paper describes the design and implementation issues of the proposed framework. Java's threading capability has been used to provide a mechanism for asynchronous invocation. One contribution of this work is its use of run-time reflection to do the remote invocation, thus eliminating the need for any byte code adjustments or a new RMI preprocessor/compiler. Another contribution is the rich set of asynchronous call alternatives it provides the client with, which are accessible through an interface very similar to that of traditional RMI calls. As the framework is implemented on the client side and requires no modification on server code, it is easily integrated with existing server software.

2 Java RMI

Java RMI provides a remote communications mechanism between Java clients and remote objects [1]. Java clients obtain references to these remote objects through a third party registry service. These references allow transparent access to the remote object's methods by mirroring the remote interface. RMI hides all execution details of communication, parameter passing and object serialization details by delegating them to 'stub' objects at both sides, on the client and the server. Method invocation is synchronous. This mode of communication may be satisfactory in applications where execution time is not critical. However, many distributed applications may benefit asynchronous invocations.

3 Asynchronous Invocation Patterns

Asynchronous invocation allows the client to continue with its computation after dispatching a call, thus eliminating the need to wait idle while its request is being process by a remote server. Several alternatives exist on how the results are passed to the client. The client may be interrupted when the results are ready, it may receive the results when it needs them, or it might not even be interested in the result. Multiple method invocations may as well be interleaved, without retrieving the response in between. There are four most commonly used techniques for providing client-side asynchrony [3].

Fire and Forget: well suited for applications where a remote object needs to be notified and a result or a return value is not required.

Sync with Server: similar to fire and forget; however, it ensures that request has been successfully transferred to the server application.

Polling: suitable for applications where a remote object needs to be invoked asynchronously, and yet, a result is required. However, the client may continue with its execution and retrieve the results later.

Result Callback: similar to Poll Object, a remote operation needs to be invoked asynchronously and a result is required. The client requests to be actively notified of the returning result.

4   Design Objectives for Asynchronous RMI Execution Framework

- **Independence of any external tools, preprocessors, or compilers**

Our main objective has been to present an execution framework that is completely compatible with standard Java, compilers, and run-time systems and does not require any preprocessing or a modified stub compiler. We have used RMI as the underlying communication mechanism and implemented asynchrony patterns on top RMI calls (as depicted in Figure 1.). Therefore, as long as a client is able to access a remote object using standard RMI, both invocation models, asynchronous /synchronous invocations, are possible. The main benefit for the developer is that he may choose the appropriate invocation model according to the needs of the application.

- **No modification of existing server software**

Another design objective is that the framework should require no modifications on the server side so that previously developed remote objects can still be accessed, now asynchronously as well. There is no necessity for a remote object to implement a particular interface or to be derived from a certain class as the framework is located on the client side.

- **Performance related concerns**

Performance issues have also been the focus of the implementation. As threading and reflection produce extra runtime overhead, special care has been taken to keep their use at minimum, so that they do not introduce a performance penalty on method execution.

5   Execution Framework Implementation

The asynchronous RMI execution model has been implemented by an execution framework (Figure 1.) which is developed in Java. It consists of a Java package itu.rmi.* containing the classes that provide the basic services for asynchronous invocations. The classes that are visible to the client are depicted in Figure 2. The execution flow of an asynchronous invocation (arrows 1 through 7 in Fig. 1.) and its implementation details are described below, assuming that a server has already registered a remote object with an RMI registry, making it available to remote clients.

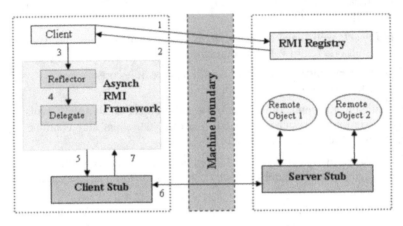

Fig. 1. Asynchronous RMI Framework Execution Flow

Initialization Phase:
1. This step involves the determination of the remote host. The client queries the lookup service *rmi registry* to retrieve a remote reference to the target remote object.
2. The lookup call returns a remote reference and results in the placement of a client stub which provides the interface to interact with the remote object.

Asynchronous Invocation Request:
3. An asynchronous invocation requires an instance of an invocation object to be created for the specific type of asynchronous call *(FireandForget, SyncWithServer, Polling, Callback)* the client wishes to make. The asynchronous call is dispatched as the client invokes the public void call(Object remoteObject, String methodName, Object params[]) overloaded call method of the invocation object with the actual parameters that specify the client stub reference, the name and the list of parameters of the remote method to be called. The client resumes execution as soon as the call method returns.

Asynchronous Invocation Processing:
4. The call method receives an invocation request and calls the appropriate method on the remote object transparently, applying the semantics of the specific type of asynchronous call. For this purpose, it uses reflection to assemble a method call during runtime. Once the method name and the argument types are resolved, they are matched with those of the incoming request to detect errors such as invoking a non-existing method, passing an incorrect number of arguments, or passing incorrect argument types to a method, raising exceptions that are caught by client. If no error exists, the call method returns after starting a service thread which handles the remainder of the invocation, allowing the client to resume execution while the asynchronous call proceeds in the new service thread. The service thread,

called a *delegate* in the our framework, is activated from a thread pool with parameters that include invocation details such as the remote object, method name, and parameters.

5. The delegate simply executes an invoke method call in its run method, (_remoteMethod.invoke (_remoteObject,_parameters);) which performs a standard RMI for the requested method over the client stub.

6. This phase involves standard RMI activity following its parameter passing semantics. The server stub passes the call request with its parameters to the server stub, which in turn, executes the method call on the remote object and returns the results back to the client stub over the network.

7. The client stub returns the result of the remote call to the *delegate*. The delegate responds differently on retrieving the result, according to the specific type of asynchronous call.

6 Types of Asynchronous Calls

Fig. 2 displays the public classes visible to user programs.

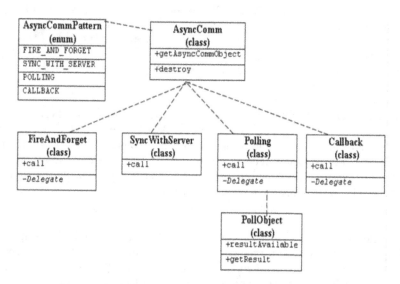

Fig. 2. Execution Framework Public Classes

The execution framework supports the four most commonly used asynchronous calls. In the following sections, we describe their execution patterns and give code samples to show how to utilize the framework for such calls, assuming the existence of the remote server objects logger, docConverter, searchEngine, and Emergency on a host with IP '192.168.1.3'.

Fire and Forget: Fire and forget is well suited for applications where a remote object needs to be notified and a result or a return value is not required. Reliability is not a concern for both sides. When the client issues such an invocation request, the call returns back to the client immediately. The client does not get any acknowledgment from the remote object receiving the invocation.

The client invokes asynchronously the log method of the remote object logger with the string parameter "my log message". The call method returns right after dispatching the delegate with the call request. Thus, the client thread and the delegate thread run concurrently, the client returning back to its execution while the delegate blocked waiting for the call to return.

```
import itu.rmi.*;
import java.rmi.*;
public class TestAsyncRMI {
public static void main(String[] args) {
  // use standard rmi to get remote reference
  Logger logger = (Logger)
            Naming.lookup ("rmi://192.168.1.3/logger");
  // get a 'fire and forget' invocation object
  FireAndForget fireAndForget = (FireAndForget)
  AsyncComm.getAsyncCommObject
                  (AsyncCommPattern.FIRE_AND_FORGET);
  // asynch call over invocation object through call method
  fireAndForget.call(logger, "log", new Object[] {"my log
      message"});
  // client continues execution immediatelyafter call returns

}
```

Sync with Server: Sync with Server is similar to fire and forget; however, it ensures that the invocation has been performed reliably. Again, a remote object needs to be notified and a result of the remote computation is not required. The difference is that, the call does not immediately return to the client but waits for an acknowledgement from the remote object to ensure that the request has been successfully transferred to the server application. Only then, control passes to the client. Meanwhile, the server application independently executes the invocation.

The client invokes asynchronously the convert method of the remote object docConverter with the input parameter msDoc. The call method blocks until the server application docConverter returns an acknowledgement that it has successfully received the request. From that point on, both the client and the server in parallel, the client returning back to its execution while the docConverter proceeds with the document conversion process.

```
import itu.rmi.*;
import java.rmi.*;
public class TestAsyncRMI {
public static void main(String[] args) {
  DocConverter docConverter = (DocConverter)
  Naming.lookup("rmi://192.168.1.3/docConverter");
  SyncWithServer syncWithServer = (SyncWithServer)
```

```
AsyncComm.getAsyncCommObject
                    (AsyncCommPattern.SYNC_WITH_SERVER);
MSDoc msDoc = new MSDoc();
```
// *asynch call over invocation object through* `call` *method, blocking until server*
// *returns an ack.*
```
boolean b = ((Boolean)syncWithServer.call(docConverter,
"convert",new Object[] { msDoc })).booleanValue();
```
   //*continue execution while server object converts the document*
```
}
```

Polling: Polling is suitable for applications where a remote object needs to be invoked asynchronously, and yet, a result is required. However, as the results may not be needed immediately for the client to proceed with its computation, the client may continue with its execution and retrieve the results later. In such a case, a poll object receives the result of remote invocations on behalf of the client. The client, at an appropriate point in its execution path, uses this object to query the result and obtain it. It may poll the object and continue with its computation if the result has not yet arrived, or it may block on the object until the result becomes available.

The client issues a polling call to the search method with the keyword "java" as the parameter. This time, the method call returns with a poll object as soon as it dispatches the delegate with the call request, allowing the client to continue with its execution while remote object processes the query and produces a result. When a result is returned, the delegate thread retrieves it in the poll object, sets a flag in the object to indicate that it is available and notifies any thread blocked on the object. The resultAvailable() method of the poll object returns a boolean value and may be checked by the client to see if a result has arrived. The client may also call the getResult()method of the poll object to get the result. However, this is a blocking call and does not return until the result actually becomes available.

```
import itu.rmi.*;
import java.rmi.*;
public class TestAsyncRMI {
public static void main(String[] args) {
  SearchEngine searchEngine = (SearchEngine)
  Naming.lookup("rmi://192.168.1.3/searchEngine");
  Polling polling = (Polling)
AsyncComm.getAsyncCommObject(AsyncCommPattern.POLLING);
```
// *asynch call over invocation object through* `call` *method- the call returns a*
// *poll object*
```
  PollObject pollObject = (PollObject) polling.call
     (searchEngine,"search", new Object[] {"java"});
```
   // *query to find out if the result of the asynchronous call is available*
```
  boolean b = pollObject.resultAvailable();
```
   // *blocking call that returns the result if it is available*
   // *or blocks the client until it becomes available and resumes it with the result*
```
List<String> result = (List<String>)
                        pollObject.getResult();
```
```
}
```

Callback: Similar to Polling, a remote operation needs to be invoked asynchronously and a result is required. However, in this case, the client needs to react to the result immediately it becomes available, not at a future time of its choice. Therefore, the client requests to be actively notified of the returning result. To this end, the client passes a callback object together with the invocation request to the execution framework. The call returns after sending the invocation to the server object and the client resumes execution. Once the result becomes available, a predefined operation on the callback object is called, passing it the result of the invocation.

Our implementation makes use of the Observer Pattern [5], therefore, callbackObject, an instance of a class which implements Observer interface is created before the client makes a call to the sendEmergency method, supplying a criterion "pressure is below 10" and a callback object callbackObject. Once the result of the remote call becomes, the update method of the observer object is invoked automatically with result parameters by the delegate using built-in method notifyObservers.

```java
import itu.rmi.*;
import java.rmi.*;
class CallbackObject implements Observer{
  public void update(Observable o, Object arg){
    // arg is the result returned by the remote object
  }
}
public class TestAsyncRMI {
public static void main(String[] args) {
   Emergency emergency = (Emergency)
   Naming.lookup("rmi://192.168.1.3/emergency");
   Callback callback = (Callback)
AsyncComm.getAsyncCommObject(AsyncCommPattern.CALLBACK);
   // create callback object
   CallbackObject callbackObject = new CallbackObject();
   // asynch call over invocation object through call method, callback object
   // also passed as a param
   callback.call(emergency, "sendEmergency", new
      Object[] {"pressure is below 10"}, callbackObject);

}
```

7 Performance Optimization

Performance of the framework has been a central concern during implementation. We tried to determine the greatest sources of runtime overhead and observed them to be related to threading facility and reflection mechanism of Java. Below, we describe the optimizations we have done.

Thread Pool: The framework transfers each new asynchronous invocation request to a new thread. Considering the overhead of spawning a new thread on each call, we optimized the interaction with the thread package and switched to using a ThreadPool

Thread Pooling Speed

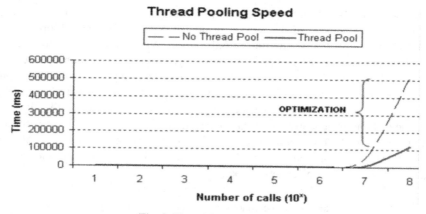

Fig. 3. Thread Pooling Speedup

which creates new threads as needed, but reuses previously created threads when they are available. Fig. 3. displays the performance gain in invocation response time, which becomes evident especially with high number of simultaneous requests.

Reflection: The second optimization we performed concerns reflection. When the call method of an invocation object receives an invocation request, it uses reflection to resolve the method name, the number of its arguments and their types. To minimize the overhead introduced by reflection, we cash the recently resolved information in private fields of the invocation object so thatsuccessive requests for a particular invocation instantly use the local data, instead of reflection lookups. Figure 4. displays speed up gained through reflection optimization.

Performance Results: We have conducted experiments in order to measure the performance of the framework and compare it with Java RMI. The test computer is

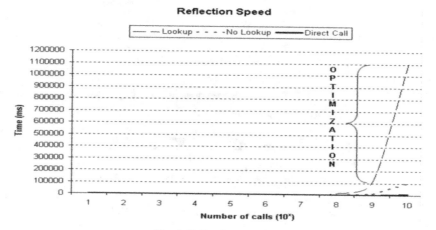

Fig. 4. Reflection speedup

Intel Core 2 Duo CPU T8300 2.4 GHz, 2GB of RAM, Windows XP Professional OS, Java build 1.6.0_11-b0. and the remote computer is Intel Pentium 4 Mobile CPU 1.70GHz, 512 MB of RAM. Java build 1.6.0_11-b03, Windows XP Professional OS.

Table 1 displays the execution cost for an asynchronous invocation of a remote method with the signature 'int add(int lhs, int rhs)' that simply adds the two input parameters and returns the result. For each invocation type, five test runs were executed and their average is reported. *Call Time* is the elapsed time for the client to make the call and resume execution. *Result Retrieval Time* is the time it takes for the result to be available. For polling type of invocation, this is the time duration until the blocking call getResult returns. For Callback, it is the duration until the update method of the observer object gets invoked.

Table 1. Asynchronous invocation execuiton costs

	Fire and Forget	Sync With Server	Polling	Callback
Call Time (ns)	3901948	11767026	3126207	2879528
Result Retrieval Time (ns)	NaN	11767026	4229923	4486045

We have implemented the remote objects introduced in Section 6 to demonstrate the different types of asynchronous calls and executed both standard RMI and asynchronous RMI calls to compare their execution time values. We assume that it takes 400 ms for the remote search engine to find a given keyword and a criterion is met every 2200 ms at the remote emergency object. Figure 6 illustrates the results, where the idle waiting state of the client issuing a standard RMI is clearly seen.

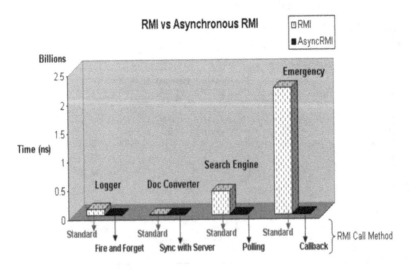

Fig. 6. Standard RMI versus Asynchronous RMI

8 Related Work

Asynchronous RMI has been the focus of several projects in literature, which usually focus only on selected aspects of the RMI, like communication performance, asynchronous invocation, or interoperability. [4] presents a system which uses the concept of a future object for asynchrony. A special compiler (armic) is used to generate stubs that handle asynchronous communication. The stubs provide asynchronous communication by wrapping each remote invocation inside a thread. Server side of the connection must also be threaded; therefore the system can not be used with remote objects already created. Furthermore, their approach is different from ours in that they do their callbacks directly from the server. In comparison, our callbacks are local. The Reflective Remote Method Invocation (RRMI) [5] is close to our approach as it makes use of reflection and provides a mechanism for asynchronous invocation. RRMI makes use of a dynamic class loader which is an extension to Java class loader (NetClassLoader) to allow client/server applications to be built. The NinjaRMI project [6] is a completely rebuilt version of RMI with extended features, including asynchronous communication. However, it is not wire compliant with standard Java RMI. It is intended to provide language extensions. The Ajents project [7] is a collection of class libraries that implement and combine several features that are essential for distributed computing using Java. However, its asynchronous communication aspect does not provide wide functionally; only the Polling pattern is implemented partially using 'future' objects.

9 Conclusion

This paper presents an execution framework which extends Java RMI to support asynchronous communication, mainly focusing on the techniques of fire and forget, sync with server, polling, and result callback. We have used RMI as the underlying communication mechanism and implemented asynchrony patterns on top of RMI calls. The threading facility and reflection mechanism of Java has made it possible for the framework to be independent of any external tools, preprocessors, or compilers. Also, as the framework requires no modifications on the server side, therefore previously developed remote objects can still be accessed asynchronously. The results of performance measurements show that, with optimizations on threading and reflection activity, the enhanced asynchronous RMI communication we have described in this paper produces a dramatic performance increase by removing unnecessary delays caused by blocking on synchronous RMI invocations.

References

1. Sun Microsystems, Inc. Java (TM) Remote Method Invocation Specification (2004)
2. Tanenbaum, A.S., Van Steen, M.: Distributed Systems: Principles and Paradigms. Pearson-Prentice Hall, ISBN:0-13-239227-5
3. Voelter, M., Kircher, M., Zdun, U., Englbrecht, M.: Patterns for Asynchronous Invocation in Distributed Object Frameworks. In: The 8th European Conference on Pattern Languages of Programs (EuroPlop 2003), Irsee, Germany, pp. 269–284 (2003)

4. Raje, R., William, J.I., Boyles, M.: An Asynchronous Remote Method Invocation (ARMI) Mechanism for Java. In: ACM 1997 Workshop on Java for Science and Eng. Comp. (1997)
5. Thiruvathukal, G.K., Thomas, L.S., Korczynski, A.T.: Reflective Remote Method Invocation. Concurrency: Practice and Experience 10(11-13), 911–926 (1998)
6. Welsh, M.: Ninja RMI: A Free Java RMI (1999),
   http://www.cs.berkeley.edu/~mdw/proj/ninja/ninjarmi.html
7. Izatt, M., Chan, P., Brecht, T.: Ajents: Towards an Environment for Parallel, Distributed and Mobile Java Applications. Concurrency: Pract. & Exper. 12, 667–685 (2000)

SNR Based Digital Estimation of Security in Wireless Sensor Networks

Adnan Ashraf[1], AbdulRauf Rajput[1], Marvie Mussadiq[2], B.S. Chowdhry[3], and Manzoor Hashmani[4]

[1] CREST Research Scholars, Mehran UET, Pakistan
[2] IT Consultant, Xevious Co.
[3] Fellow-Postdoc, Southampton University-UK
[4] Foreign Faculty Professor, Mehran UET
adnanlooking@ieee.org

Abstract. Security in wireless sensor networks (WSNs) is usually thought as privacy, auditing, intrusion detection and protection. In general, the quality of signal processing is considered as issue of middleware layers. The higher values of *signal to noise ratio* (SNR) are vital for target detection and estimation which is the most critical objective of WSN. Despite of the fact that SNR has a significant impact on objectives of WSN, not much investigation is found in literature about SNR and its security impact on such networks. The entire WSN can be rendered as useless due to SNR degradation and therefore, SNR is a prevailing security threat in WSNs. In the light of modern concepts of security, the safety should accompany the availability, scalability, efficiency and the quality parameters of inter-node communication. We show that SNR can identify suspicious activities which can exploit the performance and quality of communication in a sensor network. Also, by varying range of transmission radii and observing its impact on SNR we demonstrate that SNR-values, SNR-variance and pre-defined network threshold of SNR-variance, together can be useful in security assessment of WSN.

Keywords: Security Assessment, Digital Estimation, Signal to Noise Ratio or SNR, Wireless Sensor Network.

1 Introduction

Generally, security in network administrators' dictionaries is ranked as low, moderate and high in networks. Traditionally, these levels assume their base on security policies or descriptive rules. When requirements of these levels vary from one network application to other then there is a a common practice to understand the rule, and decide whether to apply that rule or not [1]. For example, an inventory monitoring application requires a different security level than a missile monitoring application. Different will be the security levels in the military monitoring applications during the time of war and peace. Similarly, the different levels of WSN security are suggested in these applications of physical world [2].

R. Mehmood et al. (Eds.): EuropeComm 2009, LNICST 16, pp. 35–45, 2009.

Wireless sensor network is being predicted as a pathway to the *smart network environments* (SNEs). In SNEs information resources like notebooks, i-phones and intelligent thin-clients can be replaced by intelligent sensors tied up with human fingertips. Security is still an obstacle in commercial deployments of WSN. In a WSN, the *target sensing* requires various sensors to capture different signals from different applications of the real world [3] [4]. The quality of signal is monitored by SNR values being a fundamental factor in event detection and target estimation. When signals travel from source to destination then SNR decreases with the distance [5] [6]. The entire WSN can be rendered as useless by SNR degradation and therefore, SNR is assumed as a threat for WSN security.

In this paper, we observe the SNR impact on WSN security. In our work, the impact on WSN security is calculated using discrete security assessment framework [7] [8]. We show that SNR values contribute to assess the security of a sensor network. By varying range of transmission radii and observing its impact on SNR, our simulation shows that the average, variance and threshold of SNR is useful to assess the WSN for a desired level of security. The proposed combinations of SNR based values are helpful to know the presence of such suspicious activities that may exploit the signal processing capabilities of a sensor network.

2 Problem Formulation

Various frameworks have been developed to achieve secure and efficient routing along good throughput for wireless sensor networks. High throughput does not guarantee noise free signals. Knowing that noisy signals is a threat to communication, every network tends to own some pre-defined threshold figures of signaling quality essential to achieve network objectives. Hence increasing noise is a threat to sensors' intercommunication it is imperative to know that 'how much noise a system may accept to avoid the state of *compromised security*'.

One idea to overcome this limitation is to take an optimal value of SNR. In other words, this SNR-value represents the ground capabilities of signal processing being exercised in a sensor network. No specific literature is available on SNR based security computation of WSN as security frameworks did not address this issue before. We observe by simulating a WSN and diffusing it with attacks that SNR never goes optimal. Therefore, we approach variance of SNR rather than observing SNR-threshold only. The SNR-threshold is the contour describing the maximum capabilities of signal processing that a sensor network experiences. We find our proposal of SNR-variance capable to identify odd changes in the network easily.

Traditional way of observing SNR values burdens the storage of *base station* (BS) or sink node where, every value is kept intact in order to monitor the network history [9]. In fact, every value of SNR is not important to record due to limitations in the processes of topology-building, routing-selection and memory-refreshing in a WSN. Consequently, the network behavior may dramatically change.

Consider a case, where SNR-value at one point is optimal and the change of topology suddenly routes the traffic through a noisy channel. In the next point of time, assume that WSN being a self-organized network recovers the situation fortunately, and transmits proceeding packets through a good channel. In this situation, we will not be in worry of storing SNR-values in memory of *base station* (BS). The challenge to compute the security impact for this state of network at any point of time is vital for monitoring purposes. One motive of our work is to address this challenge and analyze the security impact of such a situation on security of WSN.

One method of improving the quality of sensed value is the dense deployment of sensors. In dense deployment, many sensors are placed as close to the target as possible. This also increases the number of opportunities for the line-of-sight observations essential for accurate range estimations and SNR is improves evidently. In this case, the accurate estimation is responsibility of the algorithm used for that purpose, and this would be a big challenge.

Another way to improve reliability of network communication is to deploy sensors with enough density for multiple sensed values to be aggregated and filtered at cluster heads or at some intermediary point. The later demands efficient algorithms for distributed computations, efficient use of node memory and concise reports routed towards *base station* (BS) or sink node for estimation [10][11][12]. In our literature survey the solutions of these challenges is discussed as priority objective.

3 Literature Survey

WSNs consist of tiny nodes with low computation power and low energy resources thrown in unattended environment. When networks are adaptive with environment then the deployment part observes complex management which raises security risks in WSNs.

With the advancement of application areas, the security of WSN has been seriously questioned. The impact and nature of attacks vary among application-specific WSNs and raise the demand of uncompromised security even higher. The total security becomes utmost desire of WSN-applications due to self organizing nature, topology less infrastructure, deployment in hostile environment, limited energy, less storage and low power of computation. The existing security schemes, protocols, ciphering technologies are descriptive (rule or log based) security models and do not provide the total security in sensor networks. Shaping an optimized security is still a challenge in WSN based applications.

Many models and security frameworks have been proposed for sensing, target ranging or estimation, data aggregating, deployment mechanisms, efficient routings [5][6][10]. Some of these consider energy-levels of the network as a base of networks' strength. In a strong opinion of the majority researchers there are many network modalities that add up to the security of a network. Indeed, the problem is; how to estimate impact of each network modality on the security strength of a WSN? We find such assessment framework literature already proposed by Arain [7] [8].

David & Deborah [10] introduced a routing scheme (rumor) for power cost reduction and allow for queries to be delivered to events in the networks. This scheme builds a tradeoff between setup overhead and delivery reliability. As it is not concerned with security of the sensor network therefore, the reliability of occurrence of events is unsure.

Md & Choong [11] proposed the adoption of a probabilistic secret sharing protocols between two nodes which acknowledge each other; they incorporate these secretes with bidirectional verification and multi-path routing to multiple sink nodes to defense against attack.

Antonio et al [12] gave optimal power savings based on a small number of feedback bits. In such cases, an unwanted low power state of the network, during signal transmission or receiving causes the SNR degrading as an ultimate threat for WSN objectives.

Rajani [13] suggested a cross layer protocol design to detect the attack imposed by malicious node. He analyzed the attack using swarm intelligence algorithm, and by adding influence algorithm he improve the performance. Here again, the network performance is evaluated on the basis of average percentage of threat detection and energy consumption.

Rajani & Dr. Lisa [14] proposed novel avoiding method for sensor networks under jamming attack by using evolutionary algorithm. The performance parameters such as hops, energy, distance, packet loss, SNR, BER and packet delivery influences the decision taken in anti-Jamming techniques. The security assessment of this approach in WSN is still missing part of the research [15] [16] [17].

Arain [8] suggests the discrete security assessment framework for WSN security using network modalities of the applications' concern. Therefore, in this paper, we demonstrate that SNR based digital estimation of security of a WSN using SNR is possible in the *Discrete Security Assessment FramEwork* (DSAFE).

4 Security Estimation of Wireless Sensor Networks

Literature survey reveals that network applications demand security with highly scalable, efficient, intelligent and robust sensor environments. In addition to these security demands there exist different real world applications facing different security threats and therefore require different security levels from a WSN. Therefore, our objective of doing security estimation of a WSN is very critical for those network applications which are aimed for life saving and mission critical applications [18] [19] [20] [21]. Once, knowing the security capabilities of various WSNs a network application can choose the one that fulfills its security requirements optimally. For estimating security of WSN we worked with discrete security framework (DSAFE) which performs digital estimation of the network.

For the sake of continuity and interest of readers we give a brief introduction of digital estimation.

4.1 Theory of Digital Estimation of Security

The security defined by Arain [8] can be stated as *a set of tools and techniques for protecting assets of wireless sensor networks*. This protection is meant for all resources, hardware, processes and applications at some advanced level. Also, the author indicates that an attack is occurred in discrete manner such as damaging individual assets of a network whereas traditional security models and frameworks provide descriptive policies for security. This makes sensor networks less efficient to security threats [22] [23] [24] [25].

Indeed, we find that the policy/rule-based approaches of performing security assessment provide qualitative estimations only. These qualitative approaches are not helpful in determining those network segments having weak defense or kind of vulnerabilities. In order to develop an intelligent and adaptive network security protection system the quantitative or digital estimation of WSN security is very helpful. Such framework of digital estimation is already extracted, as [7] in recent past as shown in Table 1.

Table 1. Digital Estimation of Security using Discrete Security Assessment Framework

Segment	Parameter Name	Score	Precision (1-digit)
Network	Priority Queuing		0.2 (signed)
	Absolute Recovery		Successful Recovery ÷ Recovery Request
Sink	Penetration Level		Secure Layer- (Compromised Layer ÷ Secure Layer)
Link	Response to Attack	$0 \leq x \leq 1$	'0' or '1' known as R2A
Node	Assets Identification		(Total Nodes – Compromised Nodes) ÷ Total Nodes
	Exposure Investigation		N nodes/ Sq. Unit
Note: All values to be rounded-off to zero decimal points. The precision is removed as error.			

Using the figures in table 1, one can estimate the security strength of a given WSN in discrete fashion. It was then, followed by its evaluation strategies [9]. The discussion of evaluation strategies of D-SAFE is beyond the scope of this paper.

4.2 SNR-Based Digital Estimation of WSN

Though, many network modalities do exist for security estimation but this paper uses *signal to noise ratio* in simulations to know, merely security impact of SNR. In fact, the trend of ignoring SNR-values encouraged us to evaluate impact of SNR in WSN-security. In our strong opinion, doing digital estimation of WSN-security using SNR we may achieve following benefits.

- Controlled security level as per applications' requirements
- Development of an *intelligent security control* to work with some proactive value of network parameters
- On-demand network isolation for privacy and confidentiality from adversary nodes
- Planning of early maintenance to avoid communication-losses to assets of network and of application.
- Identification of fault in communication parameters in a WSN

In simulation, we use methodology of *Discrete-Security Assessment Framework* (D-SAFE) and a WSN simulator (i.e. JSIM). We simulate a WSN comprising 6-nodes in JSIM environment. The basic WSN model contains two target nodes for event or target sensing and broadcasting them to the next layer of 3 sensor nodes using two-hope and one-hop transmission respectively. The optimal hop-cost is also given for each node in the Fig 1. The sensing nodes are intermediate path to transport data from target node to the sink node and vice-versa.

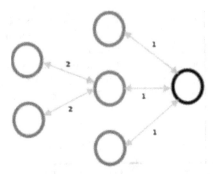

Fig. 1. Column-wise (L-R): Single (sink) node, three (sensing) nodes and two (target) nodes

Now, information like node count, SNR-values, number of hopes, data-packet size, total packet transmission time, packet loss, probability of number and type of attacks, window size and throughput is achieved from the WSN.

Referring to Fig 2, we observer that traditionally SNR values for a transmission cycle are obtained and aggregated at sinks. This indeed, burdens the limited memory resources of a wireless sensor network. Also, the recursive operations of aggregating SNR-values are not energy efficient for WSN. On the contrary, the SNR-values can be useful for real-time security estimation of sensor networks using D-SAFE.

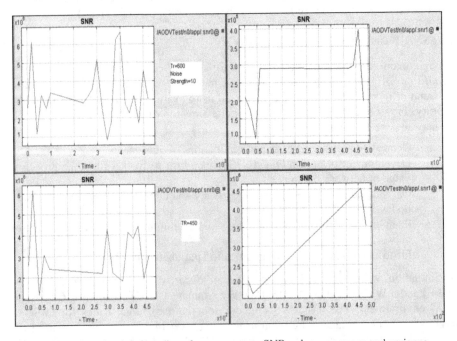

Fig. 2. A few simulated readings from numerous SNR-values, averages and variance

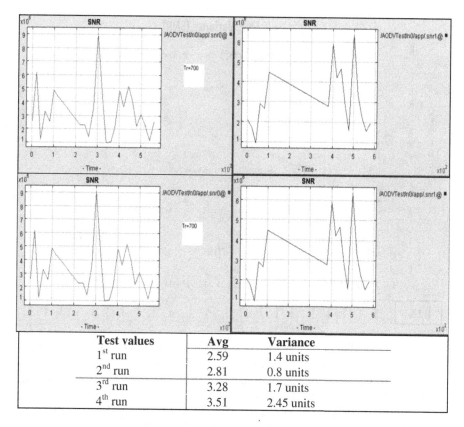

Test values	Avg	Variance
1st run	2.59	1.4 units
2nd run	2.81	0.8 units
3rd run	3.28	1.7 units
4th run	3.51	2.45 units

Fig. 2. (*continued*)

Instead of aggregating SNR-values and consuming more energy of the network in forwarding SNR information recursively, we propose that the variance of the SNR-average may be forwarded to the sink. Our proposal assumes that observation time is in accordance to the size of memory available at head node (sink, cluster-head, base station). Instead of transmitting the SNR figures alongside the data packet, the SNR-average may be calculated and retained at any part of network.

After certain duration, the variance of SNR-average is calculated and then it is transmitted over the network. In the proposed technique, calculation of SNR-variance is not performed in every time-slot and therefore it adds into total network time and total energy. For intelligent decision, the threshold of SNR-variance can be publicized among the head-nodes. We set the threshold 1.5×10^3 in all simulations of our experiments. When SNR-variance is found exceeding the threshold, then D-SAFE assumes the impact as vulnerability. Each of vulnerabilities weakens the total network strength. We recommend the use of proposed technique for the efficient use of memory.

Applying digital estimation of WSN security of D-SAFE and the proposed technique of SNR-variance the obtained result is shown in Fig 3. Also, by changing radii of random nodes and attacking the network communication in different ways we accomplish digital estimation of WSN-security.

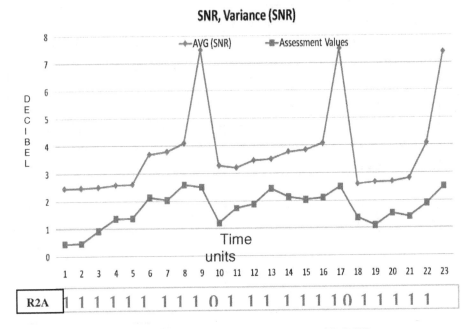

Fig. 3. Assessment graphs of SNR-variance and D-SAFE

In the Fig 3, the series of binary digits is D-SAFE assessment for its one of parameters. In D-SAFE, the SNR belongs to the *response to attack* (R2A) parameter. At two time slots (i.e. 10 and 18) the value of R2A parameter D-SAFE in [9] becomes zero. Here, we assume all values of table 1 as ideal except of R2A. Now, by substituting the resultant R2A in the following equation (1) of D-SAFE [7], the impact of SNR on WSN-security can be observed.

$$\text{Security Assessment Value} = AVG (AR + PL + R2A + AI + EI) \tag{1}$$

We know (from table 1) that R2A becomes zero during two time slots (i.e. 10th and 18th). After substituting and then converting the resultant value of D-SAFE in percentage we get 80%. This concludes in particular, that WSN offers 80% security at these two time slots. The overall security estimation of WSN in this SNR based simulation is 80% while SNR degrades. This state occurs only when variance of SNR-average exceeds the predefined threshold of SNR-variance (i.e. 1.5×10^3 in our experiment).

4.3 Analysis of Results for Accuracy of Digital Estimation

As a general observation if, any layer of WSN s' communication stack can be attacked then other WSN-layers must have protection mechanisms for sake of sensor network security. Analyzing the graphs in Fig 2 and Fig 3, we realize that SNR is too vital to be known for security even in hostile environments. We observe that the D-SAFE (Discrete Security Assessment Framework) validates the concept of separate assessment of values for each layer in WSNs.

In D-SAFE, the SNR is classified as link segment association and the detecting any abrupt change in variance alarms the situation by putting the pre-defined weight in priority queue for the parameter. Just as, in our simulation each average value of SNR represents an average of 10 SNR-values. If there are 6 SNR-average values then it means almost 60 SNR-values need to be transmitted within the network (i.e. from target node to sink node).

Our proposed technique of SNR-variance utilizes comparatively small amount of network energy as not all values are required to be sent towards sink-node. This makes the transmission of SNR-signals less recursive therefore consumes less operational energy too. On the basis of likely simulations and results, we show that using SNR-value, SNR-average, SNR-variance and threshold of SNR-variance we can identify the weaker areas in WSN. This will allow development of improved sensor networks and will enable us to predict the behavior of network components, if re-deployment is desired.

5 Conclusion and Future Work

The security estimation is a challenge for the commercialization of sensor networks. We observe that security frameworks (like D-SAFE) for discrete assessment of WSN assist for quantifying WSN-security. To enrich our assessment work we perform SNR based digital estimation of WSN-security. We also figure out the parameter (SNR) impact on security of sensor networks. As, high SNR-values don't assure for high quality communication WSNs, therefore, our work of SNR based security-estimation of WSN is helpful for determining network attacks.

We are extending our work by utilizing some energy-efficient algorithms for real-time SNR values in a WSN. Our future experiment will be in environment which may exhibit unknown circumstances. Then, by knowing SNR impact on WSN-security and behavior of sensing nodes in this environment we will tend to predict the results from redeploying sensing nodes at same location. In our strong opinion the SNR value may be used to embed demand-base quality of communication in networks-of-future. Then, it would be very useful to utilize such advanced networks for transmission of multimedia contents and video streams.

Acknowledgments. We are very much thankful to the Director and staff of NFC-IET Multan, PAKISTAN for their immense support to conduct a part of research in the vicinity. A special thanks to Sehar Khalid for supporting our work.

References

1. Ashraf, A., Mussadiq, M., Hashmani, M.: An Analytical Revelation for a Safer Network Perimeter Security. In: The proceedings of International conference on Information Networking (ICOIN 2006), Sendai-Japan (2006)
2. Muraleedharan, R., Osadciw, L.A.: Jamming Attack Detection and Countermeasures. In: Wireless Sensor Network Using Ant System. Department of Electrical Engineering and Computer Science, Syracuse University, Syracuse, pp. 13244–11240
3. AKylidiz, I.F., Su, W., Sankarasubramaniam, Y., Cayirci, E.: A survey on sensor networks. IEEE communication Magazine 40(8), 102–114 (2002)

4. Wang, D., Zhang, Q., Liu, J.: The self-protection Problem in Wireless Sensor Networks. ACM Transactions on Sensor Netwoks 3(4), Article 20 (October 2007)
5. Zou, Y., Chakrabarty, K.: Uncertainty-aware and coverage-oriented deployment for sensor networks. Journal of Parallel and Distributed Computing 64(7), 788–798 (2004)
6. Ilyas, M., Mahgoub, I.: Handbook of Sensor Networks: Compact Wireless and Wired Sensing Systems. In: LLC 2005. CRC Press, Boca Raton (2005), Library of Congress Card Number 2004043852, ISBN 0-8493-1968-4, http://ww.crcpress.com
7. Ashraf, A., Hashmani, M., Mussadiq, M., Chowdhry, B.S.: Design and Analysis of the Security Assessment Framework for Achieving Discrete Security Values in Wireless Sensor Networks. In: Canadian Conference on Electrical and Computer Engineering CCECE 2008, May 4-7, pp. 855–860 (2008)
8. Arain, A.A., Hashmani, M., Mussadiq, M., et al.: A Pretty Safe Strategy for Analyzing Discrete Security Assessment Framework in Wireless Sensor Networks. In: Book of Wireless Networks, Information Processing and Systems, November 14, 2008. CCIS, vol. 20, pp. 445–448. Springer, Heidelberg (2008)
9. Zia, T., Zomaya, A.: A security Framework for Wireless Sensor Networks. In: SAS 2006 – IEEE Sensors Application Symposium, Houston, Texas, USA, February 7-9 (2006)
10. Braginsky, D., Estrin, D.: Rumor Routing Algorithm For Sensor Networks. In: WSNA 2002, September 28, Atlanta, Georgia, USA Copyright 2002 ACM 1-58113-589-0/02/0009 (2002)
11. Abdul Hamid, M., Mamun-Or-Rashid, M., Hong, C.S.: Routing Security in Sensor Network:HELLO FLOOD Attack and Defence. In: ICNEWS (2006)
12. Marqus, A.G., Wang, X., Giannakis, G.B.: Minimizing Transmit Power for coherent Communications in Wireless Sensor Networks with Finite-Rate Feedback. IEEE Transactions on Signal Processing 56(9) (September 2008)
13. Muralee dharan, R., Ann Osadciw, L.: Jamming attack Detection and Countermeasures. In: Wireless Sensor Network Using Ant System, SPIE (2006) ISSN 0277-786X
14. Muralee dharan, R., Ann, L.: Cross Layer security protocol Using Swarm Intelligence. In: IEEE long Island System, Application and Technology conference(LISAT 2007), Farmingdale, New York (May 2007)
15. Chong, C.-Y., Kumar, S.P.: Sensor Networks: Evolution Opportunities, and Challenges. Proceedings of the IEEE 91(8), 1247–1256
16. Perrig, A., Szewczyk, R., Tygar, J.D., Wen, V., Culler, D.E.: SPINS: Security protocols for sensor networks. Wireless Networks 8(5), 521–534 (2002)
17. Kaplantiz, S.: Security Models for Wireless Sensor Networks. Conversion report, Monash University, March 20 (2006)
18. Ricadela, A.: Sensors Everywhere, January 24 (2005)
    http://informationweek.com/stories
19. Roman, R., Zhou, J., López, J.: On the security of wireless sensor networks. In: Gervasi, O., Gavrilova, M.L., Kumar, V., Laganá, A., Lee, H.P., Mun, Y., Taniar, D., Tan, C.J.K. (eds.) ICCSA 2005. LNCS, vol. 3482, pp. 681–690. Springer, Heidelberg (2005)
20. Sabbah, E., Najeed, A., Kang, K.-D., Liu, K., Abu-Ghazaleh, N.: An Application-Driven Perspective on Wireless Sensor Network Security. In: Proceedings of the 2nd ACM international workshop on Quality of service & security for wireless and mobile networks, Torromolinos, Spain (2006)
21. Park, S., Savvides, A., Srivastava, M.B.: A Simulation Framework for Sensor Networks. In: Proceedings of the 3rd ACM international workshop on modeling, analysis and simulation of wireless and mobile systems, Boston, Massachusetts, USA (2000)

22. Karlof, C., Wagner, D.: Secure Routing in Wireless Sensor Networks: Attack and Counter Measures. Ad Hoc Networks 1(2-3), 293–315 (2003)
23. Wood, A.D., Stankovic, J.A.: Denial of Service in Sensor Networks, pp. 54–62 (2002)
24. Czarlinka, A., Kundur, D.: Distributed Actuation Attacks in Wireless Sensor Networks: Implications and Countermeasures. In: Proceedings of the 2nd IEEE workshop on dependability and security in sensor networks and systems, DSSNS (2006)
25. Ngai, E.C.H., Jiangchuan Liu Lyu, M.R.: On the Intruder Detection for Sinkhole Attack in Wireless Sensor Networks Communications. In: IEEE International conference on ICC 2006, Istanbul, June 2006, vol. 8, pp. 3383–3389 (2006) ISSN:8164-9547, ISBN: 1-4244-0355-3

Quantifying the TV White Spaces Spectrum Opportunity for Cognitive Radio Access

Maziar Nekovee[1,2]

[1] BT Research, Polaris 134, Adastral Park, Martlesham, Suffolk, IP5 3RE, UK
[2] Centre for Computational Science, University College London
20 Gordon Street, London WC1H 0AJ, UK
maziar.nekovee@bt.com

Abstract. Cognitive radio is being intensively researched for opportunistic access to the so-called TV White Spaces (TVWS): large portions of the VHF/UHF TV bands which become available on a geographical basis after the digital switchover. In this paper we take a step back from the excitement surrounding TVWS, and quantitatively examine the real spectrum opportunity associated with this form of access. Using accurate digital TV (DTV) coverage maps together with a database of DTV transmitters, we develop a methodology for identifying TVWS frequencies at any given location in the United Kingdom. We use our methodology to investigate variations in TVWS as a function of the location and transmit power of cognitive radios, and examine how constraints on adjacent channel interference imposed by regulators may affect the results. Our analysis provides a realistic view on the spectrum opportunity associated with cognitive devices, and presents the first quantitative study of the availability and frequency composition of TWVS outside the United States.

Keywords: cognitive radio, dynamic spectrum access, digital dividend.

1 Introduction

Cognitive radio (CR) technology [1,2] is a key enabler for the opportunistic spectrum access (OSA) model [11,9], a potentially revolutionary new paradigm for dynamic sharing of licenced spectrum with unlicensed devices. In this operational mode a cognitive radio acts as a spectrum scavenger. It performs spectrum sensing over a range of frequency bands, dynamically identifies unused spectrum, and then operates in this spectrum at times and/or locations when/where it is not used by incumbent radio systems. Opportunistic spectrum access can take place both on a temporal and a spatial basis. In temporal opportunistic access a cognitive radio monitors the activity of the licensee in a given location and uses the licensed frequency at times that it is idle. An example of this is the operation of cognitive radio in the radar and UMTS bands. In spatial opportunistic access cognitive devices identify geographical regions where certain licensed bands are unused and access these bands without causing harmful interference to the operation of the incumbent in nearby regions.

Currently Cognitive radio is being intensively researched for opportunistic access to the so-called TV White Spaces (TVWS): large portions of the VHF/UHF

R. Mehmood et al. (Eds.): EuropeComm 2009, LNICST 16, pp. 46–57, 2009.
© Institute for Computer Science, Social-Informatics and Telecommunications Engineering 2009

TV bands which become available on a geographical basis after the digital switchover. In the US the FCC (Federal Communications Commission) proposed to allow opportunistic access to TV bands already in 2004 [3]. Prototype cognitive radios operating in this mode were put forward to FCC by Adaptrum, I^2R, Microsoft, Motorola and Philips in 2008 [12]. After extensive tests the FCC adopted in November 2008 a Second Report and Order that establishes rules to allow the operation of cognitive devices in TVWS on a secondary basis [13]. Furthermore, in what is potentially a radical shift in policy, in its recently released Digital Dividend Review Statement [4] the UK regulator, Ofcom, is proposing to "allow licence exempt use of interleaved spectrum for cognitive devices." [4]. Furthermore Ofcom states that "We see significant scope for cognitive equipments using interleaved spectrum to emerge and to benefit from international economics of scale" [4]. More recently, on February 16 2009, Ofcom published a new consultation providing further details of its proposed cognitive access to TV White Spaces [5].

With both the US and UK adapting the OSA model, and the emerging IEEE 802.22 standard for cognitive access to TV bands [6,7] being at the final stage, we can expect that, if successful, this new paradigm will become mainstream among spectrum regulators worldwide. However, while a number of recent papers have examined various aspects of cognitive radio access to TVWS in the United States [14,15,16,17,28,18,20], there is currently very little quantitative information on the *global* spectrum opportunities that may result if CR operation in TV bands becomes acceptable in other countries in the world.

To bridge this gap, we present in this paper a quantitative analysis of TV White Spaces availability for cognitive radio access in the United Kingdom. Using accurate digital TV (DTV) coverage maps together with a database of DTV transmitters, we develop a methodology for identifying TVWS frequencies at any location in the UK. We use our methodology to investigate the variations in TVWS as a function of the location and transmit power of cognitive radios, and examine how constraints on adjacent channel emissions of cognitive radios may affects the results. Our analysis provides a realistic view on the potential spectrum opportunity associated with cognitive radio access to TWVS in the UK, and presents the first quantitative study of the availability and frequency composition of TWVS outside the United States.

The rest of this paper is organised as follows. In section II we discuss in detail the operation of cognitive radio devices in the VHF/UHF TV bands. This is followed by a description of our methodology for estimating TWVS frequencies. Section III presents results of our study of the availability of TVWS in 18 locations in the UK and analyses the implications of our findings. We conclude this paper in Section V.

2   Cognitive Radio Operation in TV Bands

Broadcast television services operate in licensed channels in the VHF and UHF portions of the radio spectrum. The regulatory rules in most countries prohibit the use of unlicensed devices in TV bands, with the exception of remote control, medical telemetry devices and wireless microphones. In most developed countries regulators are currently in the process of requiring TV stations to convert from analog to digital transmission. This *Digital Switchover* is expected to be completed in the US in 2009 and in the UK in 2012. A similar switchover process is also underway or being planned (or is already completed) in the rest of the EU and many other countries around the world.

After Digital Switchover a portion of TV analogue channels become entirely vacant due to the higher spectrum efficiency of digital TV (DTV). These cleared channels will then be reallocated by regulators to other services, for example through auctions. In addition, after the DTV transition there will be typically a number of TV channels in a given geographic area that are not being used by DTV stations, because such stations would not be able to operate without causing interference to co-channel or adjacent channel stations. These requirements are based on the assumption that stations operate at maximum power. However, a transmitter operating on a vacant TV channel at a much lower power level would not need a great separation from co-channel and adjacent channel TV stations to avoid causing interference. Low power unlicensed devices can operate on vacant channels in locations that could not be used by TV stations due to interference concerns [14]. These vacant TV channels are known as TV White Spaces, or interleaved spectrum in the parlance of the UK regulator. Opportunistic operation of cognitive radios in TV bands, however, is conditioned on the ability of these devices to avoid harmful interference to licensed users of these bands, which in addition to DTV include also wireless microphones [14]. In November 2008, the FCC adopted a report setting out rules allowing licence-exempt cognitive devices to operate in TV White Spaces. In summary these rules require cognitive devices to use a combination of spectrum sensing and geolocation. The devices must be able to sense both TV signals and wireless microphones down to −114 dBm, and must also locate their position to within 50 meters accuracy and then consult a database that will inform them about available spectrum in that location. Devices without geolocation capabilities are also allowed if they are transmitting to a device that has determined its location. Cognitive devices that use sensing alone are allowed in principle. However, the FCC states that such devices will be "subject to a much more rigorous approval process" [13].

The fundamental reason why TVWS have attracted much interest is an exceptionally attractive combination of bandwidth and coverage. Signals in TV bands, travel much further than both the WiFi and 3G signals and penetrate buildings more readily. This in turn means that these bands can be used for a very wide range of potential new services, including last mile wireless broadband in urban environments, broadband wireless access in rural areas [6,7], new types of mobile broadband and wireless networks for digital homes. Furthermore, in the case of the UHF bands, the wavelength of signals in these bands is sufficiently short such that resonant antennas with sufficiently small footprint can be used which are acceptable for many portable use cases and handheld devices [15].

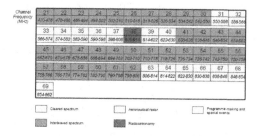

Channel Frequency (MHz)	21	22	23	24	25	26	27	28	29	30	31	32
	470-478	478-486	486-494	494-502	502-510	510-518	518-526	526-534	534-542	542-550	550-558	558-566
	33	34	35	36	37	38	39	40	41	42	43	44
	566-574	574-582	582-590	590-598	598-606	606-614	614-622	622-630	630-638	638-646	646-654	654-662
	45	46	47	48	49	50	51	52	53	54	55	56
	662-670	670-678	678-686	686-694	694-702	702-710	710-718	718-726	726-734	734-742	742-750	750-758
	57	58	59	60	61	62	63	64	65	66	67	68
	758-766	766-774	774-782	782-790	790-798	798-806	806-814	814-822	822-830	830-838	838-846	846-854
	69											
	854-862											

☐ Cleared spectrum   ☐ Aeronautical radar   ☐ Programme-making and special events

▨ Interleaved spectrum   ▨ Radioastronomy

Fig. 1. The available VHF and UHF TV spectrum in the UK after digital switchover, showing both the interleaved (TVWS) and cleared channels [4]

3 Methodology

The digital TV standard adopted in the UK and the rest of Europe is DVB-T (Digital Video Broadcasting Terrestrial) which uses 8 MHz wide frequency bands for its transmission. This is unlike the US ATSC standard where each band is 6 MHz wide. Fig. 1 shows the chart of the UK's analog TV frequency bands and how these will be divided after digital switchover into cleared and interleaved spectrum [4]. From this chart it can be seen that the total UK interleaved spectrum, which is entirely in the UHF frequency range, is 256 MHz. However, Ofcom has proposed to auction off channels 61 and 62 for licenced use [24], reducing the TV bandwidth available for access by cognitive devices to a total of 240 MHz. However the exact number and frequency composition of TVWS can vary from location to location and is determined by the spatial arrangement of DTV transmitters and their nationwide frequency planning.

The CR transmission at a given location should not cause harmful interference to TV receivers both within the coverage area of nearby transmitters, and at the edge of this area. To achieve this the CR device can transmit on the TV bands used by these transmitters only if its position is a minimum "keep-out" distance, R_{cr}, away from the edge of their coverage area [7]. Fig. 2 shows schematically a typical setup for the operation of a cognitive radio base station which operates in a given location in TV White Spaces which are available at that location.

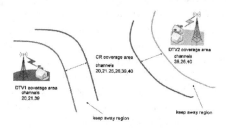

Fig. 2. Opportunistic access to interleaved TV spectrum (White Spaces) by cognitive radios

In a simplified picture, based on the pathloss model [21], the keep-out distance can be obtained as follows. Denote with R_{tv} the maximum coverage radius of the TV station, and with P_{cr} and P_{tv} the transmit power of the TV transmitter and the CR transmitter, respectively. Then, in order to avoid interference with TV receivers that are at the edge of the coverage area, we must have:

$$\frac{P_{tv}/R_{tv}^{\alpha}}{P_{cr}/R_{cr}^{\alpha}} \geq \beta_{th}, \tag{1}$$

where β_{th} is the sensitivity threshold of a TV receiver, and α is the pathloss exponent. This yields:

$$R_{cr} \geq \left(\beta_{th}\frac{P_{cr}}{P_{tv}}\right)^{1/\alpha} R_{tv}. \tag{2}$$

Consequently, a CR device at location $\mathbf{r}$ can use the frequencies associated with a TV station located at $\mathbf{R}_j$ only if $|\mathbf{r} - \mathbf{R}_j| \geq R'_j$, where

$$R'_j = \left[1 + \left(\beta_{th}\frac{P_{cr}}{P_{tv}^j}\right)^{1/\alpha}\right] R_{tv}^j. \tag{3}$$

Repeating the above procedure for every TV transmitter, one can obtain the total number of TV transmitters whose associated frequencies can be used by a CR operating with a specified transmit power, P_{cr}, at location $\mathbf{r}$, from which the total number of TVWS frequencies available for opportunistic access, $\rho(\mathbf{r}, P_{cr})$, can be obtained as:

$$\rho(\mathbf{r}, P_{cr}) = \sum_j \sum_m \Theta(|\mathbf{r} - \mathbf{R_j}| - R'_j)\delta_{mj} \tag{4}$$

where Θ is the step function and $\delta_{mj} = 1$ if a frequency f_m is used by a DTV transmitter located at R_j and zero otherwise. Furthermore the first and the second sum in the above equation are over all DTV transmitters and all DTV frequencies, respectively.

In reality coverage contours of TV transmitters are far from circular due to a combination of terrain and clutter (building, trees, etc) diffraction of radio waves, non-isotropic radiation patterns of transmitter antennas, and interference resulting from nearby DTV transmitters [22]. Furthermore, shadow fading and atmospheric effects give rise to stochastic fluctuations in the received TV signal power [22]. In our study we make use of the publicly available maps of DTV coverage in the UK [23] which were generated via computer simulations from the Ofcom's database of location, transmit power (ERP), antenna height and transmit frequency of UK's 81 main DTV transmitters. These computer simulated coverage maps are further validated and refined through measurements and direct observation by DTV users. Fig. 3 shows, as an example, the coverage map of a DTV transmitter located in the vicinity of Oxford [23].

The typical transmit power of UK's DTV transmitters ranges between 25W and 200 kW (ERP) [25]. Consequently in the case of cognitive devices with transmit powers typical of licenced-exempt usage ($\sim$ 100 mW) we have $P_{CR}/P_{TV} \ll$

1. Consequently, in this low-power limit an *upper bound for* the vacant TWVS frequencies at a given location can be directly extracted from the coverage maps of DTV transmitters, as can also be seen from Eqs.(3-4).

Our computer algorithm for obtaining such upper bounds works as follows. We use the UK National Grid (NG) coordinate system [26] in order to specify the geographical position of any location on the UK map. Given the NG coordinates of a UK location our code then maps this location onto the closest grid point on the coverage maps of DTV transmitters. For a given DTV transmitter this grid point is then evaluated to determine if it falls within the coverage area of that transmitter. If this is the case, then the frequencies associated with the transmitter are tagged as *occupied* at that location, otherwise they are tagged as *vacant*. Repeating this procedure for coverage maps of the entire 81 UK transmitters, we then obtain a list of vacant TV frequencies at a given location that can be used by a low-power cognitive device which is positioned in that location.

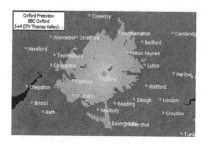

Fig. 3. Coverage map of the DTV transmitter located near Oxford is shown. The square marks the location of the transmitter. The coverage area is shown in pink [23].

In the case of high power cognitive equipments, e.g. those considered within the IEEE 802.22 standard with transmit powers as high as 4 Watts (ERP) [7], the keep-out radius associated with a cognitive radio is substantial, e.g. between $30 - 120$ km. This keep out radius need to be taken into account when estimating vacant TV frequencies at a given location. However, due to the irregular shape of TV coverage contours the required computations are very intensive. In order to reduce this computational effort, we have approximated the actual DTV coverage areas by circular disks centred at a each DTV transmitter. These disk were constructed such that each of them entirely encompassed the coverage area of the associated transmitter while also having the minimum possible surface area. With this simplification, it is then computationally straightforward to calculate from Eqs. (3-4) the vacant TV frequencies as a function of both position and transmit power of cognitive devices.

4   Results

Potential applications of TVWS devices will strongly depend on how the availability of this spectrum varies, both from location to location and as a function of transmit power of cognitive devices. The FCC, for example, is considering two classes of uses cases. The first corresponds to fixed devices with relatively high transmit power, line of sight operation and ranges up to 30 km. One expected use case for this class is broadband wireless access to rural areas, for which the IEEE 802.22 standard is being developed. A second class of use cases under consideration by the FCC are those associated with personal/portable devices which maybe nomadic or mobile [15]. In the rest of this paper we shall focus mainly on use cases corresponding to low-power cognitive access. A full analysis for the case of high transmit power devices will be presented elsewhere.

4.1   TVWS Availability and Frequency Composition

Fig. 4 summarises in a bar-chart the availability of TVWS channels for 18 major population centres in England, Wales and Scotland. The total number of channels available at each location is shown as red bar. It can be seen that there are considerable variations in the number of TVWS channels as we move from one UK location to another. For any given location, however, a minimum of 12 channels (96 MHz) are accessible to low-power cognitive devices, while the average available spectrum is just over 150 MHz.

In addition to estimating total available TVWS, it is of importance to investigate channel composition of this spectrum. In Fig. 5 we show, as an example, channel composition of TVWS in 4 cities in England: Bristol, Liverpool, London and Southampton. In this Figure vacant channels are shown as blue bars while occupied channels are left blank. As can be seen from the figure, the precise composition of TVWS channels vary greatly from location to location. In particular, both in Bristol and Liverpool most of the available channels are located in the lower end (470 − 550 MHz) of the UHF band while in the case of Southampton these channels are bunched up in the higher end of this band (630 − 806 MHz).

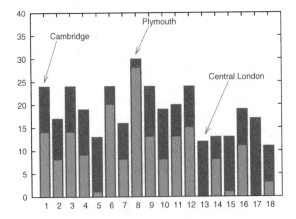

Fig. 4. Variations in the availability of TV White Spaces is shown for 18 UK locations. Results are shown before (red bars) and after (green bars) the exclusion of those vacant channels whose adjacent channels were found to be occupied by DTV transmission.

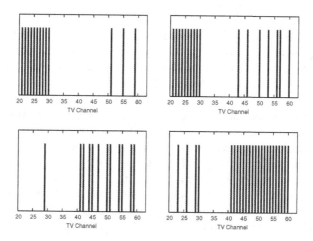

Fig. 5. The availability of TV White Space frequencies for low power cognitive radios are shown, from left to right and top to bottom, in Bristol, London, Liverpool and Southampton. Channels available for cognitive radio are shown as blue bars.

Furthermore, the available TVWS channels can be highly *non-contiguous*. This feature may greatly restrict access to TVWS by most current wireless technologies, as modulation schemes implemented in these technologies often require a contiguous portion of the spectrum. In the case of London, for example, although a total of 96 MHz spectrum is in principle available, only 16 MHz can be utilised for contiguous frequency access.

4.2   The Impact of Adjacent Channel Interference and Transmit Power

When a high power cognitive device operates in a vacant TV channel, energy leakage to adjacent channels may cause interference to TV sets that are tuned to these adjacent frequencies. To eliminate the occurrence of such adjacent-channel interference the IEEE 802.22 Working Group prescribes that if channel N is occupied by an incumbent, then cognitive devices should not only vacate this channel but they also should refrain from transmitting at channels $N \pm 1$. In addition, in the UK Ofcom has raised concerns that operation of low-power cognitive devices on a given channel may also cause adjacent-channel interference for mobile TV receivers that are in close vicinity. Consequently, even in such low-power use cases, cognitive devices may be constrained not to use vacant channels whose immediate adjacent frequencies are used for mobile TV. It is therefore of considerable interest to investigate how imposing such constraints will affect the availability of TVWS spectrum.

The total number of available TVWS after imposing the above adjacent channel constraint are shown as green bars in Fig. 6. These results are obtained by eliminating from the list of TVWS channels any vacant channel whose immediate adjacent channels were found occupied. It can be seen that imposing the constraint drastically reduces the amount of accessible spectrum in most locations considered. In particular, in the case of central London we see that with this constraint imposed there will be *no channel* available for the operation of CR devices. Averaging the results over all locations, we find that with this constraint imposed there will be only ~ 30 MHz of TV spectrum available for cognitive access.

Finally, we use the estimation approach outlined in Section III to briefly examine the impact of cognitive radio transmit power on the the availability of TVWS channels. Fig. 7 shows, as an example, variations in the number of vacant TV channels as a function of CR transmit power in the case of Manchester [27]. It can be seen that for $p_{cr} \leq 100$ mW up to 17 channels (136 MHz) are available. However, the availability decreases sharply as the transmit power is increased beyond this range. Nevertheless, there is still 40 MHz of spectrum available for CR device transmitting at 2 W, within the typical operation of future IEEE 802.22 devices.

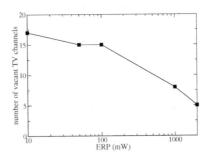

Fig. 6. Variation in the number of TVWS channels is shown as a function of transmit power, computed for the city of Manchester

5   Discussion

Opportunistic access to TV White Spaces by cognitive radios have generated much excitement recently. The research community is working intensely on addressing the remaining technology challenges, while the industry have started to identify and develop commercial exploitation cases, including (rural) broadband wireless access [6] and multimedia home networks [30,31]. Both in the US and UK regulators are establishing new policies and rules for cognitive access, while elsewhere in the world this radically new form of spectrum access is being debated. The objective of this paper was to take a step back from the excitement surrounding cognitive access to TVWS and ask the question: How much spectrum are we actually talking about?, and is this spectrum worth all the research and development effort?

To quantitatively adress these questions we developed in this paper a methodology for estimating the available UK TV White Spaces for opportunistic access by cognitive radios. Using our methodology we examined the availability of this spectrum and its channel composition in 18 UK population centres. Our analysis shows that on average $\sim$ 150 MHz of TVWS is available for access by low-power cognitive radios. This is a significant amount of spectrum, for example in comparison with the UK's 3G spectrum, which is 140 MHZ.

However, in many locations this considerable bandwidth is fragmented into many non-adjacent channels. Furthermore, the frequency composition of TVWS varies greatly from location to location. Consequently, the availability of novel spectrum pooling techniques, such as NC-OFDM [28,29] is crucial for effective utilisation of TVWS, in particular for future high bandwidth applications such as multimedia home networks. Finally, we examined the effect of constraints on adjacent channel interference imposed by regulators/standards on TVWS, and showed that such constraints drastically reduce the availability of this spectrum.

The focus of the current study was on quantifying how much spectrum could, in principle, become available for cognitive access. We did not, however, examined the mechanism by which cognitive devices can discover and utilise this spectrum. One mechanism for detecting TVWS, which has been the subject of numerous research papers [32] is sensing of primary receiver signals by cognitive devices. In particular, in order to avoid harmful interference to TV users under deep fading conditions, cognitive radios are expected to sense TV signals at extremely low signal levels. Initial studies [33,20] indicate that imposing such stringent constraints significantly reduce the utilisation of TVWS by such "oversensitive" devices. Some of our future work will focus on addressing the sensing problem from this new perspective. We are also researching scenarios involving multiple cooperative and/or competing cognitive devices operating in TVWS within the same geographical area [34]. The provision of commercial services based on cognitive radio, e.g. broadband wireless access, will inevitably involve such situations for which novel algorithms for spectrum sharing and interference control need to be developed.

References

1. Mitola, J.: Cognitive radio for flexible mobile multimedia communications. In: The Sixth international Workshop on Mobile Multimedia Communications, San Diego, CA (1999)
2. Haykin, S.: Cognitive radio: Brain-empowered wireless communications. IEEE Journal on Selected Areas in Communications 23(2), 201–219 (2005)
3. First report and notice of rulemaking in the matter of unlicensed operation in TV broadcast bands, ET Docket No. 04-186, Adopted October 18 (2006)
4. Ofcom, Digital Dividend Review, A statement on our approach to awarding the digital dividend, December 13 (2007)
5. Ofcom, Digital dividend: cognitive access, February 16 (2009)
6. IEEE 802.22 Working Group on Wireless Regional Area Networks, www.ieee802.org/22

7. Cordeiro, C., Challapali, K., Birru, D.: IEEE 802.22: An introduction to the first worldwide wireless standard based on cognitive radios. Journal of Communications 1(1), 38–47 (2006)
8. Nekovee, M.: Dynamic spectrum access – concepts and future architectures. BT Technology Journal 24(2), 111–116 (2006)
9. Nekovee, M.: Impact of cognitive radio on future management of spectrum. In: Proc. CrownCom 2008, Singapore (May 2008)
10. Nekovee, M.: Dynamic spectrum access with cognitive radio: architectures and research challenges. In: Proc. CrownCom 2006, Mykonos, Greece (May 2006)
11. Horne, W.D.: Adaptive Spectrum Access: Using the full spectrum space, Technical Report, The MITRE Corporation (2004)
12. The FCC's Office of Engineering and Technology release report on test of prototype white space devices, ET Docket No. 04-186, www.fcc.gov
13. FCC adopts rules for unlicensed use of Television white spaces, Official announcement of FCC, November 4 (2008), http://www.fcc.gov
14. Stuzra, M.A., Ghazvinian, F.: Can cognitive radio technology operating in the TV white spaces completely protect licensed TV broadcasting?, Working paper No 16, Wireless Future Program, New America Foundation.
15. Martin, F.L., Correal, N.S., Eki, R.L., Gorday, P., O'Dea, R.: Early opportunities for commercialisation of TV whitespaces in the U.S. In: Proc. CrownCom 2008, Singapore (May 2008)
16. Petty, M., et al.: Feasibility of dynamic spectrum access in underutilized TV bands. In: Proc. IEEE DySpan 2007, Dublin, Ireland (April 2007)
17. Brown, T.X., Sicker, D.C.: Can cognitive radio support broadband wireless access? In: Proc. IEEE DySPAN 2007, Dublin, Ireland (April 2007)
18. Gurney, D., Buchwald, G., Ecklund, L., Kuffner, S., Grosspietsch, J.: Geo-location database technique for incumbent protection in TV White Spaces. In: Proc. IEEE DySPAN 2008, Chicago, USA (October 2008)
19. Ahuja, R., Corke, R., Bok, A.: Cognitive radio system using IEEE 802.11a over UHF TVWS. In: Proc. IEEE DySPAN 2008, Chicago, USA (October 2008)
20. Mubaraq, M., Sahai, A.: How much white space is there? UC Berkeley, Technical Report, January 11 (2009)
21. Rappaport, T.: Wireless Communications, Principle and Practice. Prentice-Hall, Englewood Cliffs (2000)
22. DTT coverage predictions – how they are made and tested, I. Pullen, Digital News 9, 14–15 (July 1999)
23. UK FREE.TV website, www.ukfreetv.tv
24. Ofcom, Digital Dividend Review: Consultation on geographic interleaved awards 470 − 550 MHz and 630 − 790 MHz, June 12 (2008)
25. Ofcom, Digital switchover transmitter details, www.ofcom.org.uk/tv/ifi/tech/dsodetails/81plan.pdf
26. http://www.ordancesurvey.co.uk
27. Fang, Y.: Estimation of available digital TV channels for cognitive radio operation, MSc. Final Report, Telcommunication and Network Engineering, London South Bank University (2008)
28. Person, J.D., Horne, W.D.: Discontiguous OFDM considerations for dynamic spectrum access in idle TV bands. In: Proc. IEEE DySPAN 2005, Baltimore, Maryland, USA (2005)

29. Rajbanshi, R., Wyglynski, A., Minden, G.: An efficient implementation of NC-OFDM transceivers for cognitive radios. In: Proc. CrownCom 2006, Mykonos, Greece (2006)
30. CogNeA, `www.cognea.org`
31. Henry, P.: Cognitive radio for multimedia home networks, AT&T Tech View, March 16 (2009), `www.research.att.com`
32. Yucek, T., Arsalan, H.: A survey of spectrum sensing algorithms for cognitive radio applications. IEEE Communications Surveys and Tutorials 11(1), 116–130 (2009)
33. BT Technical Report (March 2009)
34. Shankar, N.S., Cordeiro, C.: Analysis of Aggregated Interference at DTV receivers in TV bands. In: Proc. CrownCom 2008, Singapore (May 2008)

Emerging Infrastructure
and Technologies II

MIMO Free-Space Optical Communication Employing Subcarrier Intensity Modulation in Atmospheric Turbulence Channels

Zabih Ghassemlooy[1], Wasiu O. Popoola[1], Vahid Ahmadi[2], and Erich Leitgeb[3]

[1] Northumbria Communication Research Lab (NCRLab), Northumbria University, Newcastle upon Tyne, UK
fary.ghassemlooy@unn.ac.uk
[2] Department of Electrical Engineering Tarbiat Modares University, Tehran, Iran
[3] Institute of Broadband Communications, TU, Graz, Austria

Abstract. In this paper, we analyse the error performance of transmitter/receiver array free-space optical (FSO) communication system employing binary phase shift keying (BPSK) subcarrier intensity modulation (SIM) in clear but turbulent atmospheric channel. Subcarrier modulation is employed to eliminate the need for adaptive threshold detector. Direct detection is employed at the receiver and each subcarrier is subsequently demodulated coherently. The effect of irradiance fading is mitigated with an array of lasers and photodetectors. The received signals are linearly combined using the optimal maximum ratio combining (MRC), the equal gain combining (EGC) and the selection combining (SelC). The bit error rate (BER) equations are derived considering additive white Gaussian noise and log normal intensity fluctuations. This work is part of the EU COST actions and EU projects.

Keywords: Atmospheric turbulence, BPSK, Free-space optics, Laser communications, MIMO systems, Subcarrier modulation, Spatial diversity.

1 Introduction

Propagating data-laden laser radiation over the atmosphere termed FSO communications is attractive for a number of reasons including unlicensed spectrum and a narrow beamwidth [1-3]. There exist global growing interest in FSO and it was extensively researched as part of the concluded EU framework 6 projects and the COST actions. Towards the end of 2008 a new COST action called IC0802 on "Propagation tools and data for integrated Telecommunication, Navigation and Earth Observation systems" was started and within this action group; our working group (consisting of around 10 participants) is involved in the optical wireless communications.

An outdoor FSO link is essentially based on line-of sight (LOS), thus, its spatial isolation from potential interferers is sufficiently maintained by its narrow beamwidth profile. But an obvious demerit of the narrow laser beamwidth is the pointing and tracking requirements in the event of misalignment. This can however be corrected using active tracking but at the cost of increased complexity and cost [3-5].

R. Mehmood et al. (Eds.): EuropeComm 2009, LNICST 16, pp. 61–73, 2009.

Fog, aerosols, rain and gases and other particles suspended in the atmosphere result in laser irradiance/intensity attenuation. The attenuation coefficient typically ranges from a few dB/km in a clear atmosphere to ~270 dB/km in a dense fog regime [4]. The huge attenuation suffered during dense fog restricts the carrier class FSO links to ~500 m [5, 6]; extending the link range in such conditions requires alternative schemes such as hybrid RF/FSO [7, 8]. Another factor that accounts for the FSO performance degradation in a clear atmosphere is the irradiance fluctuation (scintillation) and the phase fluctuation, which result from random index of refraction variations along the propagation path due to the atmospheric turbulence [3, 9, 10].

The On-Off keying (OOK) signalling format has been widely used in the commercially available FSO systems. But in channels with the atmospheric turbulence induced fading, the OOK scheme requires adaptive threshold to perform optimally [11, 12]. This fact among others has led to the increased interest in the study of SIM in FSO systems [12-14]. It has also been shown that using a fixed threshold OOK scheme results in suboptimal system, which is not only inferior to a SIM modulated FSO link but also has a BER floor [15]. In [16] the low density parity check (LDPC) coding has been explored to ameliorate the effect of scintillation on a SIM-FSO link. It is reported that the LDPC coded SIM in atmospheric turbulence achieved a coding gain of > 20 dB compared to the similarly coded OOK. In [17] the use of space-time block code with coherent and differential detection techniques has been reported to achieve a similar performance. However, invoking error control coding introduces huge processing delays and efficiency degradation in view of the number of redundant bits that will be required as outlined in [18].

In this paper the BER analysis of the SIM-FSO based multiple-input-multiple-output (MIMO) configuration in the presence of the log normal atmospheric turbulence is presented considering the following linear receiver combining techniques: EGC, MRC and SelC. Both cases of spatially correlated and uncorrelated optical field at the receivers are considered in the presence of the additive white Gaussian noise. In a related work reported in [19], the spatial diversity is considered at the receiver side for both OOK and PPM modulated FSO systems. Apart from mitigating scintillation, the MIMO system is advantageous in combating temporary link blockage by birds and misalignment when combined with a wide laser beamwidth, thereby eliminating the need for an active tracking. It also is much easier to provide independent aperture averaging with multiple separate aperture system. The terrestrial FSO is basically a LOS link with a negligible delay spread; hence inter-symbol interference (ISI) is not an issue. The rest of the paper is arranged as follows: Section 2 discusses subcarrier intensity modulation; the error performance is discussed in Section 3 while the concluding remarks are given in Section 4.

2 Subcarrier Intensity Modulation

In optical communication systems SIM is achieved by modulating the data onto a radio frequency signal, which is then used to vary the irradiance/intensity of an optical source (a continuous laser source in this case). In this work, the subcarrier is assumed to be pre-modulated using the BPSK. Other modulation methods can also be used and this is one of the major advantages of SIM. Considering weak turbulence and assuming that the log intensity l of laser radiation traversing the atmosphere obeys the normal distribution i.e. $l \sim N(-\sigma_l^2/2, \sigma_l^2)$, then the probability density function (pdf) of the intensity $I = I_o\exp(l)$ is given by [20]:

$$p_I(I) = \frac{1}{\sqrt{2\pi}\sigma_l}\frac{1}{I}\exp\left\{-\frac{\left(\ln(I/I_0)+0.5\sigma_l^2\right)^2}{2\sigma_l^2}\right\} \quad I \geq 0, \tag{1}$$

where the average received intensity $I = 0.5I_{max}$, I_{max} is the peak received laser intensity and I_0 is the received average intensity without turbulence. The σ_l^2 is a measure of the strength of laser intensity fluctuation and (1) is valid for $\sigma_l^2 < 1.2$ [20]. The instantaneous photocurrent can be modelled as [21]:

$$i_r(t) = RI(1+\xi m(t)) + n(t), \tag{2}$$

where ζ is the modulation index, R is the PIN photodetector responsivity and $n(t)$ is the additive white Gaussian noise (AWGN). Considering M subcarriers, the composite subcarrier signal during the kth symbol duration is given by:

$$m(t) = \sum_{j=1}^{M} A_j g(t-kT)d_k \cos(w_{cj}t + \varphi_j), \tag{3}$$

where $d_k \in \{-1,1\}$ for data bit '0' and '1', $g(t-kT)$ is the rectangular pulse shaping function, and T is the symbol duration. The subcarrier angular frequency and the phase are represented by $\{\omega_{cj}\}_{j=1}^{M}$ and $\{\varphi_{cj}\}_{j=1}^{M}$, respectively, while $\{A_j\}_{j=1}^{M}$ is the peak subcarrier amplitude. For the continuous wave laser transmitter to operate within its dynamic range and to avoid signal distortion due to clipping, the condition $|\zeta m(t)| \leq 1$ must always hold. Considering BPSK modulated subcarriers with non-varying amplitudes, the peak amplitude $A_j = A$. And if ζ is normalized to unity, then $A \leq 1/M$ During the kth symbol, the photocurrent is as given by:

$$i_r(t) = RI\left[1+\xi A\sum_{j=1}^{M} g(t-kT)d_k \cos(w_{cj}t + \varphi_j)\right] + n(t). \tag{4}$$

The band pass filters (BPF) in Fig.1 help separate the subcarriers and suppress any slow varying RI component in (4). The subcarrier frequencies are subsequently demodulated independently by frequency down conversion using a reference carrier signal $\cos(\omega_{cj}t + \varphi_j)$. A low pass filter (LPF) is employed to recover d_k with minimal distortion. The result per branch is an antipodal signal given by:

$$i_D(t) = \frac{d_k IR\xi Ag(t-kT)}{2} + n_D(t), \tag{5}$$

where $n_D(t)$ is the post demodulation AWGN with a variance $\sigma^2/2$. The post demodulation electrical signal-to-noise ratio (SNR_e) γ, per subcarrier is then derived from (5) as:

$$\gamma(I) = \frac{(I\xi RA)^2}{2\sigma^2}. \tag{6}$$

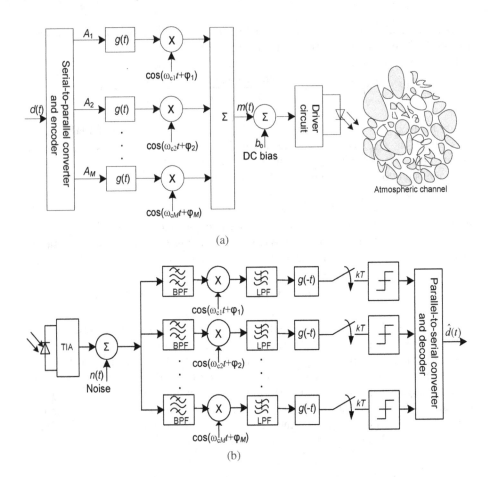

Fig. 1. SIM-FSO block diagram; (a) transmitter, and (b) receiver. TIA – Trans-impedance amplifier.

For a fixed value of ζ therefore, using multiple subcarrier increases through-put/capacity but at SNR_e penalty given by $20\log M$ dB. This suggests that multiple subcarriers should only be considered when the need for increased capacity outweighs the accompanying power penalty.

3   Error Performance

3.1   Without Diversity

For a coherently demodulated BPSK SIM operated in a channel with the atmospheric turbulence, the unconditional probability of bit error obtained by averaging the conditional error rate over irradiance fluctuation statistics is derived as [22]:

$$P_e \cong \frac{1}{\pi} \int_0^{\pi/2} \frac{1}{\sqrt{\pi}} \sum_{i=1}^{m} w_i \exp\left(-\frac{K^2 \exp(2(\sqrt{2}\sigma_l x_i - \sigma_l^2 / 2))}{2\sin^2(\theta)} \right) d\theta$$

(7)

$$\cong \frac{1}{\sqrt{\pi}} \sum_{i=1}^{m} w_i Q(Ke^{(x_i\sqrt{2}\sigma_l - \sigma_l^2 / 2)}),$$

where $K = \dfrac{R\xi I_0 A}{\sqrt{2}\sigma}$, $\{x_i\}_{j=1}^{m}$ and $\{w_i\}_{j=1}^{m}$ represent the zeros of the mth order Hermite polynomial $He_m(x)$ and the corresponding weight factors, respectively.

3.2 With Receiver Diversity

Spatial diversity is employed both at the transmitter and receiver as shown in Fig. 2. In the analysis and the subsequent sections, the single SIM-FSO is considered. First, the use of an array of N-photodetector is analysed while transmitter array is treated in the subsequent section.

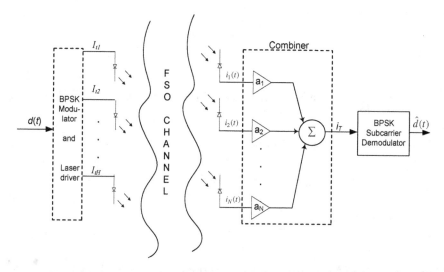

Fig. 2. $H \times N$-MIMO FSO system block diagram

We assume the spatial separation s of the photodetectors to be greater than the irradiance spatial coherence distance ρ_o (i.e. $s > \rho_o$) resulting in uncorrelated received irradiance. This assumption is realistic because ρ_o is on the order of few centimetre [20]. We also assumed that the beamwidth at the receiver is sufficiently broad to cover the entire field of view (FOV) of the N detectors. The photocurrents $\{i_{ri}(t)\}_{i=1}^{N}$ are linearly combined before being applied to the coherent demodulator to extract the transmitted data from the received subcarrier signal.

To facilitate a fair comparison between the single-transmitter-single-receiver system and the spatial diversity system, each aperture area in the photodetector array is assumed to be A_D/N, where A_D is the receiver aperture area for single-transmitter-single-receiver system. The SNR_e can thus be derived as:

$$\gamma = \frac{\left(RA\xi/2N\right)^2\left(\sum\limits_{i=1}^{N} a_i I_i\right)^2}{\sum\limits_{i=1}^{N} a_i^2 \sigma_i^2 / 2N} \le \frac{\left(RA\xi/2N\right)^2 \sum\limits_{i=1}^{N} a_i^2 \sum\limits_{i=1}^{N} I_i^2}{\sum\limits_{i=1}^{N} a_i^2 \sigma_i^2 / 2N}. \tag{8}$$

MRC

Under the MRC, the gains $\{a_i\}_{i=1}^{N} \equiv \{I_i\}_{i=1}^{N}$ resulting in the optimum SNR_e given below:

$$\gamma_{MRC}\ (\overline{I}) = \left(\frac{RA\ \xi}{\sqrt{2N}}\right)^2 \sum\limits_{i=1}^{N} \frac{I_i^2}{\sigma_i^2} \tag{9}$$

$$= \sum\limits_{i=1}^{N} \gamma_i,$$

where $\gamma_i = \left(\dfrac{RA\xi I_i}{\sqrt{2N\sigma_i^2}}\right)^2$ is the SNR for each link. The unconditional BER with the

MRC linear combining is given by [22]:

$$P_{e(MRC)} = \int\limits_{0}^{\infty} Q\left(\sqrt{\gamma_{MRC}\ (\overline{I})}\right) P_{\overline{I}}\ (\overline{I}) d\overline{I}$$

$$= \frac{1}{\pi} \int\limits_{0}^{\pi/2} [S(\theta)]^N\ d\theta \tag{10}$$

Where $S(\theta) \approx \frac{1}{\sqrt{\pi}} \sum\limits_{j=1}^{M} w_j \exp\left(-\frac{K_o^2}{2\sin^2\theta} \exp[2(x_j\sqrt{2}\sigma_l - \sigma_l^2/2)]\right)$ and $K_o = \frac{R\xi I_o A}{\sqrt{2N\sigma}}$.

Next, we consider the sub-optimum but more practical linear combining techniques.

EGC

For the EGC, gains $\{a_i\}_{i=1}^{N}$ in (8) are all made constant, thus resulting in the following SNR_e:

$$\gamma_{EGC}\ (\overline{I}) = \left(\frac{RA\xi}{\sqrt{2N\sigma}}\right)^2 \left(\sum\limits_{i=1}^{N} I_i\right)^2 < \left(\frac{RA\xi}{\sqrt{2N}}\right)^2 \sum\limits_{i=1}^{N} \frac{I_i^2}{\sigma^2}. \tag{11}$$

Thus, $\gamma_{EGC}(\bar{I}) < \gamma_{MRC}(\bar{I})$ and the unconditional BER can be obtained as [22]:

$$P_{e(EGC)} = \int_0^\infty \frac{1}{\pi} \int_0^{\pi/2} \exp\left(-\frac{K_1^2}{2\sin^2(\theta)} Z^2\right) P_Z(Z)\, d\theta dZ$$

$$= \frac{1}{\sqrt{\pi}} \sum_{i=1}^m w_i Q(K_1 e^{(x_i\sqrt{2}\sigma_u + \mu_u)})$$

(12)

where $K_1 = \dfrac{R\xi I_0 A}{\sqrt{2}\,\sigma N}$, $P_z(Z) = \dfrac{1}{\sqrt{2\pi}\sigma_u} \dfrac{1}{Z} \exp\left\{-\left(\ln Z - \mu_u\right)^2 / 2\sigma_u^2\right\}$ and

$\mu_u = \ln(N) - \dfrac{1}{2}\ln\left(1 + \dfrac{e^{\sigma_l^2} - 1}{N}\right)$ while $\sigma_u^2 = \ln\left(1 + \dfrac{e^{\sigma_l^2} - 1}{N}\right)$.

SelC

Here, the combiner samples all $\{i_{ri}(t)\}_{i=1}^N$ and selects the link with the highest SNR_e, its BER is derived as [22]:

$$P_{e(SelC)} = \frac{2^{1-N} N}{\sqrt{\pi}} \sum_{i=1}^m w_i \left[1 + erf(x_i)\right]^{N-1} Q(K_0 \exp(x_i\sqrt{2}\sigma_l - \sigma_l^2/2)),$$

(13)

3.3 Effect of Signal Correlation on the BER

For N-photodetector separated by a spatial distance less than the laser radiation spatial coherence distance (i.e. $s < \rho_0$), the received radiations are correlated. To show the effect of this on the system error performance, we consider N equally spaced photodetectors employing the optimum MRC linear combining. The unconditional BER in atmospheric turbulence is obtained by averaging (14) over the joint pdf of the intensity fluctuations.

$$P_{ec} = Q\left(\sqrt{\gamma_{MRC}(\bar{I})}\right)$$

$$= \frac{1}{\pi} \int_0^{\pi/2} \exp\left(-\frac{K_0^2}{2I_0^2 \sin^2\theta} \sum_{i=1}^N I_i^2\right) d\theta$$

(14)

Adopting the Tatarski approach [20], the correlation coefficient $\rho(s) = B_X(s)/B_X(0)$ of an optical wave in turbulent atmosphere between two points with a spatial separation s is given by:

$$\rho(s) = 1 - 2.36(ks/L)^{5/6} + 1.71(ks/L) - 0.024(ks/L)^2 +$$
$$0.00043(ks/L)^4 + \ldots$$

(15)

where $k = 2\pi/\lambda$; it can be inferred that the correlation coefficient is inversely propor-

tional to the spatial separation s for $\dfrac{s}{\sqrt{\lambda L}} < 1$ (i.e. for s less than atmospheric channel

coherence distance) from which the covariance matrix (16) is obtained.

$$
C_X = \begin{bmatrix}
\sigma_x^{\,2} & \rho\sigma_x^{\,2} & \cdot & \cdot & \rho\dfrac{s_{12}}{s_{1N}}\sigma_x^{\,2} \\[2ex]
\rho\dfrac{s_{12}}{s_{21}}\sigma_x^{\,2} & \sigma_x^{\,2} & \cdot & & \cdot \\[2ex]
\cdot & & \cdot & & \cdot \\[1ex]
\cdot & & & \cdot & \\[1ex]
\rho\dfrac{s_{12}}{s_{N1}}\sigma_x^{\,2} & \cdot & \cdot & & \sigma_x^{\,2}
\end{bmatrix},
\tag{16}
$$

where s_{ij} is the spatial separation between photodetectors i and j, $\sigma_x^{\,2} = \sigma_l^{\,2}/4$ is the log amplitude variance while ρ is the correlation coefficient between two photodetectors with spatial separation s_{12}. The joint pdf of received laser intensity is given by [9]:

$$
p_{\bar I}(\bar I) = \frac{1}{2^N \prod\limits_{i=1}^{N} I_i} \frac{1}{(2\pi)^{N/2}|C_X|^{1/2}} \exp(-\tfrac{1}{8}\beta C_X^{-1}\beta^T),
\tag{17}
$$

where $\beta = \begin{bmatrix} \ln\dfrac{I_1}{I_0} & \ln\dfrac{I_2}{I_0} & \cdot\cdot\cdot & \ln\dfrac{I_N}{I_0} \end{bmatrix}$. The expression for the unconditional

BER is then obtained as:

$$
P_e = \int_0^{\infty} p_{\bar I}(\bar I) Q(\sqrt{\gamma_{MRC}(\bar I)})d\bar I .
\tag{18}
$$

3.4 Transmitter Diversity

In this case we consider a single photodetector and multiple laser transmitters. The laser sources are assumed to be sufficiently spaced so that the photodetector receives uncorrelated laser radiations. To ensure a fair comparison and to maintain a constant power requirement, we assume that the power available for a single-transmitter system is equally shared amongst the H-laser transmitters. As such, the irradiance from each laser represents an H factor reduction compared to a single transmitter system. Another obvious approach is to assume that all the transmitters have the same power; in this case the power requirement will have to increase by a factor H [18]. Based on the former, the received photocurrent is given by:

$$
i_r(t) = \sum_{i=1}^{H} \frac{R}{H} I_i \left(1 + A\xi d_k\, g(t-kT)\cos(w_c t + \varphi)\right) + n(t).
\tag{19}
$$

Since laser arrays are only separated by a few centimetres, the phase shift experienced by the received irradiance due to path difference is therefore negligible. The SNR_e on each subcarrier can therefore be derived as:

$$\gamma_{MISO}(\bar{I}) = \left(\frac{R\xi A}{\sqrt{2}H\sigma}\right)^2 \left(\sum_{i=1}^{H} I_i\right)^2. \tag{20}$$

There exist a clear similarity between (11) and (20) hence; the unconditional BER for the multiple transmitter-single photodetector system is the same as that for the single transmitter-multiple photodetector configuration with EGC linear combining.

3.5 Transmitter Diversity-Receiver Diversity (MIMO)

In this section we consider a multiple-laser and multiple-photodetector system. In consistent with the earlier assumptions, the total transmit power is made equal to the transmit power when using a single laser to achieve the same bit rate and the combined aperture area of the N-photodetector is the same as when a single photodetector is used. The H-laser and N-photodetector are assumed spaced enough so that the received laser radiations are uncorrelated. First, we consider when the photocurrents are combined using EGC. As previously discussed, a multiple transmitter-single photodetector system with H-laser is identical to a single transmitter-multiple photodetector configuration having H-photodetector with EGC combining; thus the following represents the SNR_e assuming identically distributed irradiance:

$$\gamma(\bar{I}) = \left(\frac{R\xi A}{\sqrt{2}NH\sigma}\right)^2 \left(\sum_{i=1}^{N}\sum_{j=1}^{H} I_{ij}\right)^2 = \left(\frac{R\xi A}{\sqrt{2}NH\sigma}\right)^2 \left(\sum_{i=1}^{NH} I_i\right)^2. \tag{21}$$

This expression is the same as NH-photodetector single transmitter-multiple photodetector system employing EGC linear combining. Hence, the unconditional BER is obtained by replacing N by NH in (12).

By linearly combining the photocurrents using MRC, the individual SNR_e on each link is:

$$\gamma_i(I_i) = \left(\frac{R\xi A}{\sqrt{2}N\sigma^2 H}\sum_{j=1}^{H} I_{ij}\right)^2. \tag{22}$$

Considering the sum of independent lognormal distributed random variables as another log normal distribution [23] then the unconditional BER is derived as:

$$P_e = \frac{1}{\pi}\int_0^{\pi/2} [S(\theta)]^N d\theta, \tag{23}$$

Where $S(\theta) \approx \frac{1}{\sqrt{\pi}}\sum_{j=1}^{M} w_j \exp\left(-\frac{K_2^2}{2\sin^2\theta}\exp[2(x_j\sqrt{2}\sigma_u + \mu_u)]\right)$, $K_2 = \frac{R\xi I_0 A}{\sqrt{2}N\sigma H}$, σ_u^2 and μ_u are as previously defined except that N is now replaced by H. For an optical MIMO-FSO link under consideration therefore, the BER performance is governed by (12) with N replaced by NH for the EGC combining technique and (23) for the MRC.

3.6 Results and Discussions

The plot of (7) against the normalised electrical SNR $(RE[I]/2\sigma)^2$ is shown in Fig. 3 with $M = [1, 2, 5, 10]$, $\sigma_1^2 = 0.3$ and $\zeta = 1$. When $M = 1$ the BER curve is the same as that reported in [12]. Multiple subcarriers can therefore be used to increase the capacity but at an electrical SNR penalty defined by $20\log M$ dB. To show the effect of signal correlation, (18) is plotted in Fig. 4 for $N = [2, 3]$ and $\rho = [0, 0.1, 0.3, 0.6]$ at a turbulence level $\sigma_1^2 = 0.3$. To achieve a BER of 10^{-6}, the use of two photodetectors with $\rho = 0.3$ and 0.6 require additional ~1.8 dB and ~3.5 dB of SNR, respectively, compared to when $s > \rho_o$ (i.e. when $\rho = 0$); with three photodetectors, the additional SNR required to achieve the same BER of 10^{-6} is ~2.7 dB and ~5 dB for $\rho = 0.3$ and 0.6, respectively. This apparently shows the effect of correlated intensity and also buttresses the emphasis placed on the need for s to be greater than ρ_o in a spatial diversity system as it results in the maximum gain.

To compare the MIMO system with the single SIM benchmark reported in [12], the BER given by (23) is plotted against the normalised electrical SNR as depicted in Fig. 5 at a turbulence level $\sigma_1^2 = 0.3$ for various values of N and H. The link margin (diversity gain) resulting from the use of transmitter/receiver array is shown in Table I. A 2×2-MIMO system requires an additional ~0.4 dB of SNR compared to a 1×4-MIMO system. In the latter however, 4 photodetectors will have to be sufficiently spaced to avoid any correlation in the received signals as against 2 photodetectors in the former. Also, at the stated BER, a 4×4-MIMO based SIM-FSO link requires ~4 dB and 1 dB lower SNR compared to the single transmitter with 4 and 8 photodetectors, respectively.

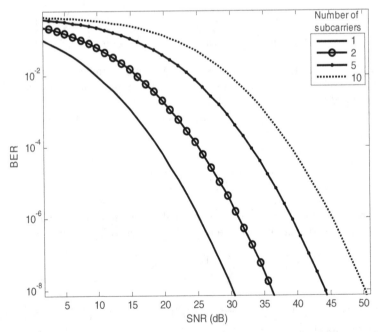

Fig. 3. BER against the electrical SNR for $M =[1,2,5,10]$ subcarriers and turbulence strength $\sigma_1^2 = 0.3$

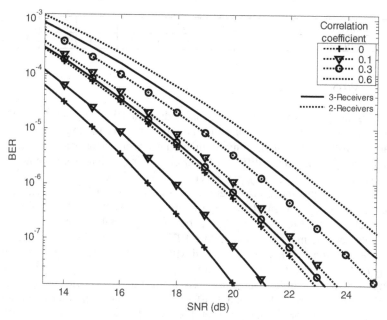

Fig. 4. BER against the electrical *SNR* at different values of correlation coefficient for number of photodetector $N = [2, 3]$ and turbulence strength $\sigma_1^2 = 0.3$

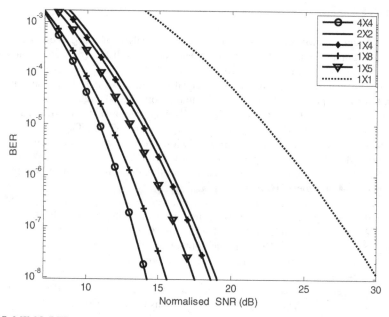

Fig. 5. MIMO BER against the electrical *SNR* for different numbers of laser and photodetector array at turbulence strength $\sigma_1^2 = 0.3$ and $M = 1$

Table 1. Link margin (diversity gain) at BER of 10^{-6} and $\sigma_l^2 = 0.3$

MIMO configuration	1x5	1x8	4x4	2x2	1x4
Link margin (dB)	10.5	12.1	13.1	9.2	9.6

4 Conclusions

We have presented an expression for the unconditional BER of $H \times N$-MIMO FSO system that uses BPSK subcarrier intensity modulation under the log normal distributed weak atmospheric turbulence environment. The error performance and the link margin (theoretical) using three different linear combining techniques have also been presented. Results showing clearly the effect of correlated received irradiance on the system error performance have also been given. In a 2-detector array and at a turbulence strength σ_l^2 of 0.3, a correlation coefficient of 0.6 results in additional ~3.5 dB of SNR to achieve a BER of 10^{-6}; this incurred power penalty increases as the received signals become more correlated. At a BER of 10^{-6}, 2 × 2-MIMO systems require ~0.4 dB additional *SNR* when compared with 1 × 4-MIMO systems. But spacing of an array of 4 photodetectors to ensure uncorrelated irradiance reception is far more demanding than spacing 2 photodetectors. Also the use of 4 × 4-MIMO to deliver the same BER of 10^{-6} requires ~4 dB and 1 dB lower SNR than using one laser source with 4 and 8 photodetectors, respectively. A 4 × 4-MIMO system is thus the preferred configuration to mitigate scintillation without increased system complexity.

References

1. Uysal, M., Jing, L., Meng, Y.: Error rate performance analysis of coded free-space optical links over gamma-gamma atmospheric turbulence channels. IEEE Transactions on Wireless Communications 5, 1229–1233 (2006)
2. Leitgeb, E., Geghart, M., Birnbacher, U.: Optical networks, last mile access and applications. Journal of optical and fibre communications reports 2, 56–85 (2005)
3. Kedar, D., Arnon, S.: Urban Optical Wireless Communication Networks: The main challenges and possible solutions. IEEE Optical communications, s2–s7 (2004)
4. Willebrand, H., Ghuman, B.S.: Free Space Optics: Enabling optical Connectivity in today's network. SAMS publishing, Indianapolis (2002)
5. Killinger, D.: Free space optics for laser communication through the air. Optics & Photonics News, 36–42 (October 2002)
6. Kim, I.I., McArthur, B., Korevaar, E.: Comparison of laser beam propagation at 785 nm and 1550 nm in fog and haze for optical wireless communications. In: SPIE Proceeding: Optical Wireless Communications III, vol. 4214, pp. 26–37 (2001)
7. Bloom, S., Hartley, W.S.: The last-mile solution: hybrid FSO radio, in AirFiber, Inc. White paper (Visited, July 2007), http://www.freespaceoptic.com/WhitePapers/Hybrid_FSO.pdf
8. Kim, I.I., Korevaar, E.: Availability of free space optics and hybrid FSO/RF systems. In: Proceedings of SPIE: Optical wireless communications IV, vol. 4530, pp. 84–95 (2001)
9. Zhu, X., Kahn, J.M.: Free-space optical communication through atmospheric turbulence channels. IEEE Transactions on Communications 50, 1293–1300 (2002)

10. Karp, S., Gagliardi, R.M., Moran, S.E., Stotts, L.B.: Optical Channels: fibers, cluds, water and the atmosphere. Plenum Press, New York (1988)
11. Huang, W., Takayanagi, J., Sakanaka, T., Nakagawa, M.: Atmospheric optical communication system using subcarrier PSK modulation. In: ICC 1993, IEEE International Conference on Communications, Geneva, May 1993, vol. 3, pp. 1597–1601 (1993)
12. Ohtsuki, T.: Turbo-coded atmospheric optical communication systems. In: IEEE International Conference on Communications (ICC), New York, pp. 2938–2942 (2002)
13. Kim, J.P., Lee, K.Y., Kim, J.H., Kim, Y.K.: A performance analysis of wireless optical communication with convolutional code in turbulent atmosphere. In: International Technical Conference on Circuits Systems, Computers and Communications (ITC-CSCC 1997), Okinawa, pp. 15–18 (1997)
14. Popoola, W.O., Ghassemlooy, Z., Leitgeb, E.: Free-space optical communication using subcarrier modulation in gamma-gamma atmospheric turbulence. In: 9th International Conference on Transparent Optical Networks (ICTON 2007), Rome, Italy, vol. 3, pp. 156–160 (2007)
15. Li, J., Liu, J.Q., Taylor, D.P.: Optical communication using subcarrier PSK intensity modulation through atmospheric turbulence channels. IEEE Transaction on communications 55, 1598–1606 (2007)
16. Djordjevic, I.B., Vasic, B., Neifeld, M.A.: LDPC coded OFDM over the atmospheric turbulence channel. Optical Express 15, 6336–6350 (2007)
17. Yamamoto, H., Ohtsuki, T.: Atmospheric optical subcarrier modulation systems using space-time block code. In: IEEE Global Telecommunications Conference (GLOBECOM 2003), New York, vol. 6, pp. 3326–3330 (2003)
18. Lee, E.J., Chan, V.W.S.: Optical communications over the clear turbulent atmospheric channel using diversity. IEEE Journal on Selected Areas in Communications 22, 1896–1906 (2004)
19. Razavi, M., Shapiro, J.H.: Wireless optical communications via diversity reception and optical preamplification. IEEE Transaction on Communications 4, 975–983 (2005)
20. Osche, G.R.: Optical Detection Theory for Laser Applications. Wiley, New Jersey (2002)
21. Gagliardi, R.M., Karp, S.: Optical Communications, 2nd edn. John Wiley, New York (1995)
22. Popoola, W.O., Ghassemlooy, Z., Allen, J.I.H., Leitgeb, E., Gao, S.: Free-space optical communication employing subcarrier modulation and spatial diversity in atmospheric turbulence channel. IET Optoelectronic 2, 16–23 (2008)
23. Mitchell, R.L.: Permanence of the log-normal distribution. Journal of the optical society of America 58, 1267–1272 (1968)

RSVP-TE Based Impairments Collection Mechanism in DWDM Network

Marco Anisetti[1], Valerio Bellandi[1], Roberto Cassata[2], Ernesto Damiani[1], and Zafar Ali[2]

[1] Università degli studi di Milano, Department of Information Technology, Italy
{marco.anisetti,valerio.bellandi,ernesto.damiani}@unimi.it
[2] Cisco System, USA

Abstract. The problem of path validation of a pure light-path in a Dense Wavelength Division Multiplexing (DWDM) optical network requires the transmission of optical impairments related parameters along the provisioned route. In this paper we propose an RSVP-TE based mechanism to collect and evaluate optical impairments measured over optical nodes along the light-path.

Keywords: DWDM, Impairments, RSVP-TE.

1 Introduction

With the development of dense wavelength-division multiplexing (DWDM), optical switches have become the key device in today's optical networks. DWDM- based meshed networks will require novel techniques of optical protection, going well beyond traditional techniques based upon redundancy at the system, card, or fiber level. It is widely acknowledged that in the next generation of optical networks (wavelength switched optical networks), redundancy will be wavelength-based. In other words, the optical infrastructure will be able to react to faults by switching wavelengths or fibers, routing connections in real time through the networks of different vendors on the optical layer. These switching capabilities will rely on a software layer implementing routing and signaling protocols. Several mechanisms for link management aimed at all-optical networks.

The Generalized Multi-protocol Label Switching (GMPLS), supports a number of mechanisms for dynamically allocating resources, providing fault protection and restoration techniques. From its beginning Generalized Multi-Protocol Label Switching (GMPLS) was intended to control wavelength switched optical networks (WSON [1]) with the GMPLS architecture document [2] explicitly mentioning both wavelength and waveband switching and equating wavelengths (lambdas) with GMPLS labels. Unfortunately GMPLS protocol suite cannot be fully exploited in photonic DWDM networks or WSON. A major problem is due to purely optical interfaces, where there is no electro-optical conversion. Nevertheless the control of WSON via GMPLS is currently under study, a further effect need to be taken into account also for the actual DWDM optical networks.

R. Mehmood et al. (Eds.): EuropeComm 2009, LNICST 16, pp. 74–82, 2009.

In fact, an optical signal progresses along its path it may be altered by the various physical processes in the optical fibers and devices it encounters. When such alterations result in signal degradation, we usually refer to these processes as "impairments". Roughly speaking, optical impairments accumulate along the path (without 3R regeneration) traversed by the signal. They are influenced by the type of fiber used, the types and placement of various optical devices and the presence of other optical signals that may share a fiber segment along the signal's path. The degradation of the optical signals due to impairments can result in unacceptable bit error rates or even a complete failure to demodulate and/or detect the received signal. Therefore, path selection and validation requires consideration of optical impairments so that the signal will be propagated from the network ingress point to the egress point with acceptable amount of degradation. In particular for enhanced path status validation, we need mechanisms that can collect all physical impairments (consisting of optical measurements such as signal power, OSNR, etc.) that affect the light-path. We propose an RSVP-TE based mechanism for collection of impairments along a light-path. The proposed technique is also suitable for optical networks that suffer of physical dysfunction due the non-ideal optical transmission medium and/or to critical situations (e.g., a fiber cut). In [3], an overview of some critical optical impairments and their routing related issues can be found. In the rest of the paper the term impairments refer to real optical measurements or estimates computed using a prediction model. The former may require mutually exclusive access to hardware to avoid interference, in which case the impairments required a blocking collection type. In the later case the impairments are collected with a non-blocking collection type. This paper addresses impairments collection for both blocking and non-blocking type leaving the definition of the collection type to as a section attribute. The description of impairments type and effects [4] is out of the scope of this paper.

2   Impairments Collection

The line path validation mechanism needs to be aware of all physical impairments (consisting of optical measurements such as signal power, OSNR, Optical Channel Monitor, etc.) that affect the light-path. Consequently this draft proposes control plane based mechanism for impairments collection. How impairments are collected (from data plane) is beyond the scope of this document.

2.1   Optical Path Validation

Our approach is in full agreement with information model [5] for path validation and in particular we refer to [1] for architectural options in which impairment validation for an optical path is defined. The validation of an optical path is assessed by collecting the physical impairments along an LSP and evaluating them. In this draft we make use of the LSP ATTRIBUTES to perform the impairments collection hop by hop along the optical path. It is important to note that collection of impairments in a blocking way requires a mutually exclusive access to the resource. Therefore the entire LSP needs to be "locked" until the collection for the impairments is completed. This implies that if another impairments collection process tries to retrieve impairments on the same node-resource already under "Administrative Impairments Locking" status, needs to be aborted. The draft uses the RSVP Admin status object to realize "LSP Administrative Impairments locking" to make sure that all nodes are ready to collect the impairments in a blocking way. Our RSVP based impairments collection protocol made the optical path validation described in [5] available. More in details the G.680 gives techniques and formulas for use in calculating the impact of a cascade of network elements. These formulations is at the base of our path validation. In the following we first define Optical Impairments collection classification, and the extensions to LSP ATTRIBUTE and RSVP Admin status objects needed to perform the aforementioned functionalities. Section 2.7 details the signaling mechanism with examples to illustrate how proposed extensions are used for impairments collection.

2.2 Optical Impairments Collection Classification and LSP Locking

Physical impairments that have effect on the light-path can be collected in two ways:

- Blocking impairments collection. In general in the case of blocking collection, the impairment collection may require a mutually exclusive access to hardware resources while performing the measurement.
- Non blocking impairments collection. A collection of physical value that can be probed in parallel at different nodes.

Consequently, every optical node can be in three states w.r.t. to a certain reserved resource: unlock, lock-requested or lock. In fact blocking collection of impairment requires the resource to be in lock state. In general this is due to the hardware limitation of optical nodes. In case of blocking collection of impairments the LSP status needs to be set to "Locked". For this purpose, we extend the Admin object [6], [7] with B bit (Blocked request bit) and C bit (block Confirm bit). Specifically, Administrative status object is extended with the following two bits for locking purpose. Following we brief explain the ADMIN status header (Figure 1) together with the aforementioned extension:

- *Reflect (R):* 1 bit. When set, indicates that the edge node should reflect the object/TLV back in the appropriate message. This bit must not be set in state change request, i.e., Notify, messages.
- *Reserved:* 25 bits. This field is reserved. It must be set to zero on transmission and must be ignored on receipt. These bits should be passed through unmodified by transit nodes.
- *Testing (T):* 1 bit. When set, indicates that the local actions related to the "testing" mode should be taken.
- *Administratively down (A):* 1 bit. When set, indicates that the local actions related to the "administratively down" state should be taken.
- *Deletion in progress (D):* 1 bit. When set, indicates that that the local actions related to LSP teardown should be taken. Edge nodes may use this flag to control connection teardown.
- *Blocking node (B):* 1 bit. When set, indicates that locking procedure is ongoing.
- *Confirm blocking (C):* 1 bit. When set, indicates that the locking procedure is successfully ongoing.

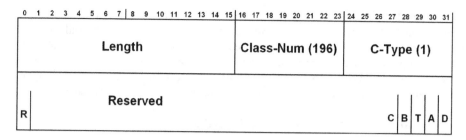

Fig. 1. The administrative Status object

During LSP locking for collection of impairments, the R bit (Reflect bit) must be set. Furthermore, if the node along the path understands B and C bits, the node must return the Admin object in the Resv Message for locking confirmation or unlocking. Since we need to block an entire LSP, any node unable to measure the required impairments must set a lock failure (unset the C bit in the Path Admin Object). The general locking procedure is defined as follows:

- Every transit node that receives the Admin status object in the Path message with B, C and R bit set needs to check if the actual status is unlock.
- In the case of unlock status, the node switches to lock-required state related to the required impairments.
- In the case of lock or lock-required states, the node forwards the Admin object message without the C bit set. This implies a lock failure.
- The Resv message performs the locking for the entire LSP in case of C and B bit set and unlocking in case of unset C bit.
- Every transit node that receives the Resv message with B and C bit set changes its status to lock.

This strategy prevents race conditions.

2.3 Optical Impairments Collection

Path validation is based on holistic analysis of the impairments collected along the path of an LSP. To signal which impairments needs to be collected we extend the LSP Attribute TLV sub-object. The impairments collection is performed as follows:

1. Source node sends a Path message with LSP Attribute object aimed to inform the transit nodes about the imminent impairments collection. The Path message also contains TLV sub-objects with required impairments.
2. Every transit node, when receives the message with LSP Attribute object, assembles the collected impairments (specified in TLV) inside a sub-TLV. The way an optical node gets knowledge of the impairments using information locally available at the node (e.g. via discovery of internal amplifiers, photodiode etc.) is out of the scope of this document.
3. Impairments collection will be executed by the returning Resv message that collects hop-by-hop impairments objects by inserting the sub-TLV inside the attached TLV. After successful forwarding of the Resv message the status of transit nodes must be switched to unlock for preventing deadlock.

In case of blocking collection of impairments the LSP lock must be obtained before impairments collection. In case of non-blocking collection type, the unavailability of certain impairments in an intermediate node must not cause the request of failure. The holistic impairments evaluation should be able to deal with missing impairments. When a transit node not in locked state receives a request for blocking collection type, an impairments collection failure (PathErr) should be sent to the Ingress node.

2.4 Impairments TLV: Collection and Recording

The proposed encoding scheme for optical impairments measurements defines a TLV associated to a particular impairments type. A TLV sub-object is encoded in an LSP REQUIRED ATTRIBUTES Object [8]. The TLV sub-object encoding for impairments Collection is shown in Figure 2

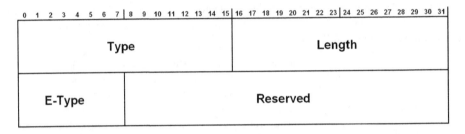

Fig. 2. TLV sub-object

The TLV header includes:

- *Type*: Collected impairments type (TBA). This can be blocking or non blocking type.
- *Length*: length of the TLV object in bytes without the 4 byte header.
- *E-type (Impairments Type, 8 bits)*: Impairments identifier encoded as per [WD6-23]. E.g., 0 for Signal power, 1 for OSNR, 2 for Pilot Tone (as blocking impairments).

This TLV defines which types of impairments (signal power, OSNR, Pilot Tone, alarm etc.) need to be collected and is carried by the Path message. A set of impairments is collected through the Resv message to allow the evaluation at the ingress node. Each item of optical impairments is collected separately. Every transit node, in the Path message, finds the impairments Collection Requested TLV and replies the impairments value in Resv using impairments recording TLV (encoded in an LSP ATTRIBUTES Object). The impairments value can be measured or estimated. Furthermore it sets the Measure Method inside this TLV according to the kind of measured media (single lambda measurement or aggregate measurement). This impairments collection improves the feasibility evaluation where network elements support at least a subset of impairments. The following TLV encodes the impairments values of the LSP associated to the impairments type defined in the impairments Collection Request TLV.

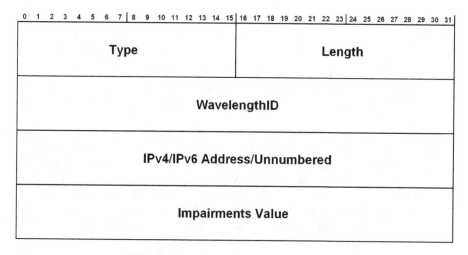

Fig. 3. Impairments recording TLV

The impairments recording TLV includes:

- *Type*: Impairments type(TBA).
- *Length*: length of the TLV value in bytes.
- *WavelengthID:* encoded as per [9]. This field identifies the wavelength. If it is measured/estimated aggregate impairments, this field is set to 0.
- *IPv4/IPv6 Address:* The address of the Node that measures the impairments.
- *Impairments Value:* Estimated or measured impairments value according to [9]. E.g., the Signal Optical Power as 32-bit IEEE 754 floating point number.

3 Signaling Procedure for Impairments Collection Using RSVP-TE

In this section we describe signaling procedures for path validation with impairments collection using examples. Consider a GMPLS LSP that has OXC1 as Ingress Node, OXC4 as Egress node with OXC2 and OXC3 in transit, as shown in Figure 4.

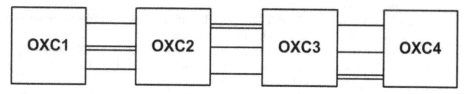

Fig. 4. Optical network scenario

In the following we consider three scenarios of impairments collection and describe signaling procedures associated with the impairments collection and how above mentioned extensions to LSP Attribute and Admin status objects are used for this purpose.

Non-blocking Collection of Impairments

The validation of an optical path is done after LSP is signalled. In case of non-blocking collection, the impairments collection follows the following procedure:

1. OXC1 node sends a Path message with Impairments Collection Request TLV aimed to inform the transit nodes about the imminent impairments collection and about the type of impairments that needs to be collected (e.g., Signal power).
2. Every transit node (OXC2,OXC3), when receives the Path message with Impairments Collection Request TLV, starts the internal impairments reading procedure and waits for the correspondent Resv message to forward the related Impairments recording TLV in the upstream flow to the ingress node OXC1. If for some reason the impairment is not available, since it is non blocking impairment, the node simply does not include the impairments measure in its own Impairments recording TLV. The holistic analysis can be performed also with a subset of the non blocking impairments.
3. Egress node OXC4 sends Resv message with Impairments Collection Request TLV containing optical impairments TLV upstream to the ingress node OXC1 and puts its own impairments value in this Impairments recording TLV.
4. Every transit node (OXC3,OXC2) inserts its own Impairments recording TLV inside Resv message in such way that ingress node collects all required impairments hop by hop.
5. OXC1 node when receives the Resv message extract the impairments recording TLV to perform holistic path validation.

Summarizing the Impairments Collection will be executed by the returning Resv message that collects hop-by-hop impairments objects upstream.

Blocking Collection of Impairments with All Nodes Ready for Impairments Collection

In this scenario the locking strategy needs to be performed first to ensure that no node in the LSP is already locked in another blocking collection. I.e., we need to be sure that all nodes along the path are ready to collect the impairments. This phase uses Admin status object in the Path and Resv message, as follows:

1. OXC1 switches to "lock-required" state and sends a Path message with Admin status object with B, C and R bit set. B bit is used to signal locking is required. C bit is used for locking confirmation. Recall it needs to be set if lock is granted, and needs to be unset otherwise.
2. Every transit node (OXC2, OXC3) that receives the Admin status object in the Path message with B, C and R bit set switches to "lock-required" state related to the required impairments.
3. Egress node OXC4 switches to lock state and forwards the Admin status object in the Resv message, resetting the R bit.
4. Every transit node (OXC3,OXC2) that receives the Resv message with B and C bit set changes its state to "locked".
5. Ingress node OXC1 when receives the Resv message with Admin status object with B and C bit set switches to "locked" state.

At the end of this procedure the entire LSP is in "locked" state and is ready for impairments collection. At this stage the Impairments Collection can be performed as described earlier. The locking is performed before impairments collection to maintain a better compatibility with the future available impairments kind that would require further action to be taken before starting the collection.

Blocking Collection of Impairments with Some Node(s) Blocked for Impairments Collection

In this scenario the locking procedure fails since some node (OXC3 in this example) is in "locked" or "lock-required" state over another LSP.

1. OXC1 switches to lock-required state and sends a Path message with Admin status object with B, C and R bit set. B bit is used to signal locking is required. C bit is used for locking confirmation. Recall it needs to be set if lock is granted, and needs to be unset otherwise.
2. OXC2 receives the Admin status object in the Path message with B, C and R bit set and switches to "lock-required" state related to the required impairments.
3. OXC3 node receives the Admin status object and, since it is already in lock or lock-required state for another LSP with the same resources, unsets the C bit. Therefore the locking procedure will fail.
4. Egress node OXC4, since the received Admin object does not have the C bit set, switches to unlock state and forwards the received Admin status object in the Resv message resetting the R bit.
5. When the other transit nodes (OXC3, OXC2) receive the Admin object in the Resv message with B bit set but with C bit unset, they switch to unlock state.
6. When the ingress node OXC1 receives the Resv message with Admin object containing B bit set and C bit unset switches to unlock.

At this stage the Locking mechanism fails since the ingress node has not received the confirmation of successful locking (C bit set).

4 Conclusion

In this paper we propose a possible solution to the problem of path validation in a pure light-path in a Dense Wavelength Division Multiplexing (DWDM) optical network via transmission of optical impairments. In particular we propose an RSVP-TE based mechanism to collect and evaluate optical impairments measured over optical nodes along the light-path. The proposed light weight mechanism can be easily integrated in the current RSVP-TE protocol making the reservation protocol impairments-aware.

References

1. Berthelon, L., Courtois, O., Garnot, M., Laalaoua, R.: Multi-wavelength fiber net works Rseaux optiques multi-longueur donde. In: Optical telecommunications 2003 (2003)
2. Bernstein, G., Lee, Y., Li, D.: A Framework for the Control ofWavelength Switched Optical Networks (WSON) with Impairments. IETF Internet Draft (2009)

3. Bernstein, G., Lee, Y.: Extending GMPLS/PCE for use inWavelength Switched Optical Networks. In: Conference on Optical Fiber communication/National Fiber Optic Engineers Conference (2008)
4. Mannie, E. (ed.): Generalized Multi-Protocol Label Switching (GMPLS) Architecture. IETF RFC3945 (October 2004)
5. Chiu Angela, L., Choudhury, G., Doverspike, R., Guangzhi, L.: Restoration Design in IP over Reconfigurable All-Optical Networks. In: Li, K., Jesshope, C., Jin, H., Gaudiot, J.-L. (eds.) NPC 2007. LNCS, vol. 4672, pp. 315–333. Springer, Heidelberg (2007)
6. Strand, J., Chiu, A.: Impairments and Other Constraints on Optical Layer Routing. RFC 4054 (May 2005)
7. ITU-T Recommendation G.680: Physical transfer functions of optical network elements (July 2007)
8. Bernstein, G., Lee, J., Li, D.: Information Model for Impaired Optical Path Validation: Work in progress (October 2008)
9. Berger, L.: Generalized Multi-Protocol Label Switching (GMPLS) Signaling Functional Description. RFC 3471 (January 2003)
10. Berger, L.: Generalized Multi-Protocol Label Switching (GMPLS) Signaling Resource ReserVation Protocol-Traffic Engineering (RSVP-TE) Extensions. RFC3473 (January 2003)
11. Farrel, A., Papadimitriou, D., Vasseur, J., Ayyangar, A.: Encoding of Attributes for Multiprotocol Label Switching (MPLS) Label Switched Path (LSP) Establishment Using Resource ReserVation Protocol-Traffic Engineering (RSVP-TE). RFC 4420 (February 2006)
12. ITU-T Recommendation G.697:Optical Monitoring for DWDM systems (2004)

MIMO-OFDM System's Performance Using LDPC Codes for a Mobile Robot

Omar Daoud[1] and Omar Alani[2]

[1] Omar Daoud, Communications and Electronics Engineering Department, P.O. Box 1,
19392 Amman, Jordan
odaoud@philadelphia.edu.jo
[2] Omar Alani, School of Electronic and Electrical Engineering, University of Leeds
Woodhouse Lane, Leeds, LS2 9JT, UK
o.y.k.alani@leeds.ac.uk

Abstract. This work deals with the performance of a Sniffer Mobile Robot (SNFRbot)-based spatial multiplexed wireless Orthogonal Frequency Division Multiplexing (OFDM) transmission technology. The use of Multi-Input Multi-Output (MIMO)-OFDM technology increases the wireless transmission rate without increasing transmission power or bandwidth. A generic multilayer architecture of the SNFRbot is proposed with low power and low cost. Some experimental results are presented and show the efficiency of sniffing deadly gazes, sensing high temperatures and sending live videos of the monitored situation. Moreover, simulation results show the achieved performance by tackling the Peak-to-Average Power Ratio (PAPR) problem of the used technology using Low Density Parity Check (LDPC) codes; and the effect of combating the PAPR on the bit error rate (BER) and the signal to noise ratio (SNR) over a Doppler spread channel.

Keywords: Low Density Parity Check (LDPC) codes, MIMO, and OFDM.

1 Introduction

Due to the rapid growth of wireless communication service, ubiquitous robotics becomes an interesting area for researchers. Although it takes several forms, this kind of robots requires a specific combination of wireless communication, user interface and signal processing techniques to assist humans in everyday tasks. Sniffer Mobile Robot (SNFRbot) is a special kind of robots, which supplies the administrator with fully monitoring capability of a dangerous environment. This monitoring is accomplished by sending live videos through Multi-Input Multi-Output - Orthogonal Frequency Division Multiplexing (MIMO-OFDM) modems to the administrator. If there are no actions taken by the administrator, the SNFRbot will act as a sub-administrator and trying to solve the situation temporarily.

Wireless link that employs multiple antennas at both ends has recently been shown to have the probability of achieving extraordinary data rates. This could be achieved in a rich scattering environment [1]. The corresponding technology is known as spatial multiplexing or BLAST and allows an increase in bit rate in a wireless radio link

R. Mehmood et al. (Eds.): EuropeComm 2009, LNICST 16, pp. 83–90, 2009.
© Institute for Computer Science, Social-Informatics and Telecommunications Engineering 2009

without additional power or bandwidth consumption [2], [3]. In a time-varying frequency-selective fading channel, the BLAST system may suffer from severe performance degradation. To avoid performance loss, OFDM may be exploited to eliminate the
inter-symbol interference (ISI) [4]. It has been shown [5], however, that OFDM suffers
from high sensitivity to non-linear distortion caused by components in the transmitter
part, such as Digital to Analogue Converters (DAC), mixers and High Power Amplifiers (HPA). Thus, the output signal will suffer from intermodulation distortion resulting
in energy being generated at frequencies outside the allocated bandwidth. Daoud *et. al.*
[6], [7] introduced a novel technique to improve the OFDM systems' efficiency by
alleviating the PAPR problem based on linear coding techniques.

This paper presents improving the proposed SNFRbot-based coded MIMO-OFDM
system by combating the PAPR problem and its effect on the BER and SNR. A detailed description of the SNFRbot architecture is given in Section 2. To confirm the
effectiveness of the proposed technique, computer simulation results are given in
Section 3, followed by conclusion in Section 4.

2   SNFRbot Architecture

Fig. 1 shows the generic architecture of SNFRbot. Generally, it consists of four layers; the sensor/video layer, software/hardware (SW/HW) layer, the wireless layer and
the administrator layer.

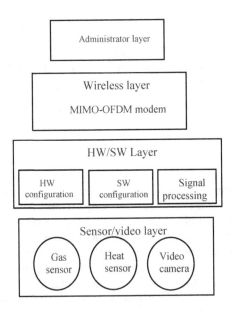

Fig. 1. Generic structure of SNFRbot

In the sensor/video layer, the SNFRbot monitors the environment's safety. If any
sudden accident happens that causes a highly deadly gases concentration or a high
temperature around, the video cam mode will be activated to send live video to the

administrator. The second layer is HW/SW layer. In this layer, both of the SNFRbot hardware and software are reconfigurable to satisfy the environment conditions, such as the SNFRbot speed. The thirds layer allows the SNFRbot to send the live videos through a coded MIMO-OFDM modem. This modem consists of four parts; Fig.2 shows the transmitter block diagram while the receiver will be as the inverse stages of the ones that are shown in Fig.2.

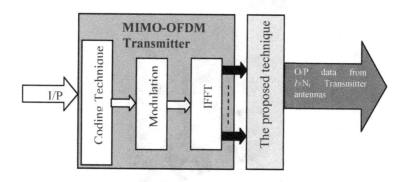

Fig. 2. Block diagram of the coded MIMO-OFDM transmitter

From Fig.2, the MIMO-OFDM transmitter consists of coding technique stage, modulation stage, the Inverse Fast Fourier Transform (IFFT) stage and the proposed stage to combat the PAPR problem. The proposed stage is summarized in the flow-chart that is shown in Fig. 3. Finally, the administrator layer, mainly it is the layer that will take actions according the received videos through the MIMO-OFDM modem.

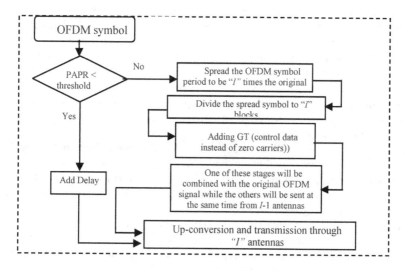

Fig. 3. The flowchart of the previously proposed work in [6] to combat the PAPR

The SNFRbot prototype is approximately in the size of 6×10^{-3} m^3 as shown in Fig.4. At this stage, it has the following parts; motor drive, a designed MIMO-OFDM modem using field-programmable gate array (FPGA), microcontroller, power supply, sensors and a video cam.

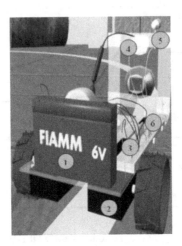

Fig. 4. The prototype of SNFRbot: 1) 6V battery, 2) motor driver, 3) microcontroller, 4) video cam, 5) heat sensor, and 6) gas sensor

In this work, the coded MIMO-OFDM modem has been built in accordance to the IEE802.11 g/n specifications to test the wireless communication of SNFRbot. It was decided to implement the algorithm in FPGA available from Xilinx [8]. The algorithm was decomposed into its functional blocks and these blocks implemented using Verilog, a well known hardware description language (HDL). 'ISE' [9], a development environment provided by Xilinx, incorporates a Verilog synthesis toolchain allowing the high-level description to be compiled and optimized. Elements of this toolchain allow the generation of a bitstream file from which the FPGA devices can be directly programmed. Furthermore, the ISE environment also provides a behavioural simulator that allows the performance of the design to be examined post-synthesis, i.e. complete with all of the routing delays and imperfections that would be present in the physical instantiation of the design in an actual FPGA. This proved to be an extremely useful tool during the implementation of this technique.

The blocks described in Fig.2 were successively implemented in Verilog HDL, each being tested and evaluated using the behavioural simulator before the next block in the chain was implemented. Additional blocks were also implemented to provide the necessary timing, synchronization and handshake signals necessary to ensure correct data transport between each block.

During the compilation and synthesis process, the ISE toolchain generates a report showing device utilisation. Once the system was implemented in Verilog HDL this report was used to determine the overall size and structure of the FPGA device required to implement this technique.

The full implementation was found to fit comfortably in a Xilinx XC2S150 part, one of the Spartan 2E series. The utilisation report indicated that approximately 75%

of the device was used. The Spartan 2E series is a mature, readily available low cost family, showing clearly that the technique can be implemented using low-cost hardware.

It is possible to reduce device utilisation still further. In the implementation used during this research, the IFFT block was implemented directly from the flow-graph to expedite development. If necessary, better, space-efficient FPGA implementations of the FFT and IFFT are available and could be used.

3   Hardware and Simulation Results

In order to verify the mathematically derived result, a MATLAB simulation program was performed and verified using a signal generator and spectrum analyser. The verification process is based on the Agilent Signal Studio Toolkit. The system parameters were:

- A uniformly distributed randomly generated data sequence was generated.
- Channel coding rate is 1/3.
- Different modulation techniques (QPSK, and 64QAM).
- IFFT size of 4k.
- Spreading rate equals to 3.
- Two different channel types; flat fading and Doppler spread channels.

For the hardware implementation and during the testing, 350 OFDM symbols were used to check the efficiency of the proposed technique. These data has been used as an input data to the proposed work block in Fig. 2. The average of the PAPR reduction ratio between the conventional and processed OFDM symbols is used in drawing the CCDF plots.

Fig. 3 shows the CCDF plots for the real part of the OFDM symbols. In this section, the model is limited to 64QAM modulation technique, coding rate equals 1/3 and a spreading rate equal to 3 for simplicity purpose. This figure is divided into three parts of CCDF plots from the designed MIMO-OFDM blocks with the proposed work, which combats the PAPR. Then the system's data rate will be improved. The first plot shows the system's efficiency without coding techniques, while the second one shows combating the PAPR using the proposed technique based turbo coding technique, and the last one shows the achieved improvement of reducing the PAPR based LDPC codes.

Fig. 4 shows the BER vs. the SNR of the QPSK modulated data, while Fig.5 shows the result of the 64QAM modulated data. Both of figures check the efficiency of the LDPC coded data in both Doppler spread and flat fading channels.

From Fig.4, the flat fading channel results give better system performance than the Doppler channel. As an example, at 6 dB SNR the BER was 3.5×10^{-2} for the flat fading channel while it was 6×10^{-1} at the same threshold for Doppler channel.

These results have been improved by changing the modulation technique to be 64 QAM. The improvement will be shown in Fig.5. From Fig.5, at the same value that has been taken previously; 6dB SNR, the BER has been improved in the flat fading situation from 3.5×10^{-2} previously to be 8.2×10^{-4}. For the Doppler channel there is also improvement. This value has been improved from 6×10^{-1} to be 1.8×10^{-1}. Thus, changing the modulation technique for the LDPC coded MIMO-OFDM system improves the system's performance.

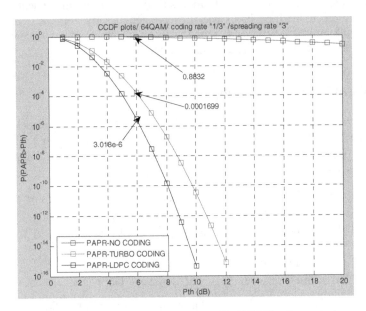

Fig. 5. The CCDF plots for the coded MIMO-OFDM hardware designs

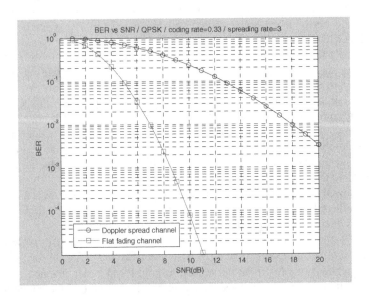

Fig. 6. The BER vs. SNR plots for the LDPC coded MIMO-OFDM simulation-based QPSK modulation technique

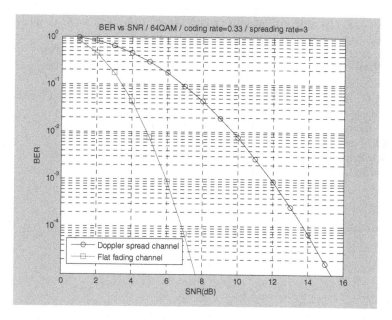

Fig. 5. The BER vs. SNR plots for the LDPC coded MIMO-OFDM simulation-based 64QAM modulation technique

4 Conclusion

The objective of this work is improving the data rate of the proposed SNFRbot robot, which can send live data to the administrator. This is fulfilled by imposing a combination between two powerful techniques; MIMO and OFDM to the wireless layer as it is shown in Fig.1. Moreover, the coded MIMO-OFDM systems performance has been improved by combating one of the OFDM drawback; PAPR. Then, the SNFRbot takes the advantage from this combination to send better resolution live videos based on one of the thirds generation (3G) mobile communication systems propositions.

From the hardware design of the previously published proposed technique, it can be concluded that it's feasible, practical and cost-effective in a real time application.

References

1. Naguib, A.F., Seshadri, N., Calderbank, A.R.: Increasing data rate over wireless channels. IEEE Signal Processing Magazine 17(3), 76–92 (2000)
2. Paulraj, A.J., Kailath, T.: Increasing capacity in wireless broadcast systems using distributed transmission/directional reception. U.S. Patent 5 345, 599 (1994)
3. Foschini, G.J.: Layered space-time architecture for wireless communication in a fading environment when using multi-element antennas. Bell Labs Tech. J., 41–59 (Autumn 1996)
4. Nee, V., Prasad, R.: OFDM wireless multimedia communications. Artech House, Boston (2000)

5. Han, S., Lee, J.: PAPR Reduction of OFDM Signals Using a Reduced Complexity PTS Technique. IEEE Signal Processing Letters 11(11), 887–890 (2004)
6. Daoud, O., Qawasmi, A.-R.: Efficient Performance of COFDM-Based DVB-T. In: IEEE SSD 2009, 6th International Multi-Conference on Systems, Signals & Devices, Tunisia (March 2009)
7. Daoud, O., Alani, O.: Reducing PAPR by utilization of LDPC code. IET Communication Proceedings 3(4), 520–529 (2009)
8. Xilinx- manufacturer of FPGA silicon and development tools,
   http://www.xilinx.com (Last accessed, 11/03/2009)
9. Xilinx ISE, http://www.xilinx.com/ise/logic_design_prod/
   webpack.htm (Last accessed, 11/03/2009)

Hybrid M-QAM with Adaptive Modulation and Selection Combining in MIMO Systems

Sang-Do Lee[1] and Young-Chai Ko[2]

[1] Telecommunication R&D Center, Samsung Electronics, Suwon, Korea
sardor.leed@samsung.com
[2] School of Electrical Engineering, Korea University, Seoul, Korea
koyc@korea.ac.kr

Abstract. In this paper, we propose a hybrid M-ary Quadrature Amplitude Modulation (M-QAM) transmission scheme that jointly uses adaptive modulation and selection combining for singular value decomposition (SVD)-based multiple-input multiple-output (MIMO) systems (AMSC-MIMO). We derive exact closed-form expressions of the performance of the proposed scheme in terms of the average spectral efficiency and the outage probability. Numerical results show that the proposed hybrid M-QAM scheme offers higher spectral efficiency and lower outage probability than the conventional adaptive modulation in MIMO systems.

Keywords: Adaptive Modulation, Variable Rate Variable Power, Selection Combining, MIMO.

1 Introduction

In order to meet the growing demand for mobile multimedia services, most of the recent wireless communication systems employ various techniques that can alleviate the adverse effect of fading channel and enhance data rate and link reliability. Diversity combining (DC) schemes are well-known techniques that can reduce the multi-path fading effect and improve the reliability of communication channels by transmitting the signal over multiple independently fading channels and coherently combining them at the receiver [1]. On the other hand, by using multiple antennas at the transmitter and receiver, multiple-input multiple-output (MIMO) technology provides powerful performance-enhancing capabilities [2,3], one of whose attractive features is the spatial-multiplexing gain over single-input single-output (SISO) systems. By taking advantage of the frequency selectivity and the time variation of fading channels, adaptive modulation (AM) is often adopted in order to increase the spectral efficiency while still meeting the bit error rate (BER) and the average transmit power constraints [4,5]. It has been shown that we can achieve higher spectral efficiency by applying AM in MIMO system (AM-MIMO) [6]. Apart from AM-MIMO, there are efforts to combine AM jointly with DC to improve both the link reliability and the spectral efficiency [7,8]. For example, [7] proposes a hybrid scheme to increase the spectral

R. Mehmood et al. (Eds.): EuropeComm 2009, LNICST 16, pp. 91–100, 2009.

efficiency of multi-channel systems by using maximal ratio combining (MRC) scheme jointly with discrete-rate adaptation. Although the MRC is optimal in the sense of output SNR, its complexity is the highest among other conventional diversity combining schemes since it requires to know the channel status of all the branches between the transmitter and receiver. To reduce the complexity, suboptimal schemes such as selection combining (SC) are often adopted with the sacrifice of the performance [9,10].

In this paper, we introduce a hybrid M-ary quadrature amplitude modulation (M-QAM) with adaptive modulation and selection combining in MIMO systems (AMSC-MIMO). The distinctive feature of AMSC-MIMO is that, while applying discrete-rate adaptation to each sub-channel of a MIMO system, it examines sub-channels whose eigenvalue gains are below the cutoff threshold, selects a sub-channel with the largest gain among them, and jointly determines the data rate and transmit power of the selected sub-channel. Note that, under suitable channel conditions, e.g., rich scattering environment, a MIMO channel can be decomposed into parallel sub-channels by singular value decomposition (SVD) and space-time pre-processing at the transmitter and receiver. In addition to the spatial multiplexing gain of SVD-based MIMO channel, the proposed scheme can exploit both the diversity gain and power loading gain to enhance the overall spectral efficiency in low SNR region, by selecting a sub-channel whose eigenvalue gain is the best among sub-channels below the threshold and enhancing the transmit power of the selected sub-channel enough to meet the required BER performance. We show in the paper that the proposed scheme increases the link gain as well as the spectral efficiency comparing to the conventional AM-MIMO scheme. In our study of the proposed scheme, we carry out performance analysis in terms of the average spectral efficiency and the outage probability assuming perfect channel state information (CSI) at both the transmitter and receiver, and then we validate our analysis from the numerical results.

This paper is organized as follows. In Section II, the channel model and the system operations under consideration are described. The performance analysis of the proposed scheme is in Sections III, and the numerical results are presented in Section IV. Finally in Section V, a brief conclusion is provided.

2   System Description

We consider a point-to-point communication model of the wireless system that has multiple transmit and receive antennas at both the transmitter and receiver.

2.1   MIMO Channel Model

Assuming frequency-flat and uncorrelated Rayleigh fading over the bandwidth of interest, we consider a MIMO system with n_T transmit and n_R receive antennas and the MIMO channel at a given time instant is represented by the channel matrix $\mathbf{H}$, each entry of which represents the complex Gaussian channel gain between the mth receive and nth transmit antenna pair, say $H_{m,n} \sim \mathcal{CN}(0,1)$. The discrete-time input-output relation over a symbol period is given by

$$\mathbf{y} = \mathbf{Hx} + \mathbf{n}, \tag{1}$$

where $E[\mathbf{nn}^H] = N_0 \mathbf{I_{n_R}}$. We assume a block fading model in which the complex channel gain remains roughly constant over each transmission slot. At each transmission slot, the transmitter sends a frame that consists of a burst of symbols and short guard intervals are periodically inserted into transmitted frames. During these guard intervals, the receiver perfectly estimates the channel state information (CSI) including the channel matrix $\mathbf{H}$ and its statistical information, which is fed back to the transmitter through a reliable link without error and delay. By applying a SVD to $\mathbf{H}$, we can express the MIMO channel as

$$\mathbf{H} = \mathbf{U\Sigma V}, \tag{2}$$

where $\mathbf{U}$ and $\mathbf{V}$ are unitary matrixes with left and right singular vectors of $\mathbf{H}$, respectively, and $\mathbf{\Sigma}$ is an $n_R \times n_T$ diagonal matrix whose main diagonal elements are the singular values of $\mathbf{H}$, $\{\sqrt{\lambda_i}\}_{i=1}^{\mathcal{R}}$. By substituting (2) into (1), we can obtain an equivalent input-output relation as

$$\mathbf{U^H y} = \mathbf{\Sigma V^H x} + \mathbf{U^H n}. \tag{3}$$

From (3), we can see that the MIMO channel is decomposed into $\mathcal{R}$ parallel sub-channels whose power gains are represented by the $\mathcal{R} \times 1$ eigenvalue vector $[\lambda_1, \cdots, \lambda_{\mathcal{R}}]^T$ and input/output symbol vectors are $\acute{\mathbf{x}} = \mathbf{V^H x}$ and $\acute{\mathbf{y}} = \mathbf{U^H y}$, respectively. The received SNR per sub-channel can be written as $\gamma_i = P_i \lambda_i / N_0$, where P_i represents the transmit power per sub-channel. According to the previous works in [11] and [6], any unordered element in the eigenvalue vector, say λ, follows the probability density function (PDF) given as

$$f_\lambda(\lambda) = \frac{1}{\mathcal{R}} \sum_{i=0}^{\mathcal{R}-1} \sum_{j=0}^{i} \sum_{k=0}^{i} \Delta_{j,k}(i, \mathcal{D}) \lambda^{j+k+\mathcal{D}} e^{-\lambda}, \tag{4}$$

where $\Delta_{j,k}(i, \mathcal{D}) = \frac{i!(\mathcal{D}+i)!(-1)^{j+k}}{(i-j)!(i-k)!(\mathcal{D}+j)!(\mathcal{D}+k)!j!k!}$. Based on (4), we can derive its cumulative distribution function (CDF) as

$$F_\lambda(x) = \int_0^x f_\lambda(\lambda) d\lambda$$

$$= \frac{1}{\mathcal{R}} \sum_{i=0}^{\mathcal{R}-1} \sum_{j=0}^{i} \sum_{k=0}^{i} \Delta_{j,k}(i, \mathcal{D}) \gamma(j + k + \mathcal{D} + 1, x),$$

$$\tag{5}$$

where $\gamma(\cdot, \cdot)$ is the lower incomplete Gamma function [12].

2.2 Mode of Operation

To enhance the spectral efficiency of the MIMO system, the transmitter adjusts data rate of each sub-channel to the instantaneous CSI. Throughout this paper, we adopt uncoded M-QAM with discrete-rate adaptation in each sub-channel and transmit power is subject to the total transmit power constraint, $P_T = \sum_{i=1}^{\mathcal{R}} P_i$. For discrete-rate adaptation, we assume the equal power allocation for every sub-channel, $P_i = P_T/\mathcal{R}$, and the received SNR range of each sub-channel is separated into $\mathcal{N}$ regions, $\{\gamma_{T_n}\}_{n=1}^{\mathcal{N}}$, each of which is associated with M_n. For uncoded M-QAM with square constellation set, $M_n = 2^{2n}$ where $n = 1, \cdots, \mathcal{N}$, and $SE_n = 2n$ bits are transmitter per symbol. When the transmission mode M_n for the ith sub-channel with $\gamma_{T_n} \leq \gamma_i < \gamma_{T_{n+1}}$ is given, the instantaneous BER can be approximated as [13]

$$BER(M_n, \gamma_i) \simeq c_1 e^{-\frac{c_2 \gamma_i}{M_n - 1}}, \tag{6}$$

where positive real values of c_1 and c_2 are set according to the BER bounds. As an example, $c_1 = 0.2$ and $c_2 = 1.6$ for $BER_T \leq 10^{-3}$ and $M_n \geq 4$. We assume that the instantaneous BER of a sub-channel is subject to an instantaneous BER constraint, $BER(M_n, \gamma_i) \leq BER_T$. Based on (6), we can obtain the required eigenvalue gain, or equivalently, the received SNR to satisfy the instantaneous BER constraint. For a given BER_T, the switching threshold for M_n-QAM can be obtained from (6) as

$$\gamma_{T_n} = \frac{M_n - 1}{K}, n = 1, \cdots, \mathcal{N}, \tag{7}$$

where $K = \frac{c_2}{\ln(c_1/BER_T)}$. Using the above definition of the received SNR per sub-channel and (7), we can write the eigenvalue gain corresponding to each switching threshold as

$$\lambda_{T_n} = \frac{N_0 \gamma_{T_n}}{P_i} = \frac{M_n - 1}{\bar{\gamma} K}, n = 1, \cdots, \mathcal{N}, \tag{8}$$

where $\bar{\gamma} = P_i/N_0$ and we define $\gamma_T = \gamma_{T_1}$ and $\lambda_T = \lambda_{T_1}$, respectively, as the cutoff threshold.

In this paper, we compare two different adaptive modulation schemes in MIMO systems, 1) the conventional AM-MIMO and 2) the proposed AMSC-MIMO, respectively.

Conventional AM-MIMO. According to the conventional M-QAM with AM-MIMO in [6], discrete-rate adaptation is applied to each sub-channel independently. While evaluating the condition of each sub-channel, the transmitter stops transmitting data stream when the received SNR of a sub-channel is below the cutoff threshold or, equivalently, $\lambda_i < \lambda_T$. We denote the sub-channel as a cutoff channel. When the received SNR of a cutoff channel is higher than the threshold, the transmitter resumes data transmission on that sub-channel. In low SNR regime, it is possible that a majority of sub-channels remain cutoff when the MIMO channel suffers from deep fading; as a result, overall spectral efficiency of AM-MIMO system is reduced significantly since the cutoff channels are just wasted without data transmission.

Proposed AMSC-MIMO. The objective of the proposed scheme is to increase overall spectral efficiency of MIMO system by maintaining appropriate data rate of cutoff channels to meet the instantaneous BER and the average transmit power constraints. To accomplish the objective, AMSC-MIMO combines discrete-rate adaptation and SC over cutoff channels. The detailed operation of AMSC-MIMO is as follows.

1. Initially, the transmitter allocates equal power $P_i^* = P_i$ for every sub-channel in the MIMO system. While performing slotted transmit operation, the transmitter obtains the perfect CSI during guard periods and determines λ_i of each sub-channel. If $\lambda_i \geq \lambda_T$, the sub-channel is treated just as in AM-MIMO and is ready for transmission right away. Otherwise, it is categorized into *cutoff channel* and is not selected for transmission.
2. Among the remaining cutoff channels, the transmitter sorts them in order of the eigenvalue gain and selects one with the highest eigenvalue gain, $\lambda_1 = \max\{\lambda_i\}_{i=1}^{\mathcal{C}}$, as the candidate channel.
3. The transmitter recursively raises the transmit power of the candidate channel by borrowing the transmit power from the last of the ordered cutoff channels, e.g., $P_1^* = P_1^* + P_{\mathcal{C}}$ and sets $P_{\mathcal{C}} = 0$ and $\mathcal{C} = \mathcal{C} - 1$, until it consumes all the remaining power of cutoff channels or until the raised power satisfies the instantaneous BER constraint, or equivalently, $P_1^* \lambda_1 / N_0 \geq \gamma_T$. In the latter case, the candidate channel is removed from the cutoff channel list and is selected for transmission with the adjusted power, P_1^*, and the transmitter repeats previous steps from 2) and selects another candidate channel among the remaining cutoff channels. In the former case, the transmitter terminates finding a candidate channel and stops further processing the cutoff channels.

From the steps above, we can observe that the proposed scheme attempts to increase the number of sub-channels that are capable of transmitting data streams, while the total transmit power still meets the constraint, $\sum_{i=1}^{\mathcal{R}} P_i \leq P_T$.

3   Performance Analysis

In this section, we obtain closed-form expressions for the performance of the proposed AMSC-MIMO in terms of the average spectral efficiency and the outage probability. For the convenience of the analysis hereafter, we assume the initial transmit power of every sub-channel is normalized as $P_i = P_T/\mathcal{R} = 1$ and, accordingly, $\bar{\gamma} = 1/N_0$ and $\gamma_i = \lambda_i/N_0$.

3.1   Eigenvalue Gain Distribution of a Candidate Channel

According to the operation of the proposed AMSC-MIMO, the ith candidate channel is defined as a cutoff channel whose eigenvalue gain denoted as $\lambda_{\mathcal{C},i}$ is the ith one among $\mathcal{C}$ cutoff channels. Thus, $\lambda_{\mathcal{C},i}$ is the $(\mathcal{C}-i+1)$th order statistic whose CDF is given by [14]

$$F_{\mathcal{C},i}(x) = \sum_{j=\mathcal{C}-i+1}^{\mathcal{C}} \binom{\mathcal{C}}{j} F_\lambda(x)^j \{1 - F_\lambda(x)\}^{\mathcal{C}-j}. \tag{9}$$

We can also obtain the PDF of the order statistic, $\lambda_{\mathcal{C},i}$, given as [14]

$$
\begin{aligned}
f_{\mathcal{C},i}(x) &= \frac{d}{dx} F_{\mathcal{C},i}(x) \\
&= \frac{F_\lambda(x)^{\mathcal{C}-i}\{1 - F_\lambda(x)\}^{i-1}}{B(\mathcal{C}-i+1,i)} f_\lambda(x),
\end{aligned} \tag{10}
$$

where $B(\cdot,\cdot)$ is the beta function [12].

Let us define an event $E_{\mathcal{C},i} = \{\frac{\lambda_T}{P_i^*} \le \lambda_{\mathcal{C},i} < \frac{\lambda_T}{P_i^*-1} | \lambda_{\mathcal{C},i} < \lambda_T\}$, and denote $\lambda_{\mathcal{C},i}^{CCH} = \{P_i^* \lambda_{\mathcal{C},i} | E_{\mathcal{C},i}\}$ as the adjusted gain of the ith candidate channel. Then, we can derive the CDF of $\lambda_{\mathcal{C},i}^{CCH}$ as

$$F_{\mathcal{C},i}^{CCH}(x) = \frac{\Pr[\lambda_{\mathcal{C},i} < \frac{x}{P_i^*}, \frac{\lambda_T}{P_i^*} \le \lambda_{\mathcal{C},i} < \frac{\lambda_T}{P_i^*-1}]}{\Pr[E_{\mathcal{C},i}]} \tag{11}$$

$$= \begin{cases} 0, & x < \lambda_T \\ \dfrac{F_{\mathcal{C},i}(\frac{x}{P_i^*}) - F_{\mathcal{C},i}(\frac{\lambda_T}{P_i^*})}{\tilde{P}}, & \lambda_T \le x < \mathcal{G}_i \lambda_T \\ 1, & \mathcal{G}_i \lambda_T \le x \end{cases},$$

where $\tilde{P} = \Pr[E_{\mathcal{C},i}]$, and $\mathcal{G}_i = \frac{P_i^*}{P_i^*-1}$. Differentiating (11) with respect to x and using (4), we can obtain the PDF of $\lambda_{\mathcal{C},i}^{CCH}$, given as

$$f_{\mathcal{C},i}^{CCH}(x) = \begin{cases} \frac{1}{\tilde{P} P_i^*} f_{\mathcal{C},i}(\frac{x}{P_i^*}), & \lambda_T \le x < \mathcal{G}_i \lambda_T \\ 0, & \text{elsewhere} \end{cases} \tag{12}$$

3.2 Spectral Efficiency

The average spectral efficiency of the proposed AMSC-MIMO system is derived as follows. At first we can write the average spectral efficiency as

$$\overline{SE}^{AMSC} = \sum_{\mathcal{C}=0}^{\mathcal{R}} SE_{\mathcal{R},\mathcal{C}} P_{\mathcal{R},\mathcal{C}}, \tag{13}$$

where $P_{\mathcal{R},\mathcal{C}}$ is the probability that there are $\mathcal{C}$-cutoff channels, and $SE_{\mathcal{R},\mathcal{C}}$ is its spectral efficiency, which can be shown as

$$P_{\mathcal{R},\mathcal{C}} = \binom{\mathcal{R}}{\mathcal{C}} F_\lambda(\lambda_T)^{\mathcal{C}} (1 - F_\lambda(\lambda_T))^{\mathcal{R}-\mathcal{C}}, \tag{14}$$

and

$$SE_{\mathcal{R},\mathcal{C}} = \sum_{k=0}^{\lfloor \frac{\mathcal{C}}{2} \rfloor} P_{\mathcal{C}}(k, \mathbf{p}_k) SE_{\mathcal{C}}(k, \mathbf{p}_k), \tag{15}$$

respectively. Note that $P_{\mathcal{C}}(k, \mathbf{p}_k)$ and $SE_{\mathcal{C}}(k, \mathbf{p}_k)$ in (15) represent the probability and the spectral efficiency of the event when k candidate channels are selected among $\mathcal{C}$ cutoff channels ($k \leq \mathcal{C}/2$), respectively. We denote $\mathbf{p}_k$ as a vector whose element represents the adjusted transmit power of a candidate channel. The vector $\mathbf{p}_k$ is drawn from a set that contains all the possible combinations of powers as its elements. For i.i.d cutoff channels, the probability, $P_{\mathcal{C}}(k, \mathbf{p}_k)$, can be derived as

$$\begin{aligned}
P_{\mathcal{C}}(k, \mathbf{p}_k) = \Pr[&P_1^* \lambda_{\mathcal{C},1} \geq \lambda_T, \ldots, P_k^* \lambda_{\mathcal{C},k} \geq \lambda_T, \\
&(P_1^* - 1)\lambda_{\mathcal{C},1} < \lambda_T, \ldots, (P_k^* - 1)\lambda_{\mathcal{C},k} < \lambda_T, \\
&(\mathcal{C} - \mathcal{P}(k))\lambda_{\mathcal{C},k+1} < \lambda_T | \lambda_{\mathcal{C},1} < \lambda_T, \ldots, \\
&\lambda_{\mathcal{C},k+1} < \lambda_T] \\
= &\left(\prod_{i=1}^{k} \frac{F_{\mathcal{C},i}(\frac{\lambda_T}{P_i^* - 1}) - F_{\mathcal{C},i}(\frac{\lambda_T}{P_i^*})}{F_{\mathcal{C},i}(\lambda_T)} \right) \\
&\times \frac{F_{\mathcal{C},k+1}(\frac{\lambda_T}{\mathcal{C} - \mathcal{P}(k)})}{F_{\mathcal{C},k+1}(\lambda_T)},
\end{aligned} \tag{16}$$

where $\mathcal{P}(k) = \sum_{i=1}^{k} P_i^*$. The spectral efficiency, $SE_{\mathcal{C}}(k, \mathbf{p}_k)$, is written as

$$SE_{\mathcal{C}}(k, \mathbf{p}_k) = \overline{SE}^{AM} + \sum_{i=1}^{k} SE_{\mathcal{C},i}^{CCH}, \tag{17}$$

where $\overline{SE}^{AM}$ is the average spectral efficiency of the conventional AM-MIMO system with $\mathcal{R} - \mathcal{C}$ independent sub-channels above the cutoff threshold, whose closed form expression has been derived in [6], as

$$\overline{SE}^{AM} = (\mathcal{R} - \mathcal{C}) \sum_{n=1}^{\mathcal{N}} SE_n \left(F_\lambda(\lambda_{T_{n+1}}) - F_\lambda(\lambda_{T_n}) \right), \tag{18}$$

and $SE_{\mathcal{C},i}^{CCH}$ is the spectral efficiency of the i-th candidate channel with transmit power P_i^*, which can be represented as

$$SE_{\mathcal{C},i}^{CCH} = \sum_{n=1}^{\mathcal{N}} SE_n P_{\mathcal{C},i,n}^{CCH}, \tag{19}$$

where the probability $P_{\mathcal{C},i,n}^{CCH}$ can be derived as

$$\begin{aligned}
P_{\mathcal{C},i,n}^{CCH} &= \Pr[\lambda_{T_n} \leq \lambda_{\mathcal{C},i}^{CCH} < \lambda_{T_{n+1}}] \\
&= F_{\mathcal{C},i}^{CCH}(\lambda_{T_{n+1}}) - F_{\mathcal{C},i}^{CCH}(\lambda_{T_n}) \\
&= \begin{cases} 1, & n = 1 \\ 0, & n \neq 1 \end{cases}.
\end{aligned} \tag{20}$$

By substituting (20) to (19), we can prove that the spectral efficiency of every candidate channel is $SE_{\mathcal{C},i}^{CCH} = SE_1$.

3.3   Outage Probability

In the conventional AM-MIMO system, outage event is defined as the case when every eigenvalue gain of the decomposed MIMO channel falls below the cutoff threshold. As a result, the transmitter cannot transmit data stream when the outage event occurs. The outage probability of the conventional AM-MIMO system can be shown as

$$P_{out}^{AM} = \Pr[\lambda_1 < \lambda_T, \cdots, \lambda_{\mathcal{R}} < \lambda_T]$$
$$= \{F_\lambda(\lambda_T)\}^{\mathcal{R}} . \tag{21}$$

In the proposed AMSC-MIMO system, outage event occurs when the largest eigenvalue gain of the decomposed MIMO channel which is multiplied by the adjusted transmit power $P_1^* = \mathcal{R}$ is below the cutoff threshold, given that every independent sub-channel falls below the cutoff threshold. The outage probability of the AMSC-MIMO system can be shown as

$$P_{out}^{AMSC} = \Pr[\max\{\lambda_i\}_{i=1}^{\mathcal{R}} < \frac{\lambda_T}{\mathcal{R}}]$$
$$= F_{\mathcal{R},1}\left(\frac{\lambda_T}{\mathcal{R}}\right) . \tag{22}$$

4   Numerical Results

Figs. 1 and 2 show the average spectral efficiency and the outage probability of two different M-QAM schemes in 2×2, 4×4 and 6×6 MIMO channels, respectively, as a function of the average SNR per sub-channel, when the target BER is set to 10^{-3}. As the number of transmit and receive antennas increase, we observe higher spatial multiplexing gain from both the conventional AM-MIMO and the proposed AMSC-MIMO. More specifically, we can notice from Fig. 1 that AMSC-MIMO shows significant enhancement of the average spectral efficiency over AM-MIMO in low SNR region, though its curve approaches that of AM-MIMO in high SNR region. From Fig. 2, we can observe that, in 2×2 MIMO channel, the AMSC-MIMO offers approximately 3 dB gain over the AM-MIMO from the perspective of the outage probability, and it offers higher performance gain as the number of antennas increases. For example, we can observe approximately 7 dB gain in 6×6 MIMO channel.

From the numerical results in this section, we can deduce that the above performance enhancements are from the fact that, by exploiting both the spatial diversity gain and the power gain in low SNR region, a candidate channel in the proposed AMSC-MIMO scheme obtains much higher output SNR than the conventional sub-channel in AM-MIMO system does.

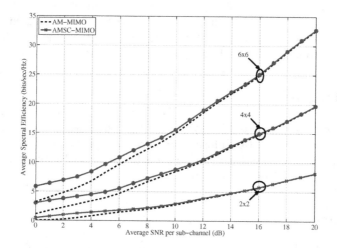

Fig. 1. The comparisons of average spectral efficiency versus the average SNR per sub-channel among the proposed AMSC-MIMO and the conventional AM-MIMO, for 2×2, 4×4 and 6×6 MIMO channels, respectively, when $BER_T = 10^{-3}$

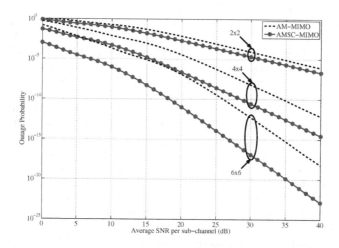

Fig. 2. The comparison of the outage probability versus the average SNR per sub-channel among the proposed AMSC-MIMO and the conventional AM-MIMO, for 2×2, 4×4 and 6×6 MIMO channels, respectively, when $BER_T = 10^{-3}$

5   Conclusion

In this paper, we proposed a hybrid M-QAM scheme that jointly uses discrete-rate adaptation and selection combining in SVD-based MIMO systems, and developed exact closed-form expressions of the performance of the proposed scheme, AMSC-MIMO, assuming perfect CSI. Our numerical results show that by exploiting both the spatial diversity gain and the power gain in low SNR region, the proposed AMSC-MIMO offers higher spectral efficiency and much lower outage probability than the conventional AM-MIMO.

Acknowledgement

"This research was supported by the MKE(The Ministry of Knowledge Economy), Korea, under the ITRC(Information Technology Research Center) support program supervised by the IITA(Institute for Information Technology Advancement)" (IITA-2009-C1090-0902-0019).

References

1. Simon, M.K., Alouini, M.-S.: Digital Communication over Fading Channels. John Wiley & Sons, Inc., Chichester (2000)
2. Paulraj, A.J., Gore, D.A., Nabar, R.U., Bolcskei, H.: An overview of MIMO communications - A key to Gigabit wireless. Proc. IEEE 92, 198–218 (2004)
3. Holter, B., Oien, G.E.: On the amount of fading in MIMO diversity system. IEEE Trans. Wireless Commun. 4, 585–595 (2005)
4. Goldsmith, A.J., Chua, S.G.: Adaptive coded modulation for fading channels. IEEE Trans. Commun. COM-46, 595–602 (1998)
5. Chung, S.-T., Goldsmith, A.J.: Degrees of freedom in adaptive modulation: A unified view. IEEE Trans. Wireless Commun. 49, 1561–1571 (2001)
6. Zhou, Z., Vucetic, B., Dohler, M., Li, Y.: MIMO systems with adaptive modulation. IEEE Trans. Veh. Technol. 54, 1828–1842 (2005)
7. Nam, H., Ko, Y.-C., Alouini, M.-S.: Spectral efficiency enhancement in multi-channel systems using redundant transmission and diversity reception. IEEE Trans. Wireless Commun. 7, 2143–2153 (2008)
8. Ko, Y.-C., Yang, H.-C., Eom, S., Alouini, M.-S.: Adaptive modulation with diversity combining based on output-threshold MRC. IEEE Trans. Wireless Commun. 6, 3728–3737 (2007)
9. Alouini, M.-S.: Adaptive and diversity techniques for wireless digital communications over fading channel. PhD thesis, California Institute of Technology (May 1998)
10. Kim, Y.G., Kim, S.W.: Optimum selection combining for M-ary signals in frequency-nonselective fading channels. IEEE Trans. Commun. 53, 84–93 (2005)
11. Dohler, M., Aghvami, H.: On the approximation of MIMO capacity. IEEE Trans. Wireless Commun. (Letter) 4, 30–34 (2005)
12. Abramowitz, M., Stegun, I.A.: Handbook of Mathematical Functions with Formulas, Graphs, and Mathematical Tables, 9th edn. Dover Publications, New York (1970)
13. Proakis, J.G.: Digital Communications, 2nd edn. McGraw-Hill, New York (1989)
14. David, H.A., Nagaraja, H.N.: Order Statistics. John Wiley& Sons, Inc., New York (2003)

Performance Analysis of a Joint Space-Time Block Codes and Channel Estimation Scheme in DL-PUSC Mode of Mobile WiMAX

Phuong T.T. Pham and Tomohisa Wada

Information Engineering Department, Graduate School of Engineering and Science,
University of The Ryukyus, 1 Senbaru Nishihara, Okinawa, 903-0213, Japan
thuphuong@lsi.ie.u-ryukyu.ac.jp, wada@ie.u-ryukyu.ac.jp

Abstract. Mobile WiMAX has emerged as a starting point of broadband mobile wireless era. Besides plenty of advantages over the prior systems, it also utilizes multiple-antenna techniques to improve the transmission quality. Although this approach has been intensively studied, there are just few published works taking into account channel estimation to obtain realistic performance. This paper studies a joint STBC and channel estimation scheme to investigate the performance of the DL-PUSC mobile WiMAX in various mobile channels. Simulation results show significant improvement, up to 8 dB gain for PER and system throughput is achieved when employing STBC.

Keywords: WiMAX, DL-PUSC, MIMO, Alamouti, MRC, Channel estimation.

1 Introduction

The IEEE 802.16e standard, often commercially regarded as mobile WiMAX (Worldwide interoperability for Microwave Access), is a stimulating technology that provides wireless access over large coverage area with high speed, high throughput and full mobility. WiMAX physical layer utilizes advanced multiple access scheme called scalable OFDMA (Orthogonal Frequency Division Multiple Access) which is derived from OFDM (Orthogonal Frequency Division Multiplexing) technique. OFDM is well known to be very efficient in utilizing the system bandwidth as well as mitigating the impairment caused by multipath frequency-selective fading channel. OFDMA multiplexes data streams from different individual users by subchannelizing the OFDM symbol and assigning each user a group of subchannels. Permuting these subchannels together, this technique can guarantee that none of the users has higher probability to suffer the severely faded channel than others. Implemented scalability supports a flexible operating bandwidth from 1.25 MHz to 20 MHz by varying the FFT size from 128 to 2048. This advantage is very important since it increases the spectral efficiency which is critical in broadband wireless network.

DL-PUSC (Downlink - Partial Usage of Subchannels), which is a particular working mode defined in [1], has received lots of interest for evaluating the system performance. This subchannelization mode assigns each user a group of subchannels consisting of several clusters. Clusters of a user are pseudo-randomly permuted

R. Mehmood et al. (Eds.): EuropeComm 2009, LNICST 16, pp. 101–112, 2009.
© Institute for Computer Science, Social-Informatics and Telecommunications Engineering 2009

among those of other users so that the system can take advantage of the frequency diversity to compete the fading channel.

Recently, the technique using multiple antennas at the transmitter and receiver called MIMO (multiple input – multiple output) has received a growing expectation to be applied to the upcoming wireless networks. MIMO technique exploits the spatial diversity to provide a significant improvement in system performance over the traditional SISO (single input – single output) approach [2]. MIMO is mainly implemented in three ways, i.e. maximizing the spatial diversity to enhance the power efficiency, increasing the capacity by using layered approach and the last one exploiting the channel knowledge feedbacked from the receiver to decompose the channel coefficient matrix by singular value decomposition [3]. Although the last scheme is proved to be able to reach the near Shannon capacity, the first one which includes several techniques such as delay diversity, space-time trellis codes, and space-time block codes (STBC) is more mature to be applied widely to practical systems. Has been vastly studied [4]-[11], STBC including the well known Alamouti scheme is one of the diversity techniques recommended by the IEEE 802.16e standard for WiMAX systems.

This paper studies applying several MIMO-STBC techniques such as maximal ratio combining (MRC), 2x1-, and 2x2- Alamouti schemes to the mobile WiMAX DL-PUSC system. Channel estimation using conventional linear interpolation technique [12] is carried out by exploiting scattered pilots in clusters rather than assuming perfectly known to obtain more practical results. Performance analysis is presented in term of packet error rate (PER) and system throughput versus signal to noise ratio (SNR) in various frequency selective fading channels. These channel models are recommended by ITU [13] for low-speed and high-speed mobile environments. Performance comparisons with SISO approach are given to show the improvement when applying MIMO techniques to the system.

In this paper, a capital letter is used to denote a frequency domain symbol, bold letter is used for a matrix or a vector whereas indexing symbol is written in italic subscript, and a ranging number is in italic capital form.

The rest of the paper is organized as follows. A brief description about DL-PUSC is given in section 2. Conventional SISO approach is introduced in section 3. MIMO-STBC including maximal ratio combining, 2x1-, and 2x2- Alamouti schemes are addressed in section 4. Channel models, simulation setup, simulation results, and discussions are presented in section 5. Finally, section 6 reviews the main aspects and concludes the paper.

2   System Overview

2.1 DL-PUSC Structure

The data structure in DL-PUSC mode is shown in fig. 1. The OFDM symbol is divided into subchannels, each user is associated to a group of subchannels. Subchannel is further partitioned into clusters and each of which contains a group of 14 consecutive subcarriers. When transmitted, clusters of different users will be permuted among themselves.

Pilot pattern in DL-PUSC is assigned cluster by cluster and designed periodic in 2-symbol period. The first symbol that carries data is considered as even and has index *0*. In each cluster, pilots are arranged at subcarriers {*4,8*} for even symbols and at subcarriers {*0,12*} for odd symbols.

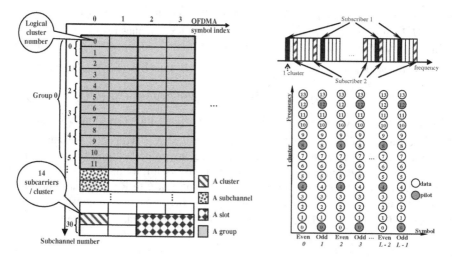

Fig. 1. Basic elements in DL-PUSC mode (left); Clusters permutation in OFDM symbol (upper right); Pilot pattern (lower right)

2.2 Signal Model

A general OFDM-MIMO transmission scheme is shown in fig. 2 in which there are *N* and *M* antennas at the transmitter and receiver respectively. In case of using SISO, the Tx diversity encoder is omitted, the channel equalizer is used instead of the Rx diversity combiner and just only one IFFT/FFT block and antenna appear at the transmitter and receiver.

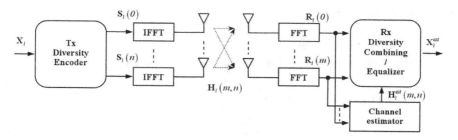

Fig. 2. Transceiver diversity OFDM system

Suppose at symbol-period *l*, processed OFDM symbols set $\{\mathbf{S}_l(n)\}$ are transmitted from the base station with all transmit (Tx) antennas to the mobile station. At the mth receive (Rx) antenna, after FFT, the received symbol is:

$$\mathbf{R}_l(m) = \sum_{n=0}^{N-1} \mathbf{H}_l(m,n)\mathbf{S}_l(n) + \mathbf{W}_l(m) . \tag{1}$$

where $\mathbf{H}_l(m,n)$ is the frequency response of the channel between the nth Tx antenna to the mth Rx antenna, $\mathbf{W}_l(m)$ is the noise at that Rx antenna, $n = 0,1,...,N-1$, $m = 0,1,...,M-1$ with N and M are the numbers of Tx and Rx antennas respectively.

In subcarrier-scale, these vectors are defined as follows. $\mathbf{R}_l(m) = [\mathbf{R}_0(m),\mathbf{R}_1(m),...,\mathbf{R}_{K-1}(m)]_l^T$, $\mathbf{H}_l(m,n) = [\mathbf{H}_0(m,n),\mathbf{H}_1(m,n),...,\mathbf{H}_{K-1}(m,n)]_l^T$, $\mathbf{S}_l(n) = [\mathbf{S}_0(n),\mathbf{S}_1(n),...,\mathbf{S}_{K-1}(n)]_l^T$, $\mathbf{W}_l(m) = [\mathbf{W}_0(m),\mathbf{W}_1(m),...,\mathbf{W}_{K-1}(m)]_l^T$ in which $[.]^T$ is matrix transpose operator and inside brackets are the correspondent values at the kth subcarrier of the lth OFDM symbol, $k = 0,1,...,K-1$ with K is the number of subcarriers in OFDM symbol, whereas l can take any value between 0 and $L-1$, L is even and denotes the number of symbols in the transmission frame.

The transfer function of the channel from Tx antenna n to Rx antenna m at the lth symbol-period is the Fourier transform of the channel impulse response $\mathbf{H}_l(m,n) = \mathbf{Fh}_l(m,n)$, where $\mathbf{F}$ is the $K \times I$ – Fourier transform matrix whose values are defined as $f_{k,i} = \frac{1}{\sqrt{K}}e^{-j2\pi\frac{ki}{K}}$, for $i = 0,1,...,I-1$, and $\mathbf{h}_l(m,n) = [\mathbf{h}_0(m,n),\mathbf{h}_1(m,n),...,\mathbf{h}_{I-1}(m,n)]_l^T$ is the I-tap discrete multipath fading channel sampled at system frequency.

In order to recover the transmitted signal, the channel transfer function must be estimated. This task is done by calculating the channel values at pilot subcarriers, which are known in advance, and interpolating all the channel values at data positions. Since the clusters of each user are not connected continuously in frequency axis, the estimation task at the receiver is carried out partially cluster by cluster. Channel should be estimated at each cluster or in a frame of several clusters connected in the time axis.

3   SISO Approach

In this case, $N = M = 1$, (1) becomes

$$\mathbf{R}_l = \mathbf{H}_l\mathbf{S}_l + \mathbf{W}_l . \tag{2}$$

At pilot positions, the least square channel values can be obtained by evaluating:

$$H_{k_p,l}^{LS} = \frac{R_{k_p,l}}{S_{k_p,l}} . \tag{3}$$

for $k_p = \{4,8\}$ at even symbols and $k_p = \{0,12\}$ at odd symbols.

Based on the pilot pattern in DL-PUSC mode, channel estimation can be performed by cascading two 1-dimension interpolations in time- and frequency-axis.

Conventional linear interpolation scheme can be utilized in both time and frequency to estimate the channel transfer function. Time interpolation as shown in fig. 3 has some differences depending on the symbol (even or odd) that the cluster belongs to, whereas frequency interpolation is performed similarly for all clusters in frame since each cluster now have 4 channel values, 2 of pilots and 2 from the time interpolation.

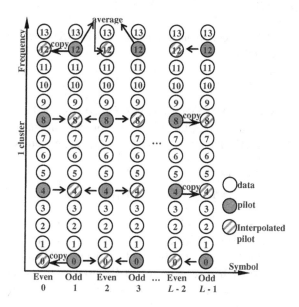

Fig. 3. Linear interpolation in time axis

Time interpolation:

$$H_{\{0,12\},l}^{est} = \begin{cases} H_{\{0,12\},l}^{LS} & l=0 \\ \dfrac{H_{\{0,12\},l-1}^{LS} + H_{\{0,12\},l+1}^{LS}}{2} & l=2,4,...,L\text{-}2 \end{cases} \quad (4)$$

$$H_{\{4,8\},l}^{est} = \begin{cases} \dfrac{H_{\{4,8\},l-1}^{LS} + H_{\{4,8\},l+1}^{LS}}{2} & l=1,3,...,L\text{-}3 \\ H_{\{4,8\},L\text{-}2}^{LS} & l=L\text{-}1 \end{cases} \quad (5)$$

Frequency interpolation:

$$H_{j,l}^{est} = \frac{\delta}{\Delta} H_{k_p,l}^{est/LS} + \frac{\Delta-\delta}{\Delta} H_{k_{p+1},l}^{LS/est}, j=k_p+1,...,k_{p+1}\text{-}1; \delta=1,...,\Delta\text{-}1, \quad (6)$$

$$\Delta=4; k_p=[0,4,8,12]; p=0,...,3.$$

When all the channel values are estimated, the original OFDM symbol can be recovered by equalizing:

$$\mathbf{S}^{est} = \frac{\mathbf{R}}{\mathbf{H}^{est}} \ . \tag{7}$$

4 STBC Approaches

There are 3 types of STBC recommended for mobile WiMAX system, i.e. MRC, 2x1- and 2x2- Alamouti schemes.

4.1 MRC ($N = 1$, $M = 2$)

In this scheme, the same OFDM symbol is transmitted from 1 Tx antenna to 2 Rx antennas. Each Rx antenna receives the data stream propagating through the channel from the transmitter to it. The received symbols at 2 Rx antennas are found as:

$$\mathbf{R}_l(0) = \mathbf{H}_l(0,0)\mathbf{S}_l(0) + \mathbf{W}_l(0)$$
$$\mathbf{R}_l(1) = \mathbf{H}_l(1,0)\mathbf{S}_l(0) + \mathbf{W}_l(1) \tag{8}$$

From (8), the method to estimate the channel and recover the user's data for each stream is identical to the SISO case. Hence, two frames of L symbols are processed in parallel and then combined together to give the final data. MRC provides an effective combining scheme in which the stream corresponding to the stronger channel contributes more than the other. This approach is expressed as:

$$\mathbf{S}^{est} = \frac{\left[\mathbf{H}(0,0)^{est}\right]^* \mathbf{R}(0) + \left[\mathbf{H}(1,0)^{est}\right]^* \mathbf{R}(1)}{\left|\mathbf{H}(0,0)^{est}\right|^2 + \left|\mathbf{H}(1,0)^{est}\right|^2} \tag{9}$$

4.2 Alamouti Schemes

For transmission using 2 Tx antennas, as indicated in the IEEE 802.16e standard, the cluster structure is slightly modified to meet the requirement for STBC schemes. The pilot insertion is changed so that their locations are arranged in period of 4 symbols rather than 2 symbols as before. This arrangement is shown in fig. 4. From now on, the time index l is used to denote 2 symbol periods.

Alamouti scheme uses multiple antennas at the transmitter and sends each processed symbol to the set of Tx antennas sequentially. The channels from all Tx antennas to the receiver during that time are assumed unchanged [5]. In the simulation reported below, the channels is modeled to change continuously over the simulation time rather than stay constant as assumed, but since their time variations are quite slow comparing to the symbol period, the processing formulas drawn out from this assumption are still proper.

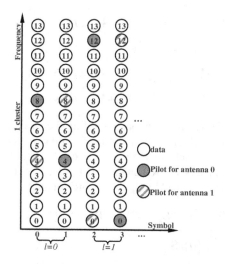

Fig. 4. Cluster structure for STBC PUSC using 2 Tx antennas

4.2.1 Alamouti 2x1 ($N = 2, M = 1$)

This scheme uses 2 antennas at the transmitter and 1 antenna at the receiver.

At symbol time $2l$ and $2l+1$, the symbols transmitted at 2 Tx antennas are defined according to the matrix $\mathbf{A} = \begin{bmatrix} \mathbf{S}_{2l}(0) & \mathbf{S}_{2l+1}(1) \\ -\left[\mathbf{S}_{2l+1}(0)\right]^* & \left[\mathbf{S}_{2l}(1)\right]^* \end{bmatrix}$, yielding the signal at the receiver:

$$\mathbf{R}_{2l}(0) = \mathbf{H}(0,0)\mathbf{S}_{2l}(0) + \mathbf{H}(0,1)\mathbf{S}_{2l+1}(1)$$
$$\mathbf{R}_{2l+1}(0) = -\mathbf{H}(0,0)\left[\mathbf{S}_{2l+1}(0)\right]^* + \mathbf{H}(0,1)\left[\mathbf{S}_{2l}(1)\right]^* . \tag{10}$$

The noise at the receiver in this scenario is ignored. Solving (10) at pilot subcarriers gives:

$$\mathbf{H}_{k_p,2l}(0,0) = \frac{\mathbf{R}_{k_p,2l}(0)\left[\mathbf{S}_{k_p,2l}(1)\right]^* - \mathbf{R}_{k_p,2l+1}(0)\mathbf{S}_{k_p,2l+1}(1)}{\mathbf{S}_{k_p,2l}(0)\left[\mathbf{S}_{k_p,2l}(1)\right]^* + \mathbf{S}_{k_p,2l+1}(1)\left[\mathbf{S}_{k_p,2l+1}(0)\right]^*}$$

$$\mathbf{H}_{k_p,2l}(0,1) = \frac{\mathbf{R}_{k_p,2l}(0)\left[\mathbf{S}_{k_p,2l+1}(0)\right]^* + \mathbf{R}_{k_p,2l+1}(0)\mathbf{S}_{k_p,2l}(0)}{\mathbf{S}_{k_p,2l}(0)\left[\mathbf{S}_{k_p,2l}(1)\right]^* + \mathbf{S}_{k_p,2l+1}(1)\left[\mathbf{S}_{k_p,2l+1}(0)\right]^*} . \tag{11}$$

4.2.2 Alamouti 2x2 ($N = 2, M = 2$)

The matrix A is used again to arrange symbols to be transmitted at the corresponding antenna. The same approach as Alamouti *2x1* system can be derived to give the receive signals at 2 Rx antennas:

$$\mathbf{R}_{2l}(0) = \mathbf{H}(0,0)\mathbf{S}_{2l}(0) + \mathbf{H}(0,1)\mathbf{S}_{2l+1}(1)$$
$$\mathbf{R}_{2l}(1) = \mathbf{H}(1,0)\mathbf{S}_{2l}(0) + \mathbf{H}(1,1)\mathbf{S}_{2l+1}(1)$$
$$\mathbf{R}_{2l+1}(0) = -\mathbf{H}(0,0)\left[\mathbf{S}_{2l+1}(0)\right]^{*} + \mathbf{H}(0,1)\left[\mathbf{S}_{2l}(1)\right]^{*}$$
$$\mathbf{R}_{2l+1}(1) = -\mathbf{H}(1,0)\left[\mathbf{S}_{2l+1}(0)\right]^{*} + \mathbf{H}(1,1)\left[\mathbf{S}_{2l}(1)\right]^{*} \tag{12}$$

By re-arranging (12) into pair of equations regarding the received signals at the same Rx antenna at symbol-time $2l$ and $2l+1$, similar formulas for calculating the channel values at pilot positions for each separate channel can be obtained. That is, the channel values at pilot subcarriers for Rx antenna 0 is given by (11), and those for Rx antenna 1 are analogously obtained by the following equations:

$$\mathbf{H}_{k_p,2l}(1,0) = \frac{\mathbf{R}_{k_p,2l}(1)\left[\mathbf{S}_{k_p,2l}(1)\right]^{*} - \mathbf{R}_{k_p,2l+1}(1)\mathbf{S}_{k_p,2l+1}(1)}{\mathbf{S}_{k_p,2l}(0)\left[\mathbf{S}_{k_p,2l}(1)\right]^{*} + \mathbf{S}_{k_p,2l+1}(1)\left[\mathbf{S}_{k_p,2l+1}(0)\right]^{*}}$$

$$\mathbf{H}_{k_p,2l}(1,1) = \frac{\mathbf{R}_{k_p,2l}(1)\left[\mathbf{S}_{k_p,2l+1}(0)\right]^{*} + \mathbf{R}_{k_p,2l+1}(1)\mathbf{S}_{k_p,2l}(0)}{\mathbf{S}_{k_p,2l}(0)\left[\mathbf{S}_{k_p,2l}(1)\right]^{*} + \mathbf{S}_{k_p,2l+1}(1)\left[\mathbf{S}_{k_p,2l+1}(0)\right]^{*}} \tag{13}$$

After calculating (11) and (13) to have channel values at pilot locations, the same channel estimation process as SISO approach can be utilized to estimate all the channel values at data positions. The original signal can be recovered by:

For Alamouti 2x1:

$$\mathbf{S}_{2l}^{est} = \left[\mathbf{H}^{est}(0,0)\right]^{*}\mathbf{R}_{2l}(0) + \mathbf{H}^{est}(0,1)\left[\mathbf{R}_{2l+1}(0)\right]^{*}$$
$$\mathbf{S}_{2l+1}^{est} = \left[\mathbf{H}^{est}(0,1)\right]^{*}\mathbf{R}_{2l}(0) - \mathbf{H}^{est}(0,0)\left[\mathbf{R}_{2l+1}(0)\right]^{*} \tag{14}$$

For Alamouti 2x2:

$$\mathbf{S}_{2l}^{est} = \left[\mathbf{H}^{est}(0,0)\right]^{*}\mathbf{R}_{2l}(0) + \mathbf{H}^{est}(0,1)\left[\mathbf{R}_{2l+1}(0)\right]^{*} + \left[\mathbf{H}^{est}(1,0)\right]^{*}\mathbf{R}_{2l}(1) + \mathbf{H}^{est}(1,1)\left[\mathbf{R}_{2l+1}(1)\right]^{*}$$
$$\mathbf{S}_{2l+1}^{est} = \left[\mathbf{H}^{est}(0,1)\right]^{*}\mathbf{R}_{2l}(0) - \mathbf{H}^{est}(0,0)\left[\mathbf{R}_{2l+1}(0)\right]^{*} + \left[\mathbf{H}^{est}(1,1)\right]^{*}\mathbf{R}_{2l}(1) - \mathbf{H}^{est}(1,0)\left[\mathbf{R}_{2l+1}(1)\right]^{*} \tag{15}$$

5 Simulation Results

5.1 Simulation Parameters

Simulation parameters are shown in table 1. Carrier frequency of 2.3 GHz is chosen, convolutional code CC(171_133) with different rates is used as channel coding. For calculating the system throughput, the OFDM symbol is assumed to carry data from 4 individual users.

Two channel models recommended by ITU for mobile environments are used to investigate the system performance.

- Model 1: ITU_Pedestrian B, speed 12 Km/h, Doppler frequency $f_D \approx 25.56$ Hz.
- Model 2: ITU_Vehicular A, speed 120 Km/h, $f_D \approx 255.56$ Hz.

These channel models are time-variant frequency-selective channels in Non Line of Sight (NLoS) conditions. The Pedestrian B (Ped.B) model is more frequency selective than Vehicular A (Veh.A) due to its longer delay spread whereas Veh.A fades faster in time due to higher moving speed. Their specific parameters are given in table 2.

Table 1. Profile parameters for DL-PUSC

Bandwidth	8.75 MHz	FFT size	1024
Sampling factor (n)	8/7	Number of used subcarriers (N_used)	840
Sampling frequency	10 MHz	Sub-carrier spacing	9.77 KHz
Number of DL symbols used in simulation	48 (2 frames)	Modulation modes	QPSK 16-QAM 64-QAM
Useful symbol time (Tb)	102.4 μs	CP ratio G	1/8
Guard Interval (Tg)	12.8 μs	Carrier frequency	2.3GHz
OFDM Symbol Time (Ts)	115.2 μs	Convolutional Coding (R_{FEC})	1/2, 2/3, 3/4, 5/6

Table 2. Profiles of channel models used in simulation

Model 1 (*Ped.B*)	Path Power(dB)	–3.9	–4.8	–8.8	–11.9	–11.7	–27.8
	Path Delay(μs)	0	0.2	0.8	1.2	2.3	3.7
Model 2 (*Veh.A*)	Path Power(dB)	–3.1	–4.1	–12.1	–13.1	–18.1	–23.1
	Path Delay(μs)	0	0.31	0.71	1.09	1.73	2.51

5.2 Simulation Results

In these simulations, signal modulated with 3 different modulation modes, i.e. QPSK, 16QAM, and 64QAM, is propagated through the Ped.B and Veh.A channel models by using SISO and STBC approaches.

Fig. 5, 6, and 7 show the performance in term of Packet Error Rate (PER) versus Signal to Noise Ratio (SNR) of each modulation mode in 2 types of channel respectively. The ideal cases (perfect channel knowledge) for SISO as well as 2x2-Alamouti are presented as references.

The results show that, in all situations, the STBC approaches always outperform the SISO scheme. The SNR gain is significantly increased from 3 to 8 dB, e.g. 64QAM at PER = 10^{-4}. Among STBC schemes, performances of MRC 1x2 and Alamouti 2x1 are almost identical since the diversity is the same, and the transmission powers in both cases are kept equal.

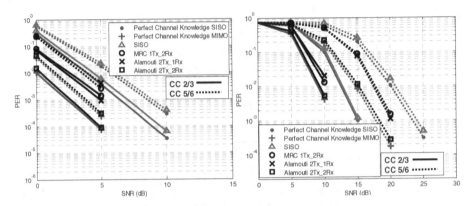

Fig. 5. PER of QPSK mode in Ped.B 12 Km/h (left) and Veh.A 120 Km/h (right)

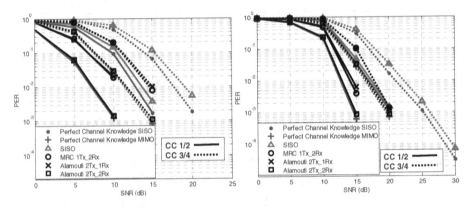

Fig. 6. PER of 16QAM mode in Ped.B 12 Km/h (left) and Veh.A 120 Km/h (right)

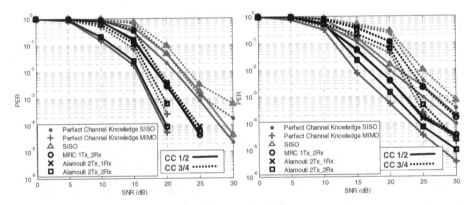

Fig. 7. PER of 64QAM mode in Ped.B 12 Km/h (left) and Veh.A 120 Km/h (right)

Fig.8 and 9 present the comparison of the throughput (Mbps) between SISO and 2x2- Alamouti schemes. In this case the OFDM symbol is shared by 4 users. System throughput is defined in [11]. Again, it can be seen that 2x2- STBC scheme gives a remarkable improvement over the SISO approach. The gain is about 6 dB in Ped.B 12 Km/h and 4 dB in Veh.A 120 Km/h at the highest throughput (64QAM 5/6).

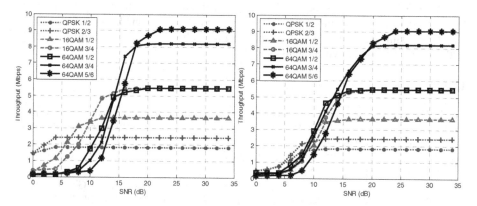

Fig. 8. SISO Throughput in Ped.B 12 Km/h (left), and Veh.A 120 Km/h (right)

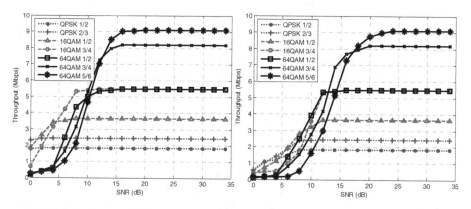

Fig. 9. 2x2- Alamouti Throughput in Ped.B 12 Km/h (left), and Veh.A 120 Km/h (right)

It should be noted that the linear interpolation method used for channel estimation works quite well thank to the pilot pattern and the cluster-size estimation. According to [14] - [15], in this setup, the Ped.B channel has a coherent time about 7.82 ms and a coherent bandwidth of 530 KHz whereas those of Veh.A model are 0.782 ms and 900 KHz respectively. From the system parameters, a cluster of 14 subcarriers covers a bandwidth of 137 KHz, and a symbol period is about 115.2 us. A block of 12 symbols, which is used for channel estimation in this simulation, spreads over 1.3824 ms of time causing a little degradation in Veh.A channel. However, in general, for this particular system, linear interpolation can ensure a good channel estimation performance.

6 Conclusion

In this paper, performance analysis of STBC in DL-PUSC mode of mobile WiMAX system has been presented. The system parameters are derived from the IEEE 802.16e-2005 standard. The channels used for simulation are the popular ITU pedestrian and vehicular models. Commonly used channel estimation technique is carried out to provide practical results. PER and system throughput performance comparison between SISO approach and several STBC schemes are presented. The STBC shows significant gain over the SISO approach in various channel conditions corresponding to the realistic mobile environments.

References

1. IEEE 802.16e-2005, Part 16: Air Interface for Fixed and Mobile Broadband Wireless Access Systems, Amendment 2: Physical and Medium Access Control Layers for Combined Fixed and Mobile Operation in Licensed Bands and Corrigendum 1 (2006)
2. Ming, J., Hanzo, L.: Multiuser MIMO-OFDM for Next-Generation Wireless Systems. Proc. of the IEEE 95(7), 1430–1469 (2007)
3. Stuber, G.L., Barry, J.R., McLaughlin, S.W., Ye, L., Ingram, M.A., Pratt, T.G.: Broadband MIMO-OFDM Wireless Communications. Proc. of the IEEE 92(2), 271–294 (2004)
4. Gesbert, D., Shafi, M., Da-shan, S., Smith, P.J., Naguib, A.: From theory to practice: an overview of MIMO space-time coded wireless systems. IEEE Journal on Selected Areas in Communications 21(3), 281–302 (2003)
5. Alamouti, S.M.: A simple transmit diversity technique for wireless communications. IEEE Journal on Selected Areas in Communications 16(8), 1451–1458 (1998)
6. Agrawal, D., Tarokh, V., Naguib, A., Seshadri, N.: Space-time coded OFDM for high data-rate wireless communication over wideband channels. In: 48th IEEE Vehicular Technology Conference, vol. 3, pp. 2232–2236 (1998)
7. Tarokh, V., Jafarkhani, H., Calderbank, A.R.: Space-time block codes from orthogonal designs. IEEE Transactions on Information Theory 47(5), 1456–1467 (1999)
8. Hsieh, F., Fan, W., Ghosh, A.: Link Performance of WiMAX PUSC. In: Proc. WCNC 2008, pp. 1143–1148. IEEE, Los Alamitos (2008)
9. Alex, S.P., Jalloul, L.M.A.: Performance Evaluation of MIMO in IEEE802.16e/WiMAX. IEEE Journal of Selected Topics in Signal Processing 2(2), 181–190 (2008)
10. Mare, K.P., Maharaj, B.T.: Performance Analysis of Modern Space-Time Codes on a MIMO-WiMAX Platform. In: Proc. WIMOB-2008, pp. 139–144. IEEE, Los Alamitos (2008)
11. Tran, M., Doufexi, A., Nix, A.: Mobile WiMAX MIMO performance analysis: Downlink and uplink. In: Proc. 19th PIMRC 2008, pp. 1–5. IEEE, Los Alamitos (2008)
12. Shen, Y., Martinez, E.F.: WiMAX Channel Estimation: Algorithms and Implementations. AN3429, Freescale Semiconductor, Inc. (2007)
13. Recommendation for ITU-R M.1225: Guidelines for evaluation of radio transmission technologies for IMT-2000 (1997)
14. Sklar, B.: Rayleigh Fading Channels in Mobile Digital Communication Systems - Part I: Characterization. IEEE Communications Magazine 35(9), 136–146 (1997)
15. Sklar, B.: Rayleigh Fading Channels in Mobile Digital Communication Systems Part II: Mitigation. IEEE Communications Magazine 35(9), 148–155 (1997)

Intelligent Transportation Systems (ITS)

The Changing Transport Datascape –
Opportunities and Challenges

John Polak

Professor of Transport Demand and Director, Centre for Transport Studies,
Imperial College London, Research Director, UK Transport Research Centre

Abstract. The safe and efficient operation of the transport system is a fundamental national requirement. This in turn depends on a wide range of analysis
and modelling tools that are used in the planning, operation and management of
transport systems and in the development and delivery of transport services.
These analysis and modelling tools have historically been constrained by data
that are severely limited in terms of their spatial, temporal and semantic granularity. We are now however, entering a period in which this datascape is under-
going profound change, with rich new types of data becoming available in
unprecedented volumes. The new transport datascape will drive innovation in
modelling and analysis tools and new transport systems and services. The aim
of this presentation is to discuss the changing nature of the transport datascape
and highlight the range of new opportunities that are emerging. The discussion
will be illustrated with examples drawn from current projects being undertaken
at Imperial College London.

R. Mehmood et al. (Eds.): EuropeComm 2009, LNICST 16, p. 115, 2009.
© Institute for Computer Science, Social-Informatics and Telecommunications Engineering 2009

Intelligent Control of Urban Road Networks:
Algorithms, Systems and Communications

Mike Smith

Department of Mathematics, University of York,
Heslington, York Y010 5DD, United Kingdom
mjs7@york.ac.uk

Abstract. This paper considers control in road networks. Using a simple example based on the well-known Braess network [1] the paper shows that reducing delay for traffic, assuming that the traffic distribution is fixed, may increase delay when travellers change their travel choices in light of changes in control settings and hence delays. It is shown that a similar effect occurs within signal controlled networks. In this case the effect appears at first sight to be much stronger: the overall capacity of a network may be substantially reduced by utilising standard responsive signal control algorithms. In seeking to reduce delays for existing flows, these policies do not allow properly for consequent routeing changes by travellers. Control methods for signal-controlled networks that do take proper account of the reactions of users are suggested; these require further research, development, and careful real-life trials.

Keywords: Intelligent Network Control, Urban Traffic Control, Capacity-maximising Control, Stability of Transport Networks, Complexity.

1 Introduction

1.1 Urban Traffic Control, Healthcare, Computing and Further Research

The problem of controlling or managing a system with many reactive "users" has been considered within studies of urban traffic control for many years; various difficulties have arisen and various solutions have been proposed. Similar difficulties arise in other fields; for example healthcare and computing both involve networks of facilities with capacity and budget constraints and many "users" who make their own decisions.

In this paper we consider only the traffic control case hoping that this case may yield insights in these other areas. In any case the author knows only about this case!

This paper considers several simple examples all designed to show that feedback loops can have a significant effect on outcomes of utilizing apparently sensible control policies or algorithms. Some examples show that other novel policies may perform much better than standard policies; because they deal with feedback better.

Novel control policies discussed here merit further research within the transport field. These policies may also be useful when healthcare and computer networks are to be managed and controlled; and so research on transferring these approaches to

R. Mehmood et al. (Eds.): EuropeComm 2009, LNICST 16, pp. 116–127, 2009.

both those fields is needed. Finally, while we have considered stability briefly in this paper, speed of reaction has not been considered in any detail. Yet speeds are now increasing rapidly in real life in many vital systems. Stability when communications and reactions are very fast merits much more attention in many fields including transport networks.

1.2 Urban Traffic Control and Traffic Assignment and the Digital Economy

Given an urban network with a given set of signal controls, a control or management change designed to benefit network users may actually make network users worse off; due to "knock on" effects which have not been properly allowed for. These knock-on effects arise as a result of the reactions of network users who are free to change their route and mode; the flow pattern can and does change in reaction to control changes. Beckmann once said: "travellers will be playing their own games while the network manager is playing his".

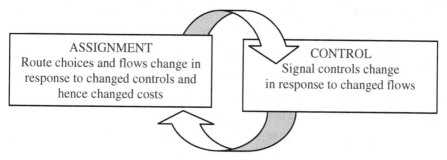

Fig. 1. The assignment–control interaction loop above is traversed indefinitely; the loop represents the interaction between a control system (where signal controls change in response to changed flows on the network according to some policy or algorithm) and an assignment system (where route-flows change toward cheaper routes as drivers respond to changed control settings and hence changed costs)

If in the loop in figure 1 traffic signal control settings are changed to achieve some aim (such as reducing the average journey time of travellers on the assumption that flows are fixed) then the following (or knock-on) change in the routes chosen by drivers (moving to cheaper routes say) may cause delays to increase instead.

Allsop in [2] first stated that route choices need to be taken into account when optimising signals and Dickson [3] gave an example to show that continually optimising signals assuming flows are fixed does not achieve the optimum result when the flows are, as is usually the case, variable.

There is as yet no reliable automatic procedure for finding (for example) a change in the control parameters of an urban traffic control system which is certain to benefit the network as a whole when the responses of divers are taken into account. This problem has been much considered; see, for example, [4, 5, 6]. Much more mathematical / computing research is needed here before real effects are felt on-street.

The digital economy is moving this problem (in both the economic sphere and the transport sphere) into a whole new era of very fast communication. *The difficulty of taking proper account of knock-on effects is multiplied when this has to be done fast.*

The speed of onset of the credit crunch is a symptom of this. Movements of international capital, reacting perhaps to excessive lending in the USA and elsewhere, have left governments to "catch up", using laborious regulatory tools, aiming to control rapidly reactive international knock-on effects. The computing power available in the digital age has improved the tools available to managers, but it has also changed forever the "game" which managers are seeking to manage or control; with uncertain consequences.

2 Considering Braess's Network

Assume first that the dotted link is not present. A total flow of 6 travels from the origin to the destination on the network of four bold-arrow links. The two route costs are equal and so no element of flow has any incentive to change route if

flow on route 1 = flow on route 2 = 3.

The average travel cost at this equilibrium is

cost of route 1 = cost of route 2 = (10.3) + (3 + 50) = 83 units.

Now assume that the dotted link has been added. If $k = 10$ (as Braess originally specified) all three routes have the same cost if

flow on route 1 = flow on route 2 = flow on route 3 = 2.

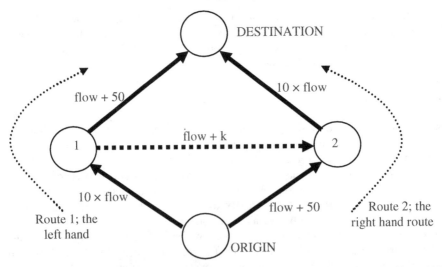

Fig. 2. The network first considered by Braess [1] to illustrate the counterintuitive effects which may arise when a network link is added to reduce congestion. Costs of traversing the links are shown: 10 × flow means that the link cost equals 10 times the flow on that link, and so on. Braess considered the effect of adding the dotted link to the basic network of four links indicated by solid arrows. See [7] for an English translation of Braess's 1968 paper.

The average travel cost at this equilibrium distribution (which we write as (2, 2, 2)) is now 10.(2+2) + 2 + 50 = 92 > 83; this is the travel cost of each route when the traffic distribution is (2, 2, 2).

In the augmented network, with the added dotted link and where k = 10, (3, 3, 0) is the optimal distribution of the total flow of 6; this distribution minimizes average or total travel cost. So the minimum average cost for this new augmented network is 83.

For the augmented network it is natural to consider the ratio of the equilibrium cost and the optimal cost, and Roughgarden [8] has called this ratio the price of anarchy. The price of anarchy for the augmented version of the Braess network is thus 92/83. Roughgarden [8] shows that if all cost functions have the form (a × flow) + b then (total cost at equilibrium flow pattern)/(total cost at optimum flow pattern) ≤ 4/3.

Valiant and Roughgarden [9] show that for large random networks (with link cost functions of the form (a × flow) + b) the ratio above approaches 4/3 with probability 1 as the number of links in the network tends to infinity; provided network loads are suitably (adversarily) chosen.

2.1   Controlling Braess's Augmented Network by Varying k in Figure 2

Consider again the augmented version of the Braess network. Consider letting k = 23 (instead of k = 10, the value chosen by Braess). It is easy to see that the flow distribution (3, 3, 0) now becomes an equilibrium with the costs of all three routes being the optimal 83. Removal of the dotted road is unnecessary; just increase its cost.

The equilibrium network performance changes as k varies in figure 2: k = 10 gives the Braess network with equilibrium (2, 2, 2) while k = 23 ensures that the dotted link is sufficiently unattractive to be unused at equilibrium and the equilibrium then becomes (3, 3, 0); as if the dotted link had indeed been removed. Let k be a "control"; if 0 ≤ k ≤ 23 then (2 + (k-10)/13, 2 + (k-10)/13, 2 − 2(k-10)/13) is the unique equilibrium flow pattern: all route costs equal 92 − 9(k-10)/13, as shown in figure 3.

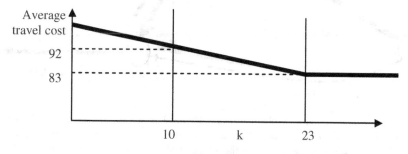

Fig. 3. The performance of the augmented Braess network versus k for non-negative k. Average travel cost at equilibrium is a decreasing function of k for 0 ≤ k ≤ 23.

3 Network Control Using Signals

In figure 4, two routes join a single Origin – Destination pair. There are two stages at the signal; the first gives green (or right of way) to route 1 and the second gives green (or right of way) to route 2. We envisage that this network is traversed day after day and that some drivers change route to a cheaper route if a cheaper route is available.

We show that changing the control policy from a standard policy to the P_0 policy (introduced in [10, 11, 12]) doubles the capacity of this network.

So suppose first that the drivers on the network in figure 4 have adjusted their routes over time so that both routes currently have equal cost; then, since route 1 is less costly than route 2 (ignoring the delays), the delay at the signal on route 1 must exceed the delay at the signal on route 2. Suppose also that flow is currently greater on route 1.

As both the flow and delay at the signal are greater on route 1 than on route 2, to reduce current delay some green-time must be swapped from the upper route to the lower route. Suppose some green-time is swapped.

This green-time swap will increase delay at the signal on route 2 and reduce delay at the signal on route 1. There is now an incentive for drivers to swap from route 2 to route 1. Suppose that some small proportion of drivers on route 2 do swap to route 1.

We are now in a similar position to that in italics two paragraphs up; and so the same argument works again (and again and again . . . .). Eventually all traffic and all available green time will become allocated to route 1. Since route 2 is twice as wide as route 1 this halves the maximum possible capacity of the network. [Differential equations may be used to make these swapping rules precise. The above argument is largely independent of swap rates and essentially depends only on swap rates being positive.]

The problem of course is similar to that in the Braess network: each green time swap reduces total delay at the signal and reduces total travel costs felt *if the flows remain fixed*. But as flows respond in the natural way to changed delays (by swapping to cheaper routes as above) then total travel costs and delays at the signal in fact increase; just as costs do in the Braess example when k is reduced. (See figure 3.)

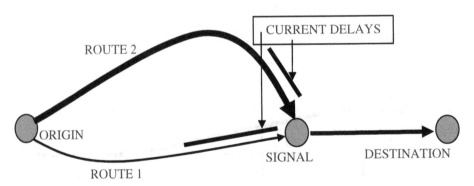

Fig. 4. A simple signal-controlled network. Route 2 is longer and (ignoring the delays at the signal) more costly than route 1. Route 2 is twice as wide as route 1 and the saturation flow at the signal for route 2 is twice the saturation flow at the signal for route 1. The signal responds to the local delays at the signalized junction. The length of each bar represents the delay felt by vehicles at the signal; as shown here these delays are currently larger on the lower route, route 1.

3.1 Designing Control Changes and the Stability of Control Systems

In designing network control changes we need to try to take account of the likely knock-on effects of our actions on future traveller choices.

This is difficult; especially if fast decisions need to be taken as in the traffic control case. Thus it is natural to look for a simple practical solution to this difficulty when control decisions are taken.

One clue is in the last simple example: here not only do delays rise as the swapping processes occur but the overall travel capacity of the network declines as the swapping processes occur. Perhaps if we aim not to minimize delay but to maximize capacity the anticipation problem will become more practically soluble and maybe even soluble *fast*. Maybe even fast enough for application to the design of real time control systems. Furthermore it may be that maximizing capacity will be quite good at reducing delays even if not minimizing delays; we are led to the P_0 control policy.

3.2 A Capacity Maximizing Control Policy or Algorithm: P_0

In this section we specify a signal control policy called P_0. If in the network shown in figure 4 the origin destination flow slowly increases from zero then at equilibrium this policy compares with standard delay minimisation as shown in figure 5 below.

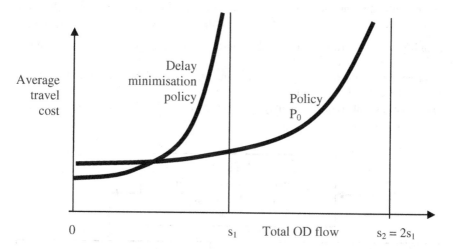

Fig. 5. Equilibrium performances of responsive delay-minimisation and P_0 policies as the total flow from the origin to the destination in figure 4 increases from zero. The capacity of the network is doubled by switching from delay-minimisation to P_0.

To specify the P_0 policy we need a little notation. Suppose that, in figure 4,

> s_1 is the saturation flow of route 1 at the junction;
> s_2 is the saturation flow of route 2 at the junction;
> d_1 is the delay felt at the junction by each vehicle traversing route 1; and
> d_2 is the delay felt at the junction by each vehicle traversing route 2.

The delays felt at this signal-controlled junction depend on both flows and green-times and this dependence is here omitted for clarity. The P_0 control policy for a junction like that in figure 4, with just two approaches, is as follows: for given flows and delays at the junction, choose green-times so that $s_1d_1 = s_2d_2$.

In figure 4 we suppose that $s_2 = 2s_1$; the P_0 policy $s_1d_1 = s_2d_2$ thus here ensures that $d_1 = 2d_2$.

We may now justify the P_0 graph in figure 5. Suppose that demand slowly increases from 0. Then initially all traffic will choose route 1 as this is shorter than route 2 and the junction delays are small because flows are small.

Eventually however as the total origin to destination flow increases junction delays will also increase; and then the difference $d_1 - d_2 = d_2 = \frac{1}{2}d_1$ also increases. Eventually $d_1 - d_2 \ (= d_2)$ will exceed Δ, the difference between the free-running costs of the two routes. When this happens the travel cost via route 1 will exceed the travel cost via route 2 and travellers will gradually switch to route 2 as the total flow increases. When delays become very high $d_1 - d_2 = d_2$ will also become very high and all travellers will be using the wider route 2, maximising the capacity of the network.

4   More Complicated Systems and Complex Systems

A more complicated interacting system arises if demand is represented, as in figure 6 above. It is then also natural to add more elements into these three boxes: for example

(1) public transport flows may be added into the assignment box to take account of travellers' choice of mode as well as route;

(2) prices and subsidies may be added into the control box to take account of changes in these "controls"; and

(3) bus routes and frequencies may be added into the demand box to take account of changes in these.

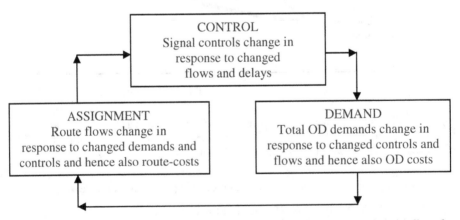

Fig. 6. Assignment–demand–control interaction: figure 1 has been expanded to allow for demand changes. This may represent a real system or a model of a real system.

In both model and real-life dynamical systems the set of equilibria is very important and it is clear that systems like that in figure 6 can get very complicated and then it may be hard to determine the set of equilibria.

However complexity is not just a question of size; as we shall see below.

4.1 A Small Complex System and a Pitchfork

In the signal controlled network shown in figure 7 below, both routes have the same undelayed travel time and the same saturation flow of s vehicles per minute at the signal. We here assume that the signal responds to traffic flows by equalizing saturation ratios.

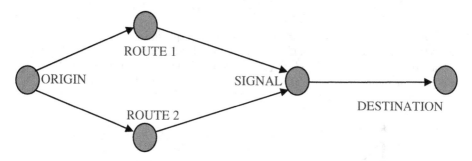

Fig. 7. The signal is adjusted to equalise the degrees of saturation at the signal for any flows along the two routes. The network is symmetrical.

Let T be the total flow from the Origin to the Destination via the two routes and let $0 < T < s$. Let X_1 be the proportion of the Origin-Destination flow which travels along route 1 and X_2 be the proportion travelling along route 2; so that $X_1 + X_2 = 1$. The flow on routes 1 and 2 will then be TX_1 and TX_2. We will consider T fixed but also we will consider different values of T (satisfying $0 < T < s$). Let G_1 be the green time proportion awarded to route 1 and G_2 be the green time proportion awarded to route 2.

Since the signal equalises the two saturation ratios at the signal, X_1, X_2, G_1, and G_2 must satisfy $X_1T/sG_1 = X_2T/sG_2$. Since G_1 and G_2 are green time proportions and so add to 1 it now follows that G_1, G_1 must be given (for any T) by:

$$G_1 = X_1 \text{ and } G_2 = X_2.$$

We further assume that the delay costs d_1 and d_2 felt at the signal by vehicles traversing routes 1 and 2 are determined by putting:

$$d_1 = BTX_1/[sG_1(sG_1 - TX_1)] \text{ and } d_2 = BTX_2/[sG_2(sG_2 - TX_2)];$$

and that the travel costs C_1 and C_2 along routes 1 and 2 are then given as follows:

$$C_1 = ATX_1 + d_1 \text{ and } C_2 = ATX_2 + d_2.$$

A and B are constants; delay cost here is identical to the second term of Webster's delay formula [13] if B is chosen to be 9/20; in this case d_1 and d_2 will be the estimated delays in minutes per vehicle.

Since $G = X$ it follows immediately that

$$C_1 - C_2 = AT(X_1 - X_2) + [BT/s(s-T)][1/X_1 - 1/X_2].$$

To find equilibria; where route costs are equal and so no traveller has any incentive to change route; we need to solve the equation $C_1 - C_2 = 0$. For any T, $X_1 = X_2 = \frac{1}{2}$ yields one solution and so is an equilibrium: are there others?

Multiply the equation $C_1 - C_2 = 0$ through by X_1X_2 and consider instead:

$$(C_1 - C_2)X_1X_2 = AT(X_1 - X_2)(X_1X_2) \ - \ [BT/s(s-T)][X_1 - X_2] = 0.$$

Now either $X_1 - X_2 = 0$ or (dividing by $X_1 - X_2$ and letting $X_2 = 1 - X_1$):

$$X_1{}^2 - X_1 + B/[As(s-T)] = 0.$$

Hence

$$X_1 = \frac{1}{2} + [\tfrac{1}{4} - B/As(s-T)]^{1/2} \text{ or } X_1 = \frac{1}{2} - [\tfrac{1}{4} - B/As(s-T)]^{1/2}.$$

There are two additional *real* roots of the quadratic equation (and so of $C_1 - C_2 = 0$) and so two additional equilibria if and only if $\frac{1}{4} - B/As(s-T) > 0$ or $T < s - 4B/As$.

The complete set of equilibrium (TX_1, TX_2) as T varies from 0 to s is shown by bold lines in figure 8. [Each "axis" of the figure also consists of equilibria, and so these are bold too.]

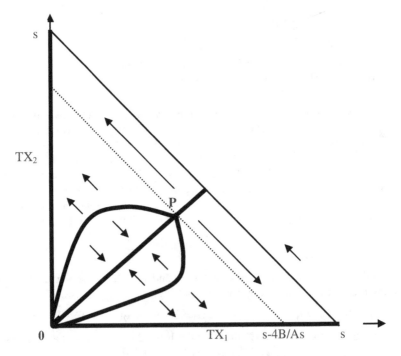

Fig. 8. Bold lines indicate the set of route-flows $TX = (TX_1, TX_2)$ which are equilibria consistent with the equisaturation policy for some T. Five branches of the equilibrium set, three of them comprising stable equilibria, converge on the origin as T becomes small. Arrows indicate the natural directions of motion of non-equilibria (for various values of T) as drivers and green-time respond to delays and saturation ratios. If X_1 is plotted against T the shape shown here becomes a pitchfork.

Let us suppose that T slowly increases from zero. If the flow pattern initially follows the central (stable) equilibrium set leading away from the origin then it will naturally carry on doing that until $T = s - 4B/As$, when the bifurcation point P is reached. As T increases beyond this point the central equilibria become unstable and the flow pattern will then naturally follow one of the long arrows and continually move toward one of the two axes.

Thus the behaviour of the system changes sharply near P. This is in part due to the change in the topological structure of the equilibrium set at this point. Consider a small circle around P: for $T < s - 4B/As$ the equilibrium set has three points within the circle and for $T \geq s - 4B/As$ the equilibrium set has just one point within the circle. Since the topological structure of the equilibrium set changes at P this point is called a *bifurcation*.

4.2 Real Life Control Systems and the Origins of Traffic Assignment

An early signal setting method for an isolated traffic signal (essentially the equisaturation method) was specified and justified by Webster [13]. TRANSYT (Robertson [14]) is a method of designing fixed time signal timings in a network.

Many cities use the traffic-responsive SCOOT control system; see Hunt [15].

Wardrop [16] introduced the equilibrium condition discussed in this paper. This is: at equilibrium, no driver has a less costly alternative route.

5   Conclusion

This paper considers control in road networks. Using a simple example the paper has shown that reducing delay on certain network links may increase delay when travellers react by changing their travel choices; and increasing delay on certain links, encouraging a more efficient equilibrium to arise, may reduce delay when travellers change their travel choices. This example is based on the Braess network [1].

Valiant and Roughgarden [9] and others suggest that Braess effects may happen in many networks; specific examples are given by Cohen and Kelly [17] and in [10].

It is shown in this paper that the Braess effect can occur in a powerful form within signal controlled networks. The overall capacity of a small network is substantially reduced by utilizing standard signal control algorithms, especially if these are used responsively. The paper has also shown that, on the other hand, the P_0 policy maximizes the capacity of this small network; Smith [12] shows that, under natural conditions, this capacity-maximising property holds in a general signal controlled network.

Stability is a vital element of any system and has been considered only very briefly here. Some general stability results have been given in Smith and van Vuren [18]. Of the six policies or algorithms considered there, the most clearly stable (allowing for the possibility of routeing changes) are all similar to P_0.

5.1   Further Work on Capacity Maximizing Policies and Bilevel Programming

These results suggest that further study of capacity-maximising control policies, embracing (1) mathematical study, (2) computer tests on larger scale model networks, (3) dynamical considerations and (4) real-life tests may all be worthwhile.

Transfer of the capacity-maximizing ideas to other fields, including perhaps healthcare networks and computer systems and the internet, also merits attention.

Finally there is a great need to extend the work described in [4, 5, 6] on bilevel optimization; and then to construct really effective computer programs optimising general networks subject to choices by stakeholders. This is certainly a grand challenge.

Acknowledgment. The author is a Researcher/Co-investigator on the FREEFLOW project. FREEFLOW is aimed at designing and implementing systems which transform road transport data into intelligence; to help travellers, operators and network managers make better (and more timely) decisions. FREEFLOW is funded by the Technology Strategy Board, the Department for Transport, the EPSRC and the partners. These partners are: Transport for London, City of York Council, Kent County Council, ACIS, Kizoom, Mindsheet, QinetiQ, Trakm8, Imperial College London, Loughborough University and the University of York. Ian Routledge is a subconsultant to the University of York and the Technical Director of FREEFLOW is Andy Graham (White Willow Consulting).

References

1. Braess, D.: Uber ein Paradoxon aus der Verkehrsplanung. Unternemensforschung 12, 258–268 (1968); English translation in [7] below
2. Allsop, R.E.: Some possibilities for using Traffic Control to Influence Trip Distribution and Route Choice. In: Proceedings of the Sixth International Symposium on Transportation and Traffic Theory, pp. 345–374. Elsevier, New York (1974)
3. Dickson, T.J.: A note on traffic assignment and signal timings in a signal-controlled road network. Transportation Research B, 267–271 (1981)
4. Smith, M.J.: Bilevel optimisation of prices and signals in Transportation Models. In: Lawphongpanich, S., Hearn, D.W., Smith, M.J. (eds.) Mathematical and Computational Models for Congestion Charging, pp. 159–199 (2006)
5. Luo, Z.Q., Pang, J.S., Ralph, D.: Mathematical programs with equilibrium constraints. Cambridge University Press, Cambridge (1996)
6. Fletcher, R., Leyffer, S.: Nonlinear programming without a penalty function. University of Dundee Numerical Analysis report NA 171 (2000)
7. Braess, D., Nagurney, A., Wakolbinger, T.: On a Paradox of Traffic Planning. Transportation Science 39(4), 446–450 (2005)
8. Roughgarden, T.: Selfish routing and the price of anarchy. MIT Press, Cambridge (2005)
9. Valiant, G., Roughgarden, T.: Braess's Paradox in Large Random Graphs. In: Proceedings of the 7th ACM Conference on Electronic Commerce (2000)
10. Smith, M.J.: A local traffic control policy which automatically maximises the overall travel capacity of an urban road network. In: Proceedings of the International Conference on Urban Traffic Control Systems, Berkeley, California (August 1979); Traffic Engineering and Control 21, 298–302 (1980)
11. Smith, M.J.: Traffic control and route choice; a simple example. Transportation Research 13B, 289–294 (1979)
12. Smith, M.J.: The existence, uniqueness and stability of traffic equilibria. Transportation Research 13B, 295–304 (1979)

13. Webster, F.V.: Traffic signal settings, Department of Transport, Road Research Technical Paper No. 39, HMSO, London (1958)
14. Robertson, D.I.: TRANSYT: a traffic network study tool. RRL Lab. report LR253, Road Research Laboratory, Crowthorne, UK (1969)
15. Hunt, P.B., Robertson, D.I., Bretherton, R.D., Winton, R.I.: SCOOT - A Traffic Responsive Method of Coordinating Signals. Transport and Road Research Laboratory Report 1014, Transport and Road Research Laboratory, Crowthorne, UK (1981)
16. Wardrop, J.G.: Some theoretical aspects of road traffic research. In: Proceedings of the Institute of Civil Engineers, Part II, vol. 1, pp. 325–378 (1952)
17. Cohen, J.E., Kelly, F.P.: A paradox of congestion in a queueing network. J. Appl. Prob. 27, 730–734 (1990)
18. Smith, M.J., van Vuren, T.: Traffic equilibrium with responsive traffic control. Transportation Science 27, 118–132 (1993)

Congestion Reduction Using Ad-Hoc Message Dissemination in Vehicular Networks

Thomas D. Hewer[1,2] and Maziar Nekovee[2,3]

[1] Department of Computer Science, University College London,
London WC1E 6BT, UK
[2] Centre for Computational Science, University College London,
London WC1H 0AJ, UK
t.hewer@cs.ucl.ac.uk
[3] BT Research, Polaris 134, Adastral Park, Suffolk IP5 3RE, UK
maziar.nekovee@bt.com

Abstract. Vehicle-to-vehicle communications can be used effectively for intelligent transport systems (ITS) and location-aware services [1]. The ability to disseminate information in an ad-hoc fashion allows pertinent information to propagate faster through the network. In the realm of ITS, the ability to spread warning information faster and further is of great advantage to the receivers of this information. In this paper we propose and present a message-dissemination procedure that uses vehicular wireless protocols for influencing traffic flow, reducing congestion in road networks. The computational experiments presented in this paper show how an intelligent driver model (IDM) and car-following model can be adapted to 'react' to the reception of information. This model also presents the advantages of coupling together traffic modelling tools and network simulation tools.

Keywords: Vehicular Networks, Modelling and Simulations, Intelligent Transportation Systems.

1 Introduction

In the realm of vehicle to vehicle communications there are several methods for the dissemination of data that are being actively researched. The use of satellite communication, such as those linked to global positioning services (GPS) offer global communication but require expensive equipment, large antennae and, due to the large distances the signal must travel, have a high latency. Cellular telephone networks offer a lower latency but are still slow when communicating with other vehicles nearby, and require cellular contracts to use the network. The scenarios presented mainly in this paper require high-speed communication that disseminates from source, which is difficult to achieve using either cellular or satellite communications.

Ad-hoc networks offer a good method to spread information outwards from an origin quickly and efficiently. It has been shown in [2] that in ad-hoc networks

R. Mehmood et al. (Eds.): EuropeComm 2009, LNICST 16, pp. 128–139, 2009.

worms spread in a epidemic pattern that can be modelled. Using such modelling techniques we can develop algorithms that allow for a change to be made to the speed, position and route of a vehicle. A further advantage of ad-hoc networking is the unlicensed use of the radio-spectrum and the recent reduction in cost for the equipment for communication. A separate leg of the research being undertaken on wireless fidelity (under IEEE standard 802.11) has been developed in the past few years specifically for vehicular ad-hoc networks (VANETs).

The simulations use both traffic modelling and message propagation to advise the vehicles of the obstacle at a greater distance than line-of-sight provides. The results show that by spreading information quickly and efficiently through the network we can develop algorithms that reduce congestion and other traffic flow effects. By coupling the telecommunications and driver model in one tool we can perform these simulations in the same runtime.

2   Simulation System

The simulation tool we use is adapted from the dynamic traffic simulator by Treiber et al. [3]. This tool uses a simple model of a two-lane roadway, but contains an advanced driver model and lane changing algorithm, MOBIL [4]. Through the addition of telecommunications and adaptions to both the intelligent driver model (IDM) and lane changing model, based on reactions to information received from an obstacle or danger, we can show that more efficient information dissemination through a network can increase system throughput and also reduce stop-and-go traffic formations.

2.1   Vehicular Modelling

To accurately model traffic behaviour, there are several key components: a driver model to develop how real people will drive under certain circumstances, a lane changing model to make realistic decisions on when would be advantageous to change lane and a roadway with rules (i.e. drive on the left in the UK).

A car following algorithm will contain at least a desired velocity, a safe time separation when following other vehicles, an acceleration and a braking criteria [3]. At each simulation time step the acceleration is calculated for each vehicle. The parameters of these models can be changed to emulate more aggressive and more considerate drivers.

When modelling vehicular networks over large areas (i.e. metropolitan areas) the flow of traffic on a single road can be seen to operate as an incompressible fluid (as later results will show) according to $Q = \rho V$, where ρ is the average density of traffic (cars/km) and V is the average velocity on the road (km/h) [5].

The IDM in the simulator follows the MOBIL model [4] which was developed by M. Treiber. MOBIL operates as a car-following model such that the acceleration and braking are defined by the distance from the car in front. The function of such an acceleration $\frac{dv}{dt}$ is as follows:

$$\frac{dv}{dt} = a \left[1 - \left(\frac{v}{v_0} \right)^\delta - \left(\frac{s^*}{s} \right)^2 \right] \tag{1}$$

where

$$s^* = s_0 + \left(vT + \frac{v\Delta v}{2\sqrt{ab}} \right) \qquad (2)$$

for acceleration on an open road a, velocity v, desired velocity v_0, distance s to front vehicle, desired dynamic distance to front vehicle s^*, velocity difference δ, a safe time delay between vehicles T, a comfortable braking value b and a minimum distance between vehicles s_0.

Lane changing algorithms add a necessary level of complexity to the IDM. In order to decide whether to change lane or not, the current acceleration must be calculated for the current lane and the acceleration in the new lane (with regards to the car behind and in front in the new lane). If the acceleration in the new lane is greater than that in the current lane, there is an advantage to be gained by changing lane.

2.2   MAC Layer Protocol

In simulating wireless fidelity networks, the majority of simulations use the IEEE 802.11 protocols [6] , as this offers the best simulation of the MAC layer functionality. The IEEE 802.11 MAC layer uses a distributed co-ordination function (DCF), which has been simulated in [7], to ensure efficient communication on the medium, and implements controls to reduce collisions. More recently the IEEE 802.11p standard has been tested in [8] specifically for inter-vehicular communications. This allows the foundation of underlying strengths in the 802.11 suite to to be enhanced for vehicular networks.

The MAC layer in the simulator operates using an adapted version of IEEE 802.11 which removes the inter-frame spacing (IFS) model, enabling equal priority to all network traffic.

The network back-off when the medium is busy X operates as follows [5]:

$$X \in 2^n \times [B_{min}, B_{max}] \qquad (3)$$

where n is the number of times it has previously had to back off in succession. B_{min} and B_{max} are the minimum and maximum possible back off time, respectively. B_{min} is often set at 0. The medium is defined busy if any car within the transmitters interference range, R_i, is currently broadcasting.

Every car within the transmission range, represented by R_c, (which is usually twice as small as the interference range) will receive the message with probability λ.

3   Algorithms

This section examines the algorithms used in the simulation. These algorithms form the basis for the work we present here and have been designed specifically for vehicle-to-vehicle and VANET scenarios.

3.1   Epidemic Message Passing Algorithm

The propagation of messages through a system requires an efficient delivery algorithm. In our simulation we use a probabilistic information dissemination protocol, which is fully defined in [5]. We assume that all vehicles know their location (via GPS technology) and that each message contains information about it's location and time of creation.

The algorithm allows for a reasonable amount of retransmission and dissemination through the network and balances the relevance of the information with the distance from the source. To this end information can disseminate quickly and efficiently and also reduce information spreading to vehicles who do not require the information (as discussed previously, this can cause more pertinent information to be lost).

The probability for rebroadcasting, P, as described by [5] is obtained from:

$$P = \begin{cases} 1 & \text{if} N_f \text{or} N_b = 0 \\ 1 - exp\left(-\alpha \frac{N_f - N_b|}{N_f + N_b}\right) & \text{otherwise.} \end{cases} \tag{4}$$

where N_f and N_b are the number of times the car has received that particular message from front and from back, respectively and α is a protocol parameter, which controls redundant transmissions. In the case of directional message propagation Eq.4 is modied such that if a message is propagating in either direction it is only kept alive by nodes near the head/tail of the group.

3.2   Lane Changing Algorithm

The existing lane change model operates by determining an advantage to be gained by changing lane and then testing if a threshold is reached by the advantage. Early incarnations of our changes to the algorithm worked to forcibly increase the advantage if a message had been received and the vehicle was in the lane with the obstacle. This has some positive effects, but can cause problems when the message propagates far back through the system. In the case of the message propagating beyond the reasonable extent of the need to change lane, this approach causes unnecessary congestion in the opposite lane to the obstacle that results in total congestion in a short time.

At the start of the simulation several static variables are applied to the model. A changing threshold is applied that indicates the increased acceleration the lane change will yield; this is set by default at 0.3ms^{-2} for cars in the field. The other value is the politeness factor which reduces the overall calculated advantage and which simulates the actual care drivers take when changing lane (i.e. the model may say it is advantageous to change lane, but the driver may be more polite or hesitant).

The basic algorithm operates by calculating a value of advantage (MyAdv), the disadvantage this causes to other (OthDisAdv) and then calculates whether a function of these values reaches a changing threshold. If the threshold is reached the vehicle changes lane.

$$MyAdv = a_{new} - a_{old} + bias \tag{5}$$

where a_{new} is the acceleration in the new lane and a_{old} is the acceleration in the old lane. Bias refers to a weighting to keep the vehicle in the slow lane, as operates in reality.

$$OthDisAdv = a_{behind(old)} - a_{behind(new)} \qquad (6)$$

where $a_{behind(old)}$ is the acceleration of the car behind in the old lane if I change lane and $a_{behind(new)}$ is the acceleration of the car behind in the new lane if I change lane. These values are then entered into the following equation to return true or false to changing lane:

$$(MyAdv - p) * OthDisAdv > Thresh \qquad (7)$$

where p is the politeness factor and $Thresh$ is the changing threshold. The form of Eq. 9 is multiplicative so the values of MyAdv and OthDisAdv have a significant impact on each other. In the following equations, these values are only calculated if the vehicle has been infected with a message. If a vehicle is ignorant it will continue to use the algorithm in Eq. 9. The initial change we made was to add a value to MyAdv in Eq. 10 as such:

$$((MyAdv + V) - p) * OthDisAdv > Thresh \qquad (8)$$

This is very much a brute force approach and as such does not truly represent real driving in a system, where the value of V would increase as the vehicle approaches the obstacle and drop to zero after the obstacle has been passed. This proportional addition to MyAdv is shown in Eq. 11 and Eq. 12:

$$Diff = \frac{Pos_{obst}}{(Pos_{me} - Pos_{obst})} \qquad (9)$$

$$((MyAdv + Diff) - p) * OthDisAdv > Thresh \qquad (10)$$

In this adaption of the original algorithm the value $Diff$ is calculated as a function of the location of the obstacle and the vehicle's distance to it. This value is capped at a maximum (currently 20) to prevent unrealistic behaviour (i.e. cutting in with zero safety headway), which means the effect is noticeable but quite subtle, when compared to the brute-force method in 8. This means that as the vehicle approaches the obstacle the incentive to change lane becomes greater, reducing the appearance of congestion at the obstacle in the same lane.

4 Simulation Studies

In this section the simulation scenarios are discussed with diagrams and presentation of the results. All the simulations were run with varying settings, so that an appreciation of all the situations that may occur (that we can control in the simulator) can be established. It is important to note, as previously mentioned, that we assume all vehicles in the simulation are equipped with the technology for message propagation. In reality this market penetration will take many years to achieve, but many car manufacturers are working on supplying this technology soon [12].

4.1   Velocity Experiments

These experiments test the effectiveness of the algorithm as vehicle velocity changes, to see if the algorithms are suited to an urban (slow) or highway (fast) environment. When ignorant (i.e. have not received the message), the cars will still attempt to change lane to avoid the obstacle, but only as part of the original lane changing algorithm, and so congestion builds up in a short amount of time, for most simulations. Below a certain network load the road will never become

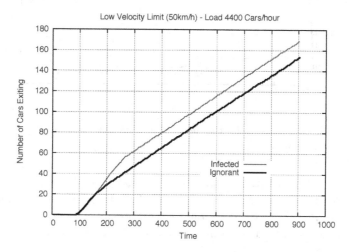

Fig. 1. Comparison of exit aggregate for infected and ignorant simulations at urban velocities (below 50km/h)

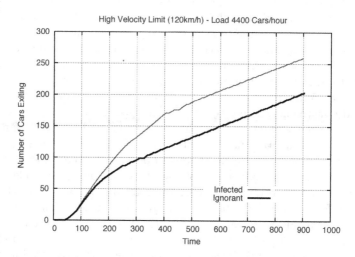

Fig. 2. Comparison of exit aggregate for infected and ignorant simulations for motorway velocities

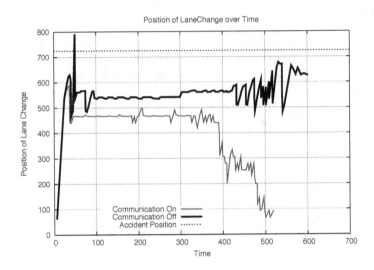

Fig. 3. Chart showing location on the field of lane changes with and without communication for experiment B

congested, so the traffic load of the experiment was varied for each experiment. The traffic load was also set low enough so that the algorithm can affect the flow of cars as, at high loads, this would not be possible. To this end there is, in any system, a critical value of traffic load after which no action can prevent or reduce congestion.

Figures Fig. 2 and Fig. 3 show the number of cars exiting the field in a simulation run as an aggregate over time. Both show an advantage for infected cars using the advanced lane changing algorithm, but the advantage is greater at higher velocities, where the vehicles have more distance between them for the same traffic load, meaning they can more easily change lane.

We found, and Fig. 2 and Fig. 3 corroborate this, that the advanced algorithm increased the time before congestion began to build up and then once congested, the infected cars still moved through the system more efficiently. By running the simulation for 15 minutes we can monitor the development of congestion in the system and how the flow is affected by the changed algorithm.

The results show some interesting behaviours, beyond the reduction of congestion in the system. By analysing the first 5-7 minutes of simulation time, we can see that the development of congestion is also slower once vehicles do start to slow down. This is because of the algorithm moving vehicles into the opposite lane to the obstacle, reducing the load on the lane with the obstacle and therefore reducing the number of stopped vehicles behind the obstacle which, when changing lane, cause a dramatic slowdown in the new lane. This reduction in stop-and-go traffic formation is also seen elsewhere in the field when the cars are infected with the warning message and switch to our adapted algorithm.

4.2   Position of Lane Change

A factor that affects the build-up of congestion in the system is related to the location of the lane change. The following results show where the lane change occurs with no communication and then using our enhanced lane change algorithm with communication active. The simulation settings were set at 4400cars/hour load, speed limit of 120km/h and a transmission range of 100m.

During the simulation the message propagates backwards towards position 0 and, with the advanced algorithm, the location of the lane-change also reduces. When the system starts to slow and traffic becomes more dense, the lane-change moves right back, causing a slower build-up of congestion and a greater amount of free traffic, as shown by Fig. 4. The initial peak of lane change position between 0-35 seconds represents the initialisation of the system, that cars can change lane very close to the obstacle due to the road being less loaded.

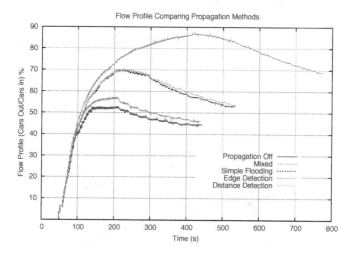

Fig. 4. Comparison of message propagation methodologies in experiment C

4.3   Transmission Method Experiments

In this experiment the available transmission methods are tested with the new algorithm, to see how they affect the overall congestion in the system. The following figure shows a simulation run until congestion is present at the origin of the field (i.e. position = 0). The values represent the proportion of cars leaving the field in relation to the cars entering $\left(\frac{CarsExiting}{CarsArriving} \right)$. This indicates how vehicles are flowing through the system, where an increase of the gradient represents free flow and a decrease represents congestion.

The models shown in Fig. 5 are simple flooding, where the message is rebroadcast just once, edge detection which is explained in section $III - A$ and distance detection, which is a different probabilistic method and a mixture of

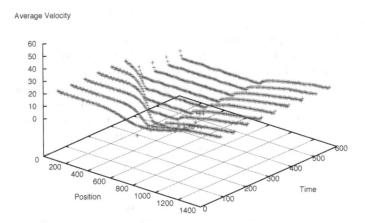

Fig. 5. Average velocities across the system without transmission

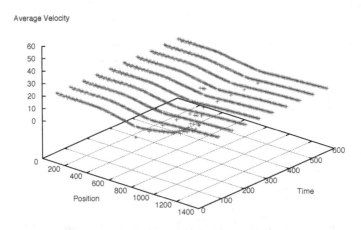

Fig. 6. Average velocities across the system with active transmission

edge and distance detection. These models are all running in the simulation, but the mixed offers the best simulation of a real epidemic protocol. The mixture of edge and distance detection algorithm, with our changes to the lane change model offers excellent results keeping near free flow until approx. 420 seconds, when the network then slows and starts to congest, but this takes longer (approx. 250 seconds from the first slowdown) than the other algorithms.

The addition of this propagation method and the changed algorithm prevents several congestion-causing situations to occur. The main situation avoided is that vehicles are unable to change lane to avoid the obstacle and begin to slow down, but then do change lane causing the cars behind to slow. This cause has been seen to initiate the build-up of congestion and by earlier warning of the obstacle the cars can change lane at a high velocity.

4.4   System Velocity

The average velocity through a system is of great importance. If a higher average velocity can be achieved the throughput will be higher than if there is much slowing of traffic. The following two figures show the average velocity calculated for intervals of 10 metres on the x axis and an interval of 30 seconds across the y axis. Each point represents the average velocity at that time/position interval.

Fig.6 shows that after an initial even velocity through the field, congestion begins to build up at the position of the obstacle between 100-200 seconds, which causes a slowdown further back to position 0. By time 330 seconds the congestion has reached position 0 and the average velocity falls from 20-25ms^{-1} to 0-5ms^{-1}.

As can be seen in Fig.7, there is a uniform average velocity before and after the obstacle during the whole period of the simulation (10 minutes). This enforces the results from the other simulations and proves there is a better flow of traffic through the network, as well as a reduction in the build-up of congestion, when effective transmission of the road condition occurs.

5   Conclusions

This paper has presented a simulation of a specific road condition, that of an accident blocking a lane on a dual carriageway. The simulation uses the coupled approach to mobility modelling and network simulation in a single process. The models and algorithms that represent the vehicles and network traffic have been implemented according to well-known and standardised models. We have shown that by adapting the algorithms when information about the accident is received via wireless transmission, we can reduce the build-up of congestion near the obstacle and improve the network throughput, both in terms of quantity of cars and average velocity.

The various algorithms we tested achieved overall improvement in the majority of cases. In some simulations the improvement was not only in the prevention of congestion overall, but by also keeping a consistent average velocity through the network, which helps to reduce the effects of stop-and-go traffic and smooth possible congestion 'waves' that emanate from the source backwards. The driver model and lane changing algorithms come from highly validated sources, and so the adaptions we have made are highly realistic and can show the effect of even simple changes (as in the brute force addition of a value to MyAdv in section $IV - C$). In order to fully test our algorithms we ran numerous tests with a wide variety of parameters, in order to test for any transient or artifactual effects. From these repetitive runs we established that most effects were long-lasting and that where those were transient, this was only due to a traffic load that was impossible to prevent congestion (as corroborated by control tests).

In the size of field simulated here we are between the microscopic and macroscopic scale of simulation, which is achieved seamlessly by the use of a coupled model of simulation. The tool we performed the simulations with was lightweight and so we could easily implement new algorithms and protocols. In order to run more complex networks we would require a more complex simulation engine for vehicle traffic. With this increase in complexity the field size will increase and therefore a more powerful network simulator is required. The proof of concept that this paper provides will lead to further work in this field, including the use of parallel and distributed computational resource.

Acknowledgement

Maziar Nekovee acknowledges the Royal Society for supporting his work through an Industry Fellowship.

References

1. Torrent-Moreno, M.: Inter Vehicle Communications, Acheiving Safety in a Distributed Wireless Environment: Challenges, Systems and Protocols. PhD thesis, Universität Karlsruhe (2007)
2. Nekovee, M.: Modeling the spread of worm epidemics in vehicular ad hoc networks. In: IEEE 63rd Vehicular Technology Conference, 2006. VTC 2006-Spring, May 7-10, vol. 2, pp. 841–845 (2006)
3. Treiber, M., Hennecke, A., Helbing, D.: Congested traffic states in empirical observations and microscopic simulations. Physical Review E 62, 1805 (2000)
4. Kesting, A., Treiber, M., Helbing, D.: General lane-changing model MOBIL for car-following models. In: Traffic Flow Theory 2007, pp. 86–94 (1999)
5. Nekovee, M., Bogason, B.: Reliable and effcient information dissemination in intermittently connected vehicular adhoc networks. In: IEEE 65th Vehicular Technology Conference, 2007. VTC2007-Spring, April 22-25, pp. 2486–2490 (2007)
6. IEEE, IEEE standard for information technology-telecommunications and information exchange between systems-local and metropolitan area networks-specific requirements - part 11: Wireless LAN medium access control (MAC) and physical layer (PHY) specifications, IEEE Std 802.11-2007 (Revision of IEEE Std 802.11-1999), pp. C1–1184 (June 12, 2007)
7. Weinmiller, J., Woesner, H., Wolisz, A.: Analyzing and improving the IEEE 802.11-MAC protocol for wireless LANs. In: Proceedings of the 4th International Workshop on Modeling, Analysis, and Simulation of Computer and Telecommunication Systems (MASCOTS 1996), pp. 200–206 (1996)
8. Yin, J., ElBatt, T., Yeung, G., Ryu, B., Habermas, S., Krishn, H., Talty, T.: Performance evaluation of safety applications over DSRC vehicular ad hoc networks. In: VANET 2004 (2003)

9. Struzak, R.: Radio-wave propagation basics. tech. rep., ICTP-ITU-URSI School on Wireless Networking for Development (2006)
10. Laasonen, K.: Radio propagation modeling. tech. rep., University of Helsinki (2003)
11. Torrent-Moreno, M.: Inter-vehicle communications: Assessing information dissemination under safety constraints. tech. rep., Institute of Telematics, University of Karlsruhe, Germany (2007)
12. Waters, D.: Connected cars 'promise safer roads'. In: BBC News 2007 (2007)

Intelligent Mobility Systems:
Some Socio-technical Challenges and Opportunities

Monika Büscher[1], Paul Coulton[2], Christos Efstratiou[2], Hans Gellersen[2],
Drew Hemment[4], Rashid Mehmood[3], and Daniela Sangiorgi[4]

[1] Centre for Mobilities Research, Department of Sociology, Lancaster University, UK
[2] Infolab, Lancaster University, UK
[3] School of Engineering, Swansea University, UK
[4] ImaginationLancaster, Institute for Contemporary Arts, Lancaster University, UK
{m.buscher,p.coulton,efstrati,hwg,d.hemment,
d.sangiorgi}@lancaster.ac.uk, R.Mehmood@swansea.ac.uk

Abstract. Analysis of socio-technical challenges and opportunities around contemporary mobilities suggests new interpretations and visions for intelligent transport systems. Multiple forms of intelligence are required (but not easily compatible), transport is too narrow a term, and innovation results in new socio-technical systems. An exploration of cumulative, collective and collaborative aspects of mobility systems, allows us to sketch challenges and opportunities in relation to practices of collaboration, communication and coordination, literacies for creativity, comfort and control, citizenship and (lack of) a sense of crisis, concluding with a discussion of methodological implications.

Keywords: intelligent mobility systems, socio-technical, collaboration.

… software will become as crucial to mobility as physical capacity …. [But] social practices will … adapt and/or appropriate particular socio-technical developments in complicated ways.
(Dennis and Urry 2008, *After the car.* [1])

1 Introduction

There is more to intelligent transport systems (ITS) than system 'intelligence', transport and technology. Ubiquitous computing, connectivity and approaches to make computing 'autonomous', self-configuring and self-healing have great potential for new forms of mobility. However, realizing this potential is a matter of appropriation, not just design and implementation. What we mean here is that everyday users – from motor manufacturers, through public-private implementation partnerships, to service providers, security agencies, and individual travelers – play an important part in shaping new socio-technical mobility systems. How they utilize technology, cope with complexity, and invent new practices is unpredictable, yet vital to innovation. This human intelligence can make or break new mobility systems.

But human and system intelligence do not mesh easily, not least because travel and movement of goods and products are socially motivated and socially organized. People actually rarely 'transport' anything – they deliver, shop, dispose of waste, meet,

R. Mehmood et al. (Eds.): EuropeComm 2009, LNICST 16, pp. 140–152, 2009.

visit, commute, travel. The practices involved are subject to ongoing 'everyday innovation'. Individualised time-space-speed rationalities often assumed by transport research are embedded in changing, dynamically coordinated social logics. For example, urban commuting patterns are defined not only by the fastest route from A to B (via C, D, E, including shops and schools), but also by dynamic 'micro-coordination' between friends and family using mobile phones [2], and more recently the use of GPS and locative media [3, 4]. Aesthetic, health and environmental considerations affect mobility behaviours [5], and people work, socialize, and relax while on the move [6]. Patterns of mobility are effects of lived social logics, complexly intertwined with economic, spatial and other calculable forms of logic.

In this paper we sketch out key challenges and opportunities that the sociality of mobility brings for the design of intelligent mobility systems. We focus on the cumulative, collective and collaborative nature of mobility systems to explore ideas for design approaches that support social practices of collaboration, communication and coordination, literacies for creativity, comfort and control, new senses and sensitivities of citizenship, and a constructive sense of crisis.

2 Cumulative, Collective, Collaborative

Many engineering and sociological perspectives look at phenomena of social order such as traffic from above. A bird's eye view is produced either literally, for example, through observation from a high vantage point [7] or figuratively, through modeling, simulation and mapping. Such detachment and abstraction seems useful not only because it makes general patterns visible, but also because it draws out multi-causal connections, for example between individual drivers' behaviours and cumulative phenomena such as traffic jams [8]. From often arduously achieved analytical vantage points, emergent phenomena can sometimes be explained by studying the interactions between relatively simple rules of individual behaviour. Social science can contribute to this explanatory effort and the design of intelligent mobility systems through specifying underlying rules, identifying types of individuals [9], as well as by developing theoretical models.

More recently, debates around the 'digital economy' have suggested that apart from 'mindlessly' cumulative (but potentially hugely consequential) emergent phenomena there are also more creative and constructive collective phenomena. An example of 'collective intelligence' [10] is the massive multi-player effort involved in the 2003 alternate reality game (ARG) 'We love bees' [11]. At its height, the ARG puzzle of a kidnapped beekeeper brought together more than 600,000 participants from across the globe. To solve the puzzle they used Web 2.0 Internet technologies and mobile phones to communicate, instantiating, according to Leadbeater, a novel form of collaboration: mass innovation. What is remarkable about this emerging form of collective sense-making and action is that it is 'not an anarchic free-for-all; it was organized, but without a division of labour imposed from on high'. New mobility service models such as car clubs, lift share or lets schemes build on and develop such practices and are extending more conventionally conceived ideas of ITS [12].

We appreciate these contributions and their relevance to developing new intelligent mobility systems and services. However, mobile methods of research – for example ethnographic participant observation with mobile workers [13] and experimental implementations of prototype technologies in technology design and art [5, 14, 3] – place researchers in amongst drivers, pedestrians, players. Changing perspective like this raises critical new questions: How do participants on the ground understand, orient and contribute to the orderliness of mobile societies [Garfinkel, in 15]? They do not have a view from above, so order must manifest on the ground as well. How? What is the relationship between order on the ground and order as seen from above? What implications does the fact that order is made in motion have for the design of intelligent mobility systems? These are complex questions that go to the heart of our understanding of sociality, technology, and mobility. In research on human-computer interaction, computer supported cooperative work and participatory design, questions like these have given rise to a powerful concept of 'situated action' and design approaches that seek to support its operation [16]. Actions are situated in the sense that they are contingent, negotiated in communication and collaboration with others, and in interaction with environments, material artefacts and technologies. Studies show that plans, rules, models, theories are important resources for, but not sufficient descriptions of, situated action. Drawing on this work, we can highlight key aspects of the sociality of mobility 'on the ground'. After presenting these as a cluster, we will draw out challenges and opportunities for designers of new mobility systems.

Key aspects of the sociality of mobilities on the ground:

- *Scenic intelligibility.* People can often tell what other people are doing or are going to do by looking. Recognition of, and the ability to fit into, social scenes – for example, different cultures of driving when travelling – are practical, sequentially, spatially organised achievements [17]. For instance, by observing a car's orientation to other cars, drivers can make remarkably precise judgments about the 'kind of person' another driver is, whether they are planning to overtake, are attentive or tired, amicable or aggressive [15]. Social relations are, so to speak, made in the gaps between vehicles [15], documenting creative contextual reasoning rather than simple rule following behaviour.

- *Accountability.* Scenic intelligibility relies on the fact that actions (and, to a degree, intentions, motivations, emotions) are 'account-able', that is, observable and reportable [18] – not just retrospectively to determine culpability for failures, but also in real time through embodied conduct, which (sometimes involuntarily) accounts for what people are doing, thinking, intending to do (see also [19]). Studying behaviour in public places, for example, Goffman describes how pedestrians 'diagnose' opportunities for passage between lone walkers and parties, identifying 'vehicular units' [20], 'whose coordinated gait accountably achieves their "togethering"' [21]. Technologically augmented 'embodied' conduct (with e.g. spoilers, indicators, engine sound) allows the subtly meaningful negotiation of proximity, speed and orientation.

- *Phenomenal field.* Accountability in environments designed for mobility and inhabited in motion, also has an experiential dimension. For example, people experience speed not only by looking at their in-car instruments, but also through sensing their own movement and other vehicular units' speeds. The resulting negotiation locally defines 'normal speed' – often in line with official limits, but also open to drift, depending on perceived safety and circumstance.

Today the world 'mediated by technology is known in no less immediate a fashion than is any other experiential life world' [15], and the resulting 'phenomenal field' is an intersubjective field, that is, it is experienced as sufficiently the same for everyone (allowing for cultural, biographical, or physiological differences), where principles of reciprocity of perspective and experience apply [22]. Reciprocity means that if I changed place with you, I would see what you see and experience what you experience. These principles matter enormously in the actively produced order of mobility on the ground, because they make others' behaviour intelligible, predictable, anticipatable.

- *Indexicality*. Actions are 'indexed' by and meaningful in relation to context. For example, a slow driver turning on his left indicator on a wider stretch of a narrow road with no turn-offs is likely to be inviting cars stacked up behind him to pass, rather than indicating that he will turn left at the next turn. A flash of left-right-left indicator lights by a passing driver can be read as a 'thank you' in response, rather than an emergency warning or a confusion over where to turn. Indexicality is an immensely powerful resource for creating order on the ground.
- *Reflexivity*. Action is made meaningful prospectively and retrospectively, shaping context as it unfolds. For example, a glance in the rear mirror may reveal the driver left behind above waving and shouting, revealing the indicator signal to have actually been meant as a request for help. Retrospectively, it defines the context of the situation as troublesome rather than easy, revealing 'context' to be a fluid effect of action rather than a fixed 'container' for action.

Against this backdrop, mobilities emerge as locally organized, practical, collaborative achievements. They are ordered, but through contingent, embodied and emplaced situated reasoning and action rather than rule following and internalized cultural consensus. This explains how traffic can remain (relatively) orderly even when people do not follow rules or when unforeseen events occur, and it illuminates how unspoken cultural traffic conventions in different countries can be intelligible (enough) for safe driving. Indeed it highlights how traffic is in important and constructive ways as much a matter of 'making it up as we go along' as it is of following rules. From this appreciation, two key challenges/opportunities arise.

2.1 Intelligent Mobility Systems: Key Challenges/Opportunities

Firstly, designers need to move from a concept of rule governed behaviour to an appreciation of contingent social and material practices of creating order on the ground, and a notion of mobility rather than transport systems. The user profile currently inscribed in ITS technology (individual, rational, planning) and a unit to be 'transported' is inadequate. Rather than just being concerned with getting to and from locations, people (as well as goods and products) are mobilized in and through situated action. Everyday practices intersect so intricately with technologies, material environments and artefacts as to come together as socio-technical systems of mobility. Such a move is challenging, not least because of the complexity it introduces. However, shifting the focus from transport to mobilities also highlights powerful opportunities for design to support social and material practices and intersections between different forms and modes of mobility, most significantly the convergence of physical and virtual mobilities brought about through growing use of the Internet, mobile phones and locative media, also when on the move.

Secondly, in view of the varied manifestations of human intelligence in mobility systems, it is fruitful to move from a focus on computational 'intelligence' to approaches that support and integrate multiple intelligences. These should include:

- *Situated human sense-making practices*: drawing on approaches of augmenting human intellect [23], we call for approaches that support people in managing the scenic and phenomenological intelligibility of mobile societies.
- *(More extrovert) system reasoning*: given the complexity of future mobility systems, automation, context awareness, and self-configuration are critical tools. However, these forms of system intelligence need to be designed in a way that supports alignment with human intelligence [24].
- *Intelligence production*: the efficiency and flexibility of intelligent mobility systems depends on rich, live information. Automatic sensing and data collection is useful, but not enough because there can never be enough data, it is hard to know what to sense, sensors fail, and many activities cannot easily be sensed by machine sensors. Moreover, the cost of installation/commissioning of distributed ad hoc sensing is high.
- *'Global' sense making or qualculation*: The concept of 'qualculation' [47] describes the combination of calculation and qualitative judgement enabled by sensing technologies, data collection and computation. It builds on the actuarial calculations undertaken by insurance and marketing companies and their representational practices to make sense of phenomena that are 'too far, too small, too fast, or too slow, or even too big to be experienced by us as we are presently constituted' [25]. With Thrift, we argue that socio-technical innovation opens up possibilities to 'constitute ourselves' differently. In other words, we argue that people can acquire new sensitivities, sensibilities and practices that allow them to sense and make sense of cumulative and collective phenomena.

We now begin to develop these ideas through discussion of collaboration, communication, coordination, literacies for creativity, comfort and control, new senses and sensitivities of citizenship, and a constructive sense of crisis.

3 Collaboration, Communication, Coordination

Collaboration, communication and coordination are becoming increasingly important as products, goods and people are becoming more mobile. Practices of micro-coordination between people could be better supported by providing more, more reliable, accurate, real time, and credible information for people to plan, manage and coordinate their journeys. The main challenge in informed travel is to identify the right balance between intelligence provided by the infrastructure and the volume and form of information delivered to travelers, in order to allow intelligent decisions.

Existing travel information systems, such as electronic signage on motorways, are designed to consider travelers as crowds, lacking personalised information, format and delivery. Moreover, most advanced traffic management systems rely on a centrally controlled infrastructure and information source. These two characteristics hinder the development of trust and credibility in such systems. Indeed, a travel information system that delivers information unrelated to someone's journey, gradually becomes 'noise' for the traveler. As shown by Foo and Abdulhai [26] the reaction of drivers to electronic signage messages decreases over time, showing a potential distrust of the displayed messages. An information system that relies on a single source of information (for example the Highway Agency is the primary source for reporting congestions or accidents in the UK) is at risk of becoming untrustworthy. Incidents where wrong or inaccurate information is delivered by the single information source, would damage trust levels on the system as a whole.

An opportunity is to consider recent trends in mobile computing, for example, context-aware applications and participatory sensing, along with trends in internet technology, for instance, user generated content and social networking applications. Location based applications are the most common examples of context-aware applications [27] but context aware systems may also include attributes such as user preferences, time or proximity of other users to adapt their behaviour [28]. The concept of participatory sensing is a more recent phenomenon and describes systems in which users actively participate in a project as 'sensors' [29]. Moreover, by visualizing the connection between the measurements and the measurers, a sense of community can be supported, as illustrated in *comob*, a mobile phone application developed by two locative media artists to map spatial relationships between family, friends, or community sensing groups [30]. Web 2.0 technologies such as social networking sites and user generated content allows information to be shared among users in a reliable manner. In particular, social dynamics that operate in many on-line communities and content sharing sites have been shown both to scale to very large numbers and to ensure users are able to develop appropriate internal trust practices.

Cost-savings are an important incentive; it costs road network operators to plan/commision/de-commision sensors on the road while it is relatively cheap to have sensors in cars and mobile devices. Further, higher precision/granularity of information can be achieved from distributed sensing. But the combination of such technologies also has the potential to allow the design of real-time travel information systems that are built around relationships between people. For example: "if particular travel information is provided by my colleagues I will trust it'. Moreover, as we will discuss further below, by turning individual users into a source of information, designers can develop more flexible models for privacy control: 'I will share my location with my family, and, when arranging a meeting, with my colleagues'. Aggregation of information on a community level can help develop a constructive sense of crisis (see below): 'What is the carbon footprint of my neighborhood?'.

Primary challenges for context awareness and participatory community sensing are the development of mechanisms to collect and deliver the right information in the right context. Intelligence lies in the discovery of each person's context and the correct filtering and presentation of the delivered information.

4 Literacies of Mobility: Creativity, Comfort and Control

Creativity, comfort and control are perhaps the most important aspects of contemporary mobility systems, which are built around fossil fueled, steel bodied, individually

owned and predominantly individually used cars and lorries [1]. Creativity, comfort
and control have many different aspects, reaching from the cultural creativity in
expressing status and individuality through car ownership, to discourses of safety,
privacy and cocooning comfort, and notions of flexibility and control over one's destinations on the open road. In this paper, we focus on one particular aspect that cuts
across creativity, comfort and control: embodied literacies of mobility. How do people probe, explore, perceive, make sense of technologies of mobility? How do they
find their bearings amongst them? How does this allow them to be creative, make
themselves comfortable, put themselves in control? How can technology design
support attempts to develop literacies and find one's bearings? By specifying chal-
lenges/opportunities and design initiatives that arise at this juncture, we can concre-
tize and develop our suggestions for design.

Mark Weiser's pioneering vision for 'ubiquitous' computing [31] has been extremely powerful in this regard. Its 'highest ideal to make a computer so imbedded, so
fitting, so natural, that we use it without even thinking about it' and Weiser's call to
make the computer 'invisible' have been enthusiastically embraced by technology
designers, most often literally. For all the right reasons – for example, to protect car
drivers from complexity overload – designers seek to hide computing by embedding it
in devices and environments, making it 'autonomous', self-healing, and context-
aware [28]. These approaches can be powerful, but they can also – paradoxically –
impede what they seek to support by undermining principles of intersubjectivity and
reciprocity as well as practices of making sense of the phenomenal field. For example,
if speed is sometimes, for some drivers controlled automatically (e.g. through proximity sensing), practices of negotiating embodied accountabilities are disrupted. But
Weiser's main concern was not invisibility per se, but 'invisibility-in-use', synony-
mous with the phenomenological notion of 'ready-to-hand' [32], meaning that users
should be able to focus on their activities rather than on their technologies.

To achieve 'invisibility-in-use', it is becoming increasingly clear that approaches
to design more 'extrovert' forms of system reasoning that support situated sense-
making practices rather than black-box function are required, echoing early calls for
computer-based coaching to enable computer users to 'diagnose' machine capabilities
[33]. Bellotti et al [24], for example, highlight the challenges of 'making sense of
sensing systems'. Drawing inspiration from analyses of situated interaction between
people, they focus on problems of addressing embedded systems, mutual attention
and alignment, noticing and addressing accidents, and they seek to sensitise designers
to the challenges of human-computer interaction. In a similar vein, drawing directly
on Weiser's work, Chalmers [34] proposes 'seamful design', revealing system 'su-
tures' (for example, between areas where location information is or is not available),
and Dourish [35] calls for 'accountable' computing:

> Accountability, in this sense, means that the interface is designed so as to pre-
> sent, as part of its action, an "account" of what is happening. The goal of the
> account is to make the action of the system concrete as part of an ongoing inter-
> action between the system and the user. So, the account should not simply be an
> abstract description of the system's behavior, but rather an explication ...

However, not surprisingly, given situated sociality of mobility practices discussed
above, accountability in this sense is exceedingly hard to design 'into' intelligent

mobility technologies. Anderson et al [36] articulate how autonomy undermines the little 'natural' accountability that computing systems have (by way of deterministic behaviours). Most notably they argue that appropriate or 'recipient designed' accounts (accounts that are sensitive to recipients' indiosyncracies and context) are required to 'explicate' in ways that are relevant and understandable in specific use situations. This is impossible in encounters of man and machine, where asymmetries of sentience place technology at a disadvantage in the reflexive production of recipient designed moves [33]. Anderson et al appreciate this difficulty and recommend participatory engagement with prospective end users, because this will give designers at least an idea of the kinds of accounts that would be required and in what kinds of situations.

We build on this research, but, given the inherent difficulties of understanding function from the design of interfaces, and of designing appropriate accounts, we shy away from notions of human-computer 'interaction' and 'accountable' computing, and a focus on interface design. Instead, we study the 'diagnostic' methods of how people make material artefacts, environments and technologies within their phenomenal fields 'speak', how they notice, act in line with, and create order in human-technology engagement. We describe this as supporting people in making computing 'palpable' [36]. Such diagnostic practices are critical to people's ability of finding their bearings or moorings, act creatively, and find comfort and control [37].

5 Citizenship

Sharing of mobility-related data and experiences, automatically sensed or manually contributed in social networks opens opportunities for intelligent mobility systems, leveraging users as intelligent sensors. At the same time, concerns that already exist regarding the storage, processing and dissemination of personal information in social networks become amplified by the increasing inclusion of detailed movement data. Users may willingly grant operators almost unlimited use of mobility pattern data, in exchange for the benefit of enhancing their social and their mobility experience. For example, while the use of locative media clearly has the potential to accidentally share information with someone, it is the automated categorization that poses the biggest threat. Beresford and Stajano [38] have shown how even anonymous traces can yield the identity of users when combined with profile information. Krumm [39] analysed GPS data from 172 drivers and was able to infer a home address in 13% of all cases, and names in 5%. Bettini, Wang and Jajodia [40] have thus argued that location history can act as a quasi-identifier of users. One of the key challenges of creating desirable intelligent mobility systems is the fact that by making the mapping, tracking, interrogating of movement in physical and digital spaces possible, we not only enable 'intelligent' mobility behaviour, but also enable large scale, potentially intrusive surveillance. This could erode civil liberties and people's privacy.

Clearly, this threat should be addressed and some promising approaches are emerging. Many technical approaches to preserve location privacy have been proposed - from separation of who from where and when in mobility data (e.g., k-anonymity, [41]), to obfuscation by blurring detail in the data [42]. However these approaches generally assume a dichotomy in the use of location data, as either authorized or unauthorized. The act of sharing mobility-related data is then reduced to a binary decision: friends are granted access, strangers are blocked. Yet, privacy is not just about anonymisation or confidentiality, it is a "boundary negotiation process" (Altman, in [43]). Dourish, whose call for 'accountable' computing pioneered the use of computational reflection to support human-computer interaction is exploring how it might support people in understanding privacy [44] in pervasive computing.

An important challenge is to understand sharing practices for mobility-related data, and to develop usable technologies that support the negotiation of privacy. Social science studies are beginning to address these questions, examining how people are developing new sensitivities and senses in engagement with new mobile technologies, and new social practices of managing privacy of their digitally augmented mobile bodies more effectively. Licoppe [45], for example, describes emergent practices of managing co-proximity in his observations of a community of mobile game players in Japan, where users tried to manage the implications of being tracked and thus visible to unknown fellow players. People would go to great lengths to acknowledge the possibility of face-to-face meetings when two players happened to be close, but also employed elaborate excuses for why such meetings could not happen. Design, policy and practice should engage with such studies and support such emergent practices.

6 A Sense of Crisis?

Cumulative or collective effects of situated action within mobility systems (such as congestion, air pollution and climate change) are ill understood by those causing them, and only partially understood by those studying them. This makes it difficult to change practices and design strategies, policies, technologies, infrastructures to bring about desirable effects and avoid or mitigate undesirable ones. A key problem in moving intelligent mobility systems forward is the fact that with creeping troubles such as congestion, air pollution or climate change, people often struggle to establish a sense of crisis until it is too late, which can also be seen in histories of environmental crises [46]. Thus, not only can we never know enough to reliably 'engineer' new socio-technical mobility systems, but without a constructive sense of crisis, we also lack motivation. Without a sense of crisis (and a sense of the possibility of constructive action) acceptance and investment in intelligent mobility system technology and behaviour change will be too patchy to make the 'critical mass' needed for a working intelligent mobility systems. The rejection of the 2008 Transport Innovation Fund application in Manchester is a potent example.

Community sensing that combines quantitative with qualitative located data and data analysis through 'qualculation' [47] promises some leverage here. Approaches such as the comob collaborative measuring initiative, or Christian Nold's urban emotion maps [see 30] resonate powerfully with ideas of 'reality mining', coined by Eagle et al [48], who carried out the largest experiment to date on machine learning from mobile phone data. A key challenge for research and socio-technical innovation is to move beyond people as data collectors, to people collectively making sense of data that is 'reality-mined'. For example, providing home energy data could be used not just so that energy supplies can be improved in some way, but so that personal energy-consuming practices can be understood/reflected upon in the context of consumption at many layers, from family to friends to community. With a view to mobility systems, social positioning methods used to study people's movements by tracking their mobile phones could inform not only planning decisions [49], but also everyday micro-coordination of mobility.

7 Discussion and Methodological Considerations

In this paper our aim was to sketch out key socio-technical challenges and opportunities for designing intelligent mobility systems and to motivate and enable designers to work with, rather than against, situated reasoning and everyday creativity. Mobility systems are nested socio-technical systems, with often contradictory forces at work, positive and negative feedback, and ripple effects for every attempt to constrain or enable collaboration, creativity, comfort or control, citizenship and sense-making practices. A key challenge is to juggle these forces and effects. This cannot be done through conventional 'design and implement' approaches. Iterative, collaborative design, using a 'living laboratory' approach [50] enables experimental appropriation or 'colonization' and shaping of prototype mobility systems. However, in the context of mobility, particular challenges arise: of engaging diverse stakeholder communities and large numbers of members of the public in such design endeavours. A closer look at playful collaborations can inform methods of engagement that address these challenges.

Leadbeater's analysis of the ARG 'We love bees' is inspiring for design, but somewhat superficial. He appreciates the work of the game's designers in creating the incentives and conditions for collaboration, but mainly celebrates the creative power of spontaneously self-organised mass innovation. However, on closer inspection, the relationship between the design (and the designers) of the game and the players is more complex and revealing for the design of new intelligent mobility systems technologies and services. McGonigal, one of the game's designers, reports how the collaboration between the players was very carefully orchestrated by a group of meta-players or 'puppet-masters', who strategically instructed and informed participants [51]. But far from being all-powerful masters, the puppetmasters were drawn into engaging encounters with their players. McGonigal describes the art of playing with players 'without making them feel like mere puppets'. It was not a matter of puppet-masters' pulling people's strings: 'we could give the players a set of instructions—but clearly we could not predict or dictate how they would read and embody those instructions. We were absolutely not in control of our players' creative instincts'. She also asks 'How do you develop the puppet master-player relationship into a collaborative one, and what real-time recourses do you have to actively manage that relationship?' and describes her team's strategies. Drawing inspiration from this approach, we would like to argue that 'living laboratories' for intelligent mobility systems may not just be understood as a means to the end of designing more effective intelligent mobility systems. They may actually describe a permanent state of socio-technical innovation that places an emphasis on the process of collaborative design and accepts that any resulting systems will be temporary and subject to everyday innovation in a way that should be supported as well as guided.

Acknowledgements

We thank the participants in the workshop 'Alternative mobility futures' (Lancaster Centre for Mobilities Research, 17th March 2009), with whom we are currently writing alternative mobility scenarios: Gareth Matthews, James Tomasson, Julien McHardy, Martin Pedersen, Bashar Al Takrouri, Paula Bialski, John Delap, Javier Galetrio Garcia, Anil Namdeo, Tom Roberts, Jen Southern, Agnieszka Strzeminska, Paul Upham, Laura Watts, Matt Wilson, and John Urry.

References

1. Dennis, K., Urry, J.: After the car. Polity, London (2008)
2. Ling, R., Yttri, B.: Nobody Sits at Home and Waits for the Telephone to Ring: Micro and Hyper-Coordination Through the Use of the Mobile Phone. In: Katz, J., Aakhus, M. (eds.) Perpetual contact: Mobile communication, private talk, public performance. Cambridge University Press, Cambridge (2002)
3. Hemment, D.: Locative Arts. In: Malina, R. (ed.) Leonardo, vol. (39:4), pp. 348–356. MIT Press, Cambridge (2006)
4. Southern, J.: Lines of flight. In: ISEA (2009)
5. Bamford, W., Coulton, P., Walker, M., Whyatt, D., Davies, G., Pooley, C.: Using Mobile Phones to Reveal the Complexities of the School Journey. In: MOBILEHCI 2008, Amsterdam, Netherlands, September 2-5 (2008)
6. Lyons, G., Jain, J., Holley, D.: The use of travel time by rail passengers in Great Britain. Transportation Research Part A 41, 107–120 (2007)
7. Whyte, W.: The social life of small urban spaces. Project for Public Spaces (1980)
8. Resnick, M.: Turtles, termites, and traffic jams. Explorations in massively parallel microworlds. MIT Press, Cambridge (1994)
9. Jensen, M.: Passion and heart in transport — a sociological analysis on transport behaviour. Transport Policy 6, 19–33 (1999)
10. Levy, P.: Education and training: New technologies and collective intelligence. Prospects 17(2), 249–263 (1997)
11. Leadbeater, C.: We-think. Mass innovation, not mass production. Profile Books, London (2008)
12. Meroni, A., Sangiorgi, D., Simeone, G.: Intelligent mobility system sector scenarios: Service design to foster sustainable mobility within urban areas. In: Emergence Conference, Pittsburgh (September 2007)
13. Laurier, E.: Doing Office Work on the Motorway. Theory, Culture & Society 21(4-5), 261–277 (2004)
14. Büscher, M., Kristensen, M., Mogen, P.: When and How (not) to Trust IT? Supporting Virtual Emergency Teamworksen. International Journal of Information Systems for Crisis Response and Management 1(2), 1–15 (2009)
15. Lynch, M.: 'Appendix: The linear society of traffic'. In: Scientific practice and ordinary action. Cambridge University Press, Cambridge (1993)
16. Suchman, L.: Human-machine reconfigurations. Cambridge University Press, Cambridge (2007)
17. Jayyusi, L.: Toward a Socio-logic of the Film Text. Semiotica 68(3/4), 271–296 (1988)

18. Garfinkel, H.: Studies in ethnomethodology. Polity, London (1967)
19. Dekker, S.: Ten Questions About Human Error. Erlbaum, Hillsdale (2005)
20. Goffman, E.: Relations in public. Harper & Row, New York (1971)
21. Mondada, L.: Emergent focused interactions in public places: A systematic analysis of the multimodal achievement of a common interactional space. Journal of Pragmatics (2008)
22. Schutz, A.: On phenomenology and social relations. The University of Chicago Press, Chicago (1970)
23. Engelbart, D.C.: Augmenting human intellect: A conceptual framework. Stanford Research Institute Summary report (1962)
24. Bellotti, V., Back, M., Edwards, W.K., Grinter, R.E., Henderson, A., Lopes, C.: Making sense of sensing systems: Five questions for designers and researchers. In: Terveen, L. (ed.) Proceedings of CHI 2002, pp. 415–422 (2002)
25. Harré, R.: Creativity in science. In: Dutton, D., Krausz, M. (eds.) The concept of creativity in science and art. M. Nijhoff, The Hague (1981)
26. Foo, S., Abdulhai, B.: Evaluating the impacts of changeable message signs on traffic diversion. In: Proceedings of IEEE Intelligent Transportation Systems Conference (ITSC 2006), pp. 891–896 (2006)
27. Cheverst, K., Davies, N., Mitchell, K., Efstratiou, C.: Using Context as a Crystal Ball: Rewards and Pitfalls. Personal Technologies Journal 5(1), 8–11 (2001)
28. Dey, A.: Understanding and using Context. Personal and Ubiquitous Computing 5(1), 4–7 (2001)
29. Burke, J.E., Hansen, D., Parker, M., Ramanathan, A., Reddy, N., Srivastava, S.,, M.: Participatory sensing. In: Proceedings of ACM Sensys World Sensor Web Workshop (2006)
30. Southern, J., Speed, C.: Comob (2009), http://www.comob.org.uk/
31. Weiser, M.: The computer for the 21st century. ACM SIGMOBILE Mobile Computing and Communications Review 3(3), 3–11 (1999)
32. Heidegger, M.: Being and time. Blackwell, London (1962)
33. Suchman, L.: Human-machine reconfigurations. Cambridge University Press, Cambridge (2007)
34. Chalmers, M.: Seamful Design and Pervasive computing Infrastructure. In: Proceedings of the Pervasive Computing 2003 Workshop 'At the Crossroads: The Interaction of HCI and Systems Issues in Pervasive computing' (2003)
35. Dourish, P.: Where the action is: The Foundations of Embodied Interaction. MIT Press, Cambridge (2001)
36. Andersen, P. (ed) PalCom Deliverable 54: Open architecture. (2007), http://www.ist-palcom.org/publications/deliverables/Deliverable-54-[2.2.3]-open-architecture.pdf
37. Büscher, M., Mogensen, P.: Matereal methods. In: Büscher, M., Goodwin, D., Mesman, J. (eds.) Ethnographies of diagnostic work. Dimensions of transformative practice, Palgrave (forthcoming, 2009)
38. Beresford, A.R., Stajano, F.: Location Privacy in Pervasive Computing. IEEE Pervasive Computing Magazine 2(1), 46–55 (2003)
39. Krumm, J.: Inference Attacks on Location Tracks. In: LaMarca, A., Langheinrich, M., Truong, K.N. (eds.) Pervasive 2007. LNCS, vol. 4480, pp. 127–143. Springer, Heidelberg (2007)
40. Bettini, C., Wang, X.S., Jajodia, S.: Protecting Privacy Against Location-Based Personal Identification. In: Jonker, W., Petković, M. (eds.) SDM 2005. LNCS, vol. 3674, pp. 185–199. Springer, Heidelberg (2005)

41. Gruteser, M., Grunwald, D.: Anonymous Usage of Location - Based Services Through Spatial and Temporal Cloaking. In: First ACM/USENIX International Conference on Mobile Systems, Applications, and Services (MobiSys 2003), pp. 31–42. ACM Press, San Francisco (2003)
42. Duckham, M., Kulik, L.: A Formal Model of Obfuscation and Negotiation for Location Privacy. In: Gellersen, H.-W., Want, R., Schmidt, A. (eds.) PERVASIVE 2005. LNCS, vol. 3468, pp. 152–170. Springer, Heidelberg (2005)
43. Palen, L., Dourish, P.: Unpacking "privacy" for a networked world. In: Proceedings of CHI 2003 (2003), http://www.ics.uci.edu/~jpd/publications/2003/chi2003-privacy.pdf
44. De Paula, R., et al.: In the Eye of the Beholder: A Visualization-based Approach to System Security. Int. J. Human-Computer Studies (63) 1-2, 5–24
45. Licoppe, C.: Recognizing mutual 'proximity' at a distance: Weaving together mobility, sociality and technology. Journal of Pragmatics 41 (in press)
46. Mosley, S.: The Chimney of the World, 2nd edn. Routledge, New York (2008)
47. Thrift, N.: Movement-space: The changing domain of thinking resulting from the development of new kinds of spatial awareness. In: Non-representational theory. Routledge, London (2008)
48. Eagle, N., Pentland, A., Lazer, D.: Mobile Phone Data for Inferring Social Network Structure. In: Liu, H., et al. (eds.) Social Computing, Behavioral Modeling, and Prediction, pp. 79–88. Springer, Heidelberg (2008)
49. Ahas, R., Mark, Ü.: Location Based Services – New Challenges for Planning and Public Administration. Futures 37, 547–561 (2005)
50. Schumacher, J., Niitamo, V.P. (eds.): European Living Labs. A new approach for human centric regional innovation. Wissenschaftlicher Verlag, Berlin (2008)
51. McGonigal, J.: The puppetmaster problem: Design for real world, mission based gaming. In: Harrigan, P., Wardrip-Fruin, N. (eds.) Second Person. MIT Press, Cambridge (2006)

iRide: A Cooperative Sensor and IP Multimedia Subsystem Based Architecture and Application for ITS Road Safety

Muslim Elkotob and Evgeny Osipov

Department of Computer Science and Electrical Engineering
Luleå University of Technology, SE–97187 Luleå, Sweden

Abstract. In this paper we present iRide (intelligent ride), an IP Multimedia Subsystem (IMS) application for warning drivers about hazardous situations on the road. iRide takes real-time information about road conditions and traffic situations from a wireless sensor network installed directly in the road surface. Upon logging to the iRide system, users start to receive periodic updates about the situation on the road along their route ahead. iRide is able to predict hazardous situations like slippery surface or dangerous distance to the nearest car and help drivers avoid accidents. We describe the service and the supporting network architecture of iRide. We discuss the major challenges associated with designing an IMS application for ITS, an intelligent transport system. Having a prototype implementation working on a small scale, we take it to the next step to perform system dimensioning and then verify the feasibility of having such a system using OPNET simulations.

1 Introduction

In this paper, we describe a new solution associated with the design of one part of a communication framework for a cooperative road infrastructure system (CRIS). CRIS aims at making the road surface intelligent and is being developed in the scope of the iRoad project comprising a constellation of Swedish governmental, industrial and academic partners [8]. iRide is based on road marking units (RMU) containing a set of sensors measuring instantaneous properties of the road. They are connected to a microcontroller with a low-power radio transceiver. RMUs are joined to form a wireless sensor network.

When it comes to warning a driver about a hazardous situation beyond the visibility of on-board safety systems and the line of sight of the driver, we chose the IP Multimedia Subsystem (IMS). In this article, we present iRide, an IMS application and the supporting communication architecture for preventive hazard warning in the iRoad CRIS. Information about road conditions is collected in the network of on-road sensors and transmitted via a 3G backhaul link to the IMS servers for real time processing and hazard analysis. iRide updates users about the situation ahead their route. To the best of our knowledge, iRide is among the first attempts to apply the IMS framework in the context of ITS.

R. Mehmood et al. (Eds.): EuropeComm 2009, LNICST 16, pp. 153–162, 2009.

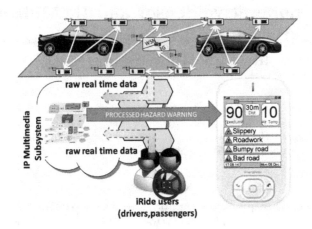

Fig. 1. iRide actors and information flow

This paper is structured as follows. In Section 2 we overview the major design challenges when developing the iRide application. In Section 3 we present the iRide service logic and network architecture with some insights on performance requirements and evaluation. Section 4 provides an extensive overview of related work. Section 5 is a discussion of future and an outlook on subsequent research and development for iRide. We conclude the paper with Section 6.

2   Design Space and Solution Outline

In Figure 1, the high level logic behind the iRide application is illustrated including a screenshot of the client-side midlet on a smartphone. The wireless sensor network (WSN) formed by intelligent road marking units (RMU) installed directly in the road surface is able to continuously monitor road properties. Information observed by the sensors is transmitted wirelessly over multiple hops to a gateway to a 3G network. Inside the WSN, data is transmitted using low power radio technology. Currently, the iRoad RMUs are equipped with IEEE 802.15.4-based radio transceivers. The 3G modem is installed on a road side unit (smart sign, fence, camera pole). In [1] the feasibility of such transmission in real-time was demonstrated. A WSN-3G gateway forwards raw data over the IMS infrastructure to the iRide application server (AS) for further processing. iRide users entering the intelligent road area login to the system from their mobiles.

The functional logic behind the iRide warning application is shown in Figure 2. The system jointly processes the information about road conditions and car motion. The results of this processing are prognoses of hazardous situations. The system can determine when the speed of an iRide user is too high for a currently slippery road or that the distance to the ahead going car is decreasing too fast and there is a risk of collision. When such an event is detected, iRide sends a warning to the respective users. For our implementation, we used the Mobile Java Communication Framework (MJCF)[10].

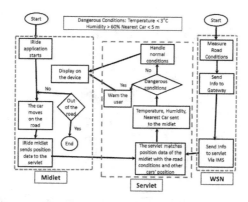

Fig. 2. iRide service logic

3   iRide Design and Implementation

This section presents several important aspects for iRide design and implementation. One is the service logic where the major states and the transitions leading to them are outlined. Another aspect is the data representation and information flow. Then the signaling flow within the iRide system is discussed.

3.1   iRide IMS Architecture and Service Logic

The iRide service logic and architecture are illustrated in Figures 2 and 3 respectively. An essential part of the iRide application is the multi-hop wireless sensor network integrated with a wireless infrastructure connecting IMS clients to the main system (Figure 3). The raw data from each road marking unit is transmitted and then via a GPRS or 3G modem to a radio access network (RAN). In the application server data is entered into the database indexed by the coordinates of the RMUs. Data from the user terminal travels a similar RAN-GGSN-AS path. WSN and IMS client information paths meet at the IMS control plane. Table 1 shows the data involved in the prediction of hazardous situations in iRide.

   The data in Table 1 is transmitted to the application server using SIP protocol messages. The IMS client displays the right audio-visual primitive to the iRide user based on the command received from the application server. The iRide process on the application server predicts hazardous situations by doing joint processing of data received from the client's midlet and the WSN. Upon arrival, all messages are time-stamped at the server. We achieve virtual synchronization between the WSN and mobile terminal clocks. The set of events and the corresponding warning signals generated by the servlet are shown in Table 2. The distance parameter D is calculated by the servlet for every pair of back-to-back cars based on the position information supplied periodically by the midlets. Our servlet maintains two lists of X and Y coordinates one for each direction of the intelligent road. When a new car enters the appropriate segment, its coordinates are appended to the tail of the list. In this way, the order of records in the list

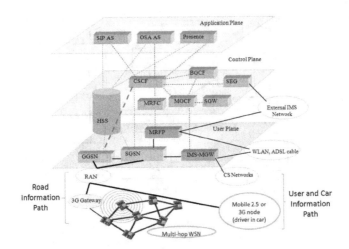

Fig. 3. IMS architectural model of iRide

Table 1. *iRide* data table

Data	Function and Purpose	Source of data
Msg_id	Midlet identifier for sorting requests	terminal
Road_unit_id	RMU identifier for the servlet	road
Km_no	Absolute position of RMU on the road	road
T	Temperature of the road surface	road
H	Humidity around the car	road
Pos	Position of a car on the intelligent road	terminal

indicates the relative position of the cars on the road. The servlet process goes periodically through each list in a round robin manner, calculates the Euclidean distance between each pair of cars, and checks sensor measurements.

A snapshot of the current iRide IMS client implementation is shown in Figure 1. The color scheme of the graphical warning profile and the intensity of the appropriate audio warnings depend on how critical the situation is. We also animate the relative position of the iRide user to the closest car in front or behind (whichever is more critical) and show the actual distance numerically. The warning profile includes graphical primitives for road signs associated with particular iRide signals, such as "slippery road", "bumpy road", etc. Some information can be supplied into the system by road authorities such as "road work".

3.2 iRide Implementation Details in MJCF

In MJCF, midlets use a complex data structure called a record store which is responsible for Authentication Authorization and Accounting (AAA) as well as

Table 2. iRide events and actions in the prototype implementation

Events	Warning or Danger alerts
$T \leq 3°C$	Warning: slippery road
$D \leq 5m$	Danger: minimum distance too small
$H \geq 70\%$	Warning: limited visibility due to fog
$(H \geq 70\%)\&\&(5m \leq D \leq 15m)$	Danger: critical distance in bad visibility conditions
$(T \leq 3°C)\&\&(5m \leq D \leq 15m)$	Danger: critical distance on slippery road
$(H \geq 70\%)\&\&(T \leq 3°C)\&\&$ $(5m \leq D \leq 15m)$	Danger: critical distance on slippery road with limited visibility

IMS presence information for iRide users. A servlet on the backend handles the record store data in a watcher-list. For midlet-servlet communication, we create a class called MessageProtocol whose simple attributes contain the data shown in Table 1. iRide communication is implemented using the MJCF built-in IMS methods publish, unPublish, setNote and the IMS class geoPriv. The setNote method is used to convey the current presence status. The geoPriv class on the servlet is used to update the location coordinates of the midlet. Once the midlet updates its state information, it calls the publish method. Upon exiting the application, the unPublish method is called. The message sequence chart in Figure 4 summarizes the signaling used in iRide.

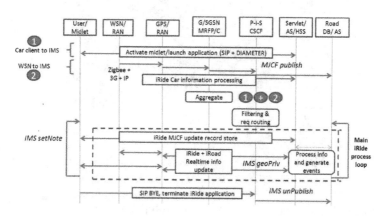

Fig. 4. Message sequence chart and signaling flow

3.3   iRide System Requirements

Here we dimension the bottleneck performance regions of the IMS architecture for worst case iRide scenarios. The road is split into segments each of which is assigned an iRide server process responsible for tracking and warning all vehicles. The major iRide IMS bottleneck is the Call Session Control Function (CSCF) proxy, the place where requests from individual users meet. If the frequency of user requests exceeds the CSCF capacity, iRide will be unable to provide continuous service to all users. The performance of the CSCF proxy can be significantly improved by adding extra processing units (blades) [7], [13]. Assume an iRide covered road segment of 100 km. Taking an average of 10 cars per 50 m (totally crammed road), we have 20000 cars in the segment. The smallest iRide cycle for information update for each user is 5 seconds. We used an average SIP message size of 800 bytes and 3 messages per transaction causing the arrival rate of iRide requests at the CSCF proxy to be about 4000 requests per sec (rqps). Downlink traffic for warnings gives an additional 2000 rqps. The total load on the proxy sums up to 6000 rqps. The fastest CSCF proxy known to us has eight blades and preemptive FCFS request scheduling; it is able to process up to 2500 rqps [7]. Therefore we need three such proxies to ensure continuous service.

3.4   iRide Estimated Performance

Figure 5 shows the topology we constructed using the OPNET [11] simulator. It includes several data gateway machines that aggregate ZigBee traffic and 3G traffic from road units and drivers in the vicinity of a particular subnet (labeled mobile subnet). All road and user traffic is aggregated into a main iRide data gateway and then sent via the core network towards a load balancer that dispatches requests to 3 CSCF units.

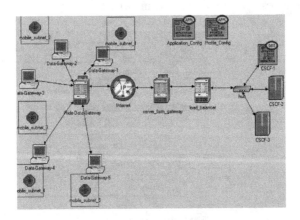

Fig. 5. OPNET middle tier and backend topology network for iRide

iRide relies mainly on SIP-based instant messaging and small file transfer that contains images or audio warnings. Dainotti et al. [6] have classified traffic and its behavior when it comes to identifying invariance in the behavior of TCP-based applications such as SMTP and HTTP. According to the statistical traffic analysis studies conducted, above 80% of all traffic has a lognormal distribution for inter-packet arrival times. This means that with comparable packet sizes for iRide system messages going through the access network, IP core, and into the IMS system, data traffic will have a single-tailed lognormal distribution. With

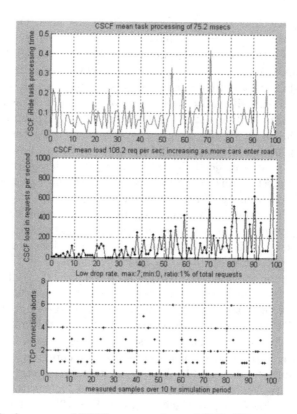

Fig. 6. Performance of CSCF server units and TCP-SIP sessions in iRide

1% packet loss rate in the IP backbone, we obtain a connection abortion count in the range [1-7]. With the load balancer acting as a dispatcher and sending requests to the CSCF module with the least load, the load exerted on a single CSCF module was increasing over the 10 hr simulation period but still having the bulk of load values in the range of 0-200 tasks per second (Figure 6).

The overall delay cycle of a message in iRide is 200 msecs in each direction plus 100 msecs processing delay adding up to half a second. A car moving at 80 kmh covers 11 meters in that time; at 100 kmh it covers 14 meters. This is the sensitivity range of iRide. A warning has to be issued when the critical distance approaches the calculcated values if moving at the respective speeds.

Having presented the iRide IMS architecture, service logic, signaling flow, and an overview of system requirements and dimensioning, we move on to the next section where we discuss related work in the areas of IMS and ITS.

4   Related Work

iRide, which uses information from a wireless sensor network together with an IMS infrastructure for improving road safety, is a new use-case scenario for IMS.

In this section, we analyze some related work in the area. One line of work concerns integrating new access technologies with IMS such as cable in [9]. In the scope of iRide, the challenge is to integrate a WSN with IMS. We conjecture that native support for WSN/3G gateways in the IMS architecture is essential for future IMS-ITS related applications. Blum et al. [4] focus on service creation and delivery for SMEs within IMS-based environments and following a Software Oriented Architecture (SOA) paradigm. Bachmann et al. [3] point out IMS client development challenges. While designing and implementing the iRide service architecture, we used some experiences from [2]. In contrast to the results of the existing ITS related projects [5], [14], [12], we do not require any hardware or sophisticated mechanisms in the car. iRide only requires that its users have smartphones able to run the iRide Java midlet.

Steuer et al. [17] present a connectivity management solution for vehicular telemedicine applications in heterogeneous networks. The solution is relevant to iRide because it involves communication between vehicles (ambulances) and the closest medical center in order to remotely handle a stroke by the time paramedics arrive on the spot. Williams et al. [19] survey the state of the art in ITS indicating that it has become a key feature to have reliable bi-directional links between a vehicle and an infrastructure. GLIDE (Green Light Determining System), ERP (Electronic Road Pricing System), and EMAS (Expressway Monitoring and Advisory System) are discussed. Singapore is used as a showcase in the paper. Furthermore, some standardization efforts in the ITS area are outlined, including the ISO TC204 WG1 on System Architecture initiative and WG4 on Automatic Vehicle Identification. In the V2I (vehicle to infrastructure) area, the paper outlines key projects including: CVIS [12], SAFESPOT [14], and COOPERS [5] (Europe) and SMARTWAY [16] (USA).

The Idris automatic vehicle detection and classification patented technology and software [15] uses in-ground loop technology recording inductance as a vehicle passes over, whereas we use vibration sensors as a way to detect passing vehicles. Idris includes a Single Stopped Vehicle (SSV) algorithm to automatically detect when a vehicle abruptly stops and disrupts the normal flow of traffic. iRide has at its core, a car warning system which is based on a near-distance detection algorithm we used in our implementation.

5   Discussion and Further Work

In iRide, key information elements are road surface conditions (humidity, temperature) and positions of cars. We considered a rather simplified case where either all iRide users are equipped with GPS-enabled smart phones or a specialized device in the car communicates this information to user terminals.

Future work will include methods of getting position information for cars where no GPS support is available. Information will be acquired directly from the road that is able to detect vehicles by observing the vibrations in the asphalt and changes in the magnetic field of the environment. The feasibility of such passive autonomous detection of vehicles is described in [18]. Another issue associated with current cooperative ITS and tracking of cars in safety applications is revealing the car's identity and the associated privacy issues. In iRide we do not detect driver identity, thus preserving user privacy. IMS treats the client side with the driver's device as a Java midlet (IMS client) with a unique process id coupled to the backend side Java servlet on the application server. This property of iRide gives some hope for wider acceptance of the application.

The IMS architecture and framework provides methods that allow good joint handling of the two sets of data in iRide. IMS has a mature evolving architecture but still needs some adjustments to be suitable for integration with new access technologies (e.g. WSN in iRide) and safety-critical applications (e.g. ITS). Openness, modularity, and interworking are the key success factors needed for ITS to work properly with IMS and our paper together with its proof-of-concept implementation is an eye-opener. We would also like to acknowledge the efforts of the whole development team that contributed to iRide which includes besides us authors Giuseppe Lisi and Jonas Innala.

6   Conclusions

The IP Multimedia Subsystem can be applied to many different domains such as conversational, content-delivery, and real-time multimedia interactive services for entertainment and health-care. In the area of intelligent vehicular transportation systems, IMS has not yet been widely applied to the best of our knowledge. We presented an original design and proof-of-concept implementation of iRide, an IMS application for early warning of drivers about hazardous situations on the road. When using IMS in connection with ITS, several architectural and technical challenges appear. A particular challenge addressed in iRide is the merging of two sets of information, one from the wireless sensor network and one from the cars themselves. While developing iRide, we identified a spectrum of issues that need to be resolved before using the application on real roads. We however conclude that all these technological issues are possible to solve and the overall usage of IMS in the context of intelligent transport systems is feasible.

References

1. Hessler, A., Westhoff, D., Osipov, E.: Encrypted persistent data storage for asynchronous wireless sensor networks. In: 13th Annual International Conference on Mobile Computing and Networking, 2007. ACM Mobicom demo. (2007)
2. Alhezmi, A., Elkotob, M., Mrohs, B., Rack, C., Steglich, S.: Next generation service architectures: Challenges and approaches. In: ASWN 2006: Proceedingsof the Sixth International Workshop on Applications and Services in Wireless Networks, Berlin, Germany. Fraunhofer IRB Verlag (2006)
3. Bachmann, A., Motanga, A., Magedanz, T.: Requirements for an extendible IMS client framework. In: MOBILWARE 2008: Proceedings of the 1st international conference on MOBILe Wireless MiddleWARE, Operating Systems, and Applications, ICST, Brussels, ICST (Institute for Computer Sciences, Social-Informatics and Telecommunications Engineering), pp. 1–6 (2007)

4. Blum, N., Magedanz, T., Stein, H.: Service creation & delivery for sme based on soa / ims. In: MNCNA 2007: Proceedings of the 2007 Workshop on Middleware for next-generation converged networks and applications, pp. 1–6. ACM, New York (2007)
5. COOPERS Integrated Project. Co-operative systems for intelligent road safety (2008), http://www.coopers-ip.eu/ (accessed 2009-01-12)
6. Dainotti, A., Pescape, A., Ventre, G., Jubin, J.: A packet-level characterization of network traffic. In: Proc. Globecom 2008 (December 2008)
7. Ghosh, P., Roy, N., Basu, K., Das, S., Wilson, P., Das, P.: A case study-based performance evaluation framework for cscf processes on a blade-server. In: ICNS 2007: Proceedings of the Third International Conference on Networking and Services, Washington, DC, USA, p. 87. IEEE Computer Society, Los Alamitos (2007)
8. iRoad. Project web site (2009), http://www.iroad.se/ (accessed 2009-01-12)
9. Mani, M., Crespi, N.: How ims enables converged services for cable and 3g technologies: a survey. EURASIP J. Wirel. Commun. Netw. 8(3), 1–14 (2008)
10. Mobile Java Communication Framework. Ericsson ims innovation development framework (2009), http://www.imsinnovation.com/ (accessed 2009-01-13)
11. OPNET. Opnet simulator (2009), http://www.opnet.com/ (accessed 2009-03-15)
12. CVIS Integrated Project. Cooperative vehicle infrastructure systems (2008), http://www.cvisproject.org/ (accessed 2009-01-12)
13. Rajagopal, N., Devetsikiotis, M.: Modeling and optimization for the design of ims networks. In: ANSS 2006: Proceedings of the 39th annual Symposium on Simulation, Washington, DC, USA, pp. 34–41. IEEE Computer Society, Los Alamitos (2006)
14. SAFESPOT Integrated Project. Co-operative systems for road safety: Smart vehicles on smart roads (2008), http://www.safespot-eu.org/ (accessed 2009-01-12)
15. IDRIS Diamond Consulting Services. Idris automatic vehicle detection and classification technology (2009), http://www.idris-technology.com (accessed 2009-01-12)
16. SMARTWAY. Project web site (2009), http://www.epa.gov/smartway (accessed 2009-01-12)
17. Steuer, F., Geithner, T., Kaschwig, T., Bür, K., Albayrak, S.: A connectivity management system for vehicular telemedicine applications in heterogeneous networks. In: TridentCom 2008: Proceedings, ICST, Brussels, Belgium, pp. 1–10 (2008)
18. Birk, W., Lundberg Nordenvaad, M.: Surface mounted vehicle property sensing for cooperative road infrastructre systems. In: ITS World Congress (submitted 2009)
19. Williams, B.: What's new in intelligent transport systems standards. Synthesis Journal, 51–58 (2008)

DVB-T/H Portable and Mobile TV Performance in the New Channel Profiles Modes

Tomáš Kratochvíl

Department of Radio Electronics, Brno University of Technology,
Purkyňova 118, 61200 Brno, Czech Republic
kratot@feec.vutbr.cz

Abstract. This paper deals with an experimental laboratory assessment of new channel profile modes in the transmission of DVB-T/H portable and mobile TV over fading channels. These new profiles called PI (Pedestrian Indoor), PO (Pedestrian Outdoor), VU (Vehicular Urban) and MR (Motorway Rural) are originally from the Celtic Wing TV project. The DVB-T/H performance was tested in a laboratory environment using R&S test and measurements equipments. The results of the BER before and BER after Viterbi decoding and MER (Modulation Error Rate) were evaluated as the objective criteria for the DVB-T/H portable and mobile TV reception.

Keywords: digital terrestrial television, portable TV, mobile TV, profile mode, fading channel, DTT, DVB-T/H.

1 Introduction

The DVB-T (Digital Television Broadcasting – Terrestrial) [1] [2] and DVB-H (Digital Television Broadcasting – Handheld) [3] [4] are technical standard that specifies the framing structure, channel coding and modulation for digital terrestrial television (DTT) broadcasting. They are flexible systems that allow networks in SFN (Single Frequency Network) to be designed for the delivery of a wide range of services, from LDTV (Low Definition), over SDTV (Standard Definition) to HDTV (High Definition). They both allow fixed, portable, mobile and even handheld reception. It is in conjunction with standard DVB-H for mobile TV terminals that was built on the proven mobile performance of DVB-T.

With focus on portable and mobile TV implementation aspects it is most important to determine the reception environment. The option "stationary" is associated with reception by a rooftop outdoor antenna to fixed receiver. The "portable" means that the device can easily be carried or taken from one point to another. It contains omni directional antenna and it operates in a nomadic mode (not operated while moving fast). The "mobile" means reception while moving at high speeds in cars, buses, trains etc. In the context of DVB-H, portable antenna reception is defined as the reception at no speed or very low speed (walking speed, approx. 3 km/h) and mobile antenna reception is defined as the reception at medium to high speed (no walking speed, approx. 30 km/h and higher up to 100 km/h in vehicular traffic).

R. Mehmood et al. (Eds.): EuropeComm 2009, LNICST 16, pp. 163–174, 2009.
© Institute for Computer Science, Social-Informatics and Telecommunications Engineering 2009

Mobile reception suffers from all impairments relevant for portable reception (noise AWGN, multipath reception, narrowband interferers etc.) [5]. In addition Doppler shift is experienced and the properties of the transmission channel change over time. Doppler shift results in a frequency shift of the received OFDM (Orthogonal Frequency Division Multiplex) carriers as a function of the speed and the direction of the movement. The receiver has to track channel variations in time and frequency (channel estimation) and it must handle noise-like distortions. It must be correctly synchronized in a mobile channel (guard interval for coarse timing, scattered pilots for fine timing and continual pilots for frequency synchronization) and the received field strength and *C/N* (Carrier-to-Noise) have to be sufficient [6].

The paper is organized as follows: After a short introduction the standard and new channel profiles for portable and mobile environment are presented. Then the laboratory environment is presented including its setup for portable and mobile TV transmission. After that the experimental results are commented including the figures of bit error rates during the mobile TV transmission. These results were achieved by using a professional and reference test and measurement system made by Kathrein and classical mobile TV receiver (handheld device by Nokia). The conclusion makes a short evaluation of results and it deals with practical implementation in mobile TV environment. The reference list contains not only relevant DVB and ETSI documents, textbooks and reports, but it is also supplemented with previous works of the author.

2 Standard and New Channel Profiles Modes

The terrestrial propagation channel is considered to be frequency selective because of their respective coherence bandwidths. A frequency selective fading is classically characterized through a Power Delay Profile (PDP) which gives the relative time of arrival, the relative power and the type (Ricean or Rayleigh distribution, spectrum) of each group of unresolved echoes (also called taps).

The performance of the DVB-T system has been simulated during the development of the standard [2] with two channel models - for fixed reception (F1) and portable reception (P1), respectively. These profiles are included in Annex B of quoted ETSI standard as DVB-T channel characteristics as RC20 ANX B and RL20 ANX B. These are theoretical channel profiles for simulation without Doppler shift. For DVB-H transmission analysis the P1 channel with twenty paths is convenient and it was used in [8] for *C/N* performance evaluation. For practical implementations profiles with reduced complexity have been used successfully. In many cases it is sufficient to use only six paths with the highest amplitude. Primary profiles for realtime simulation with Doppler shift (mobile channel simulations) are presented in [7]. These profiles are included in Annex K of quoted ETSI technical report as DVB-T channel characteristics. Three channel profiles were selected to reproduce the service delivery situation in a mobile environment. Two of them reproduce the characteristics of the terrestrial channel propagation with a single transmitter – for typical urban reception (TU6), typical rural area reception (RA6). The third one reproduces the situation coming from an SFN operation of the DVB-T network (0dB echo profile).

Previous profiles are for real time simulation with Doppler shift (mobile channel simulation). For DVB-H transmission analysis the TU6 channel is convenient and it

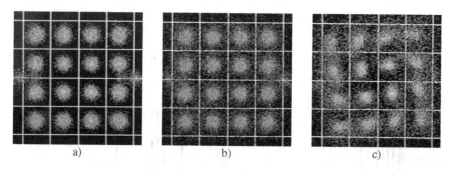

Fig. 1. DVB-T/H constellation analysis a) Gaussian channel (noise AWGN), b) Rayleigh channel with 20 paths P1 without Doppler shift (RL20 ANX B), c) Vehicular Urban VU30 channel with Doppler shift. The figures are real measurement examples of portable and mobile TV environment influence on 16-QAM constellation (C/N in the channel was approx. 20 dB).

was used in [8] for *C/N* performance evaluation. This profile reproduces the terrestrial propagation in urban area. It is made of delayed six paths and having wide dispersion in delay and relatively strong power. Influence of the channel type and presence of the Doppler shift on DVB-T/H constellation of 16-QAM is in Fig. 1 as an example.

To conclude, standard portable and mobile channel models for DVB-T/H are defined in [2] [7] [8]. These models were used for the effective simulation in digital terrestrial television transmission and partly in GSM (Global System for Mobile Communications) tests. The mobile channel TU-6 could be used. This profile reproduces the terrestrial propagation in an urban area. It has been defined by COST 207 as a TU6 (Typical Urban) profile and is made of 6 paths having wide dispersion in delay and relatively strong power. But using the TU6 channel profile leads to some difficulties. At low speeds (e.g. pedestrian movement), the TU6 is not well adapted and creates more demanding than real pedestrian movement conditions. New channels models were developed to manage these difficulties. The portable indoor (PI) and portable outdoor (PO) channel models with 12 paths have been developed for describing the slowly moving handheld reception (at speed 3km/h) indoors and outdoors. The channel models are based on measurements in DVB-T/H SFN and have paths from two different transmitter locations. The indicated Doppler frequency of 1.69 Hz is corresponding 3 km/h velocity at 666 MHz [8].

There were used new fading channel profiles models presented in Celtic Wing TV project report [9] for the experimental transmission. The basis of the new channel models were real measurement data, which was acquired from extensive DVB-H field measurements. The measured data was studied extensively and parameters such as total excess delay, delay spread, number of taps, power delay profiles, K-factors and Doppler spread were obtained. The derivation of the tapped delay line models was based on average PDP determined from the impulse response of four different channel types. Finally, these channels are PI3 (Pedestrian Indoor at speed 3km/h, see Fig. 2a), PO3 (Pedestrian Outdoor at speed 3 km/h, see Fig. 2b), VU30 (Vehicular Urban at speed 30 km/h, see Fig. 3a) and MR100 (Motorway Rural at speed 100 km/h, see Fig. 3b) with 12 paths and Doppler spectrum characteristics [9].

Pedestrian Indoor channel with 12 paths

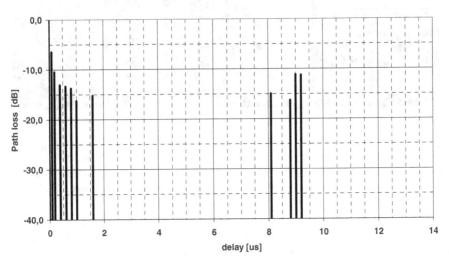

a) PI3 channel model impulse response *Path loss* $_{PI3}$ = *f(delay)*

Pedestrian Outdoor channel with 12 paths

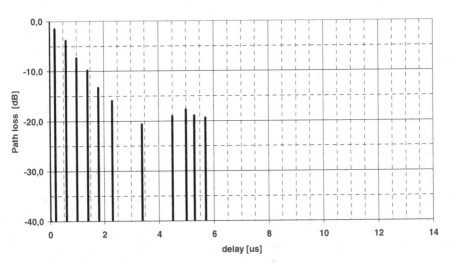

a) PO3 channel model impulse response *Path loss* $_{PO3}$ = *f(delay)*

Fig. 2. DVB-T/H portable channel profiles and their impulse responses performance a) PI3 (Pedestrian Indoor, 3 km/h), b) PO3 (Pedestrian Outdoor, 3 km/h). Direct path and all the indoor or outdoor echoes are formed by using Gaussian Doppler Spectrum. Actual Doppler shift in both pedestrian channels and TV channel C39 (618 MHz) is approx 1.71 Hz (related to the velocity of light and transmitted frequency).

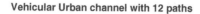

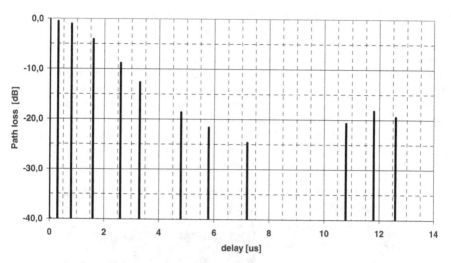

a) VU30 channel model impulse response *Path loss* $_{VU30}$ = f(*delay*)

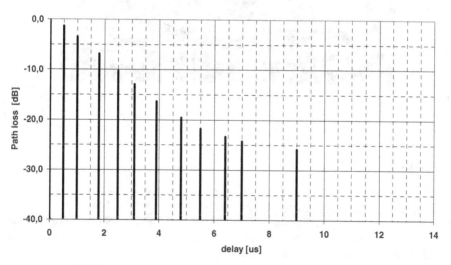

a) MR100 channel model impulse response *Path loss* $_{MR100}$ = f(*delay*)

Fig. 3. DVB-T/H mobile channel profiles and their impulse responses performance a) VU30 (Vehicular Urban, 30 km/h), b) MR100 (Motorway Rural, 100 km/h). Direct paths are formed by using Gaussian Doppler spectrum and all the mobile echoes are formed by Classical (Rayleigh) spectrum. Actual Doppler shift in urban and rural channels and TV channel C39 (618 MHz) are approx 17.17 Hz and 57.26 Hz, respectively (related to the velocity of light and transmitted frequency).

3 Laboratory Transmission Setup

Experimental testing of the DVB-T/H portable and mobile TV transmission in the new channel profiles was realized in the laboratory environment. The transmitter and receiver test beds (see Fig. 4) were consisted of DVB-T/H test transmitter R&S SFU with noise generator and fading simulator up to 20 paths, MPEG-2 TS generators included in SFU and external R&S DVRG, reference test receiver Kathrein MSK-33, DVB-T receiver (STB, set-top box) and DVB-H receiver (mobile phone).

There was tested transmission of the variable content possible for portable and mobile reception of digital television: e.g. SDTV service MPEG-2 MP@ML stream (portable reception) and LDTV service MPEG-4 Part 10 stream (mobile reception). There were also used the new fading channel profiles models – Pedestrian Indoor, Pedestrian Outdoor, Vehicular Urban and Motorway Rural.

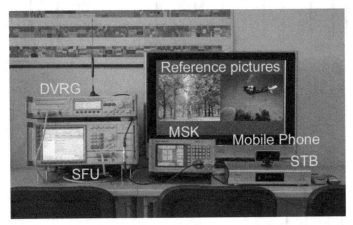

Fig. 4. Laboratory environment for DVB-T/H transmission: DVB-T/H transmitter R&S SFU, MPEG-2 TS (Transport Stream) player R&S DVRG, DVB-T reference test receiver Kathrein MSK-33, DVB-T set-top box Topfield with LCD TV screen and DVB-H mobile phone Nokia.

4 Experimental Results

System parameters of the analyzed DVB-T/H transmission were set to a configuration of 16-QAM, OFDM mode 2k or 8k with one of the code rates 1/2 (higher robustness) or 2/3 (lower robustness). The transmitted data were MPEG-2 TS (Transport Stream) statistically multiplexed with several programs compressed with MPEG-2 and MPEG-4 AVC and data rate of the stream from 5.1 up to 14.5 Mbit/s.

Table 1. DVB-T/H in a new channel profiles and its minimal C/N in dB performance details

Mode	Code rate	Channel profiles				
		AWGN	PI3	PO3	VU30	MR100
2k	1/2	10.0	12.2	13.1	14.2	15.0
2k	2/3	10.2	14.3	15.1	16.3	17.0
8k	1/2	10.2	12.8	13.6	N/A	N/A
8k	2/3	10.6	14.8	15.4	N/A	N/A

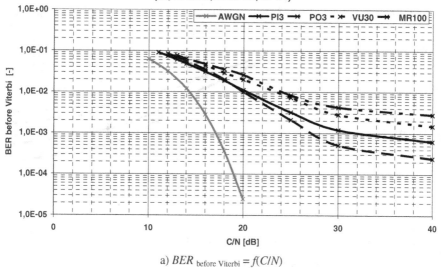

a) $BER_{\text{before Viterbi}} = f(C/N)$

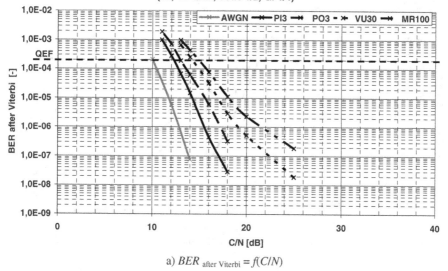

a) $BER_{\text{after Viterbi}} = f(C/N)$

Fig. 5. DVB-T/H portable and mobile TV performance in the new fading channel models – PI3 (Pedestrian Indoor, 3 km/h), PO3 (Pedestrian Outdoor, 3 km/h), VU30 (Vehicular Urban, 30 km/h) and MR100 (Motorway Rural, 100 km/h). Setup details: RX level 60 dBuV, channel C39 (618 MHz), 8 MHz channel bandwidth, OFDM mode 2k, non-hierarchical modulation 16-QAM, code rate 1/2, guard interval 1/4.

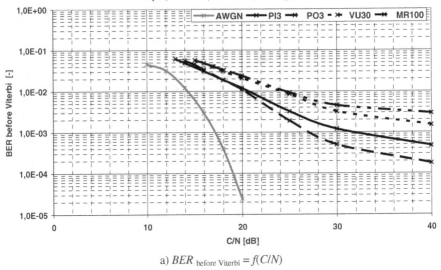

a) $BER_{\text{before Viterbi}} = f(C/N)$

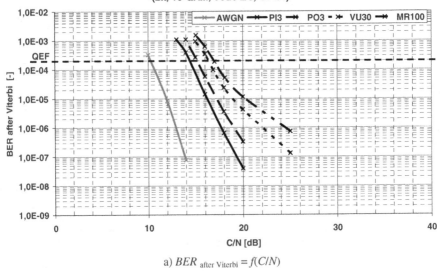

a) $BER_{\text{after Viterbi}} = f(C/N)$

Fig. 6. DVB-T/H portable and mobile TV performance in the new fading channel models - PI3 (Pedestrian Indoor, 3 km/h), PO3 (Pedestrian Outdoor, 3 km/h), VU30 (Vehicular Urban, 30 km/h) and MR100 (Motorway Rural, 100 km/h). Setup details: RX level 60 dBuV, channel C39 (618 MHz), 8 MHz channel bandwidth, OFDM mode 2k, non-hierarchical modulation 16-QAM, code rate 2/3, guard interval 1/4.

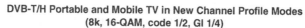

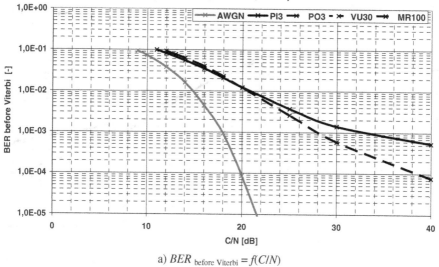

a) $BER_{\text{before Viterbi}} = f(C/N)$

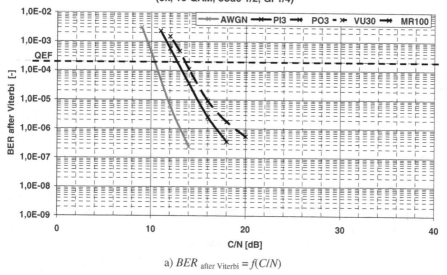

a) $BER_{\text{after Viterbi}} = f(C/N)$

Fig. 7. DVB-T/H portable and mobile TV performance in the new fading channel models – PI3 (Pedestrian Indoor, 3 km/h), PO3 (Pedestrian Outdoor, 3 km/h), VU30 (Vehicular Urban, 30 km/h) and MR100 (Motorway Rural, 100 km/h). Setup details: RX level 60 dBuV, channel C39 (618 MHz), 8 MHz channel bandwidth, OFDM mode 8k, non-hierarchical modulation 16-QAM, code rate 1/2, guard interval 1/4. (Note: VU30 and MR100 N/A).

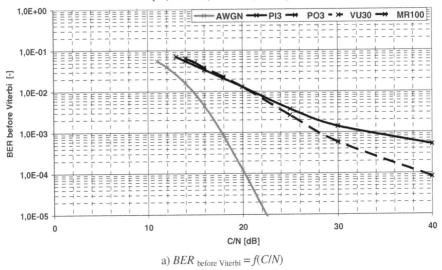

a) $BER_{\text{before Viterbi}} = f(C/N)$

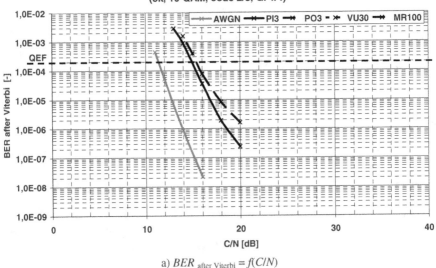

a) $BER_{\text{after Viterbi}} = f(C/N)$

Fig. 8. DVB-T/H portable and mobile TV performance in the new fading channel models - PI3 (Pedestrian Indoor, 3 km/h), PO3 (Pedestrian Outdoor, 3 km/h), VU30 (Vehicular Urban, 30 km/h) and MR100 (Motorway Rural, 100 km/h). Setup details: RX level 60 dBuV, channel C39 (618 MHz), 8 MHz channel bandwidth, OFDM mode 8k, non-hierarchical modulation 16-QAM, code rate 2/3, guard interval 1/4. (Note: VU30 and MR100 N/A).

The minimal C/N (Carrier-to-Noise Ratio) in dB in all laboratory transmission experiments was determined at which the channel BER (Bit-Error Rate) before Viterbi for the code rate of 1/2 or 2/3 is equal or less than 3.10^{-2}. Then the further BER after Viterbi decoding of inner error protection is equal or less 2.10^{-4}. This condition finally leads to error-free signals QEF (Quasi Error Free) at the input of the MPEG-2 TS demultiplexer and final BER after RS decoding is equal or less than 1.10^{-11} [7].

These evaluation criteria were used in last decade and they are valid if the channel is not time varying and burst errors do not occur. The recent works modified the criteria to additional ESR (Erroneous Second Ratio) and FER (Frame Error Rate). The first criterion is the ratio between the number of correct blocks and the total number of blocks transmitted. It was established due to the burst errors sensitivity in indoor portable reception. The second criterion was used in DVB-H analysis and the FER is the ratio of uncorrected frames during an observation period. FER is usually evaluated as FER5 where threshold ratio is 5%. These criteria should better correspond with time varying channels in case of portable and mobile reception.

The results for DVB-T/H transmission with portable and mobile reception environments and required minimal C/N ratio in dB based on QEF determination are shown in the Tab 1. The results were measured using reference test receiver Kathrein MSK-33. Detailed results of referenced BER before Viterbi decoding and BER after Viterbi decoding (BER before RS decoding) for portable and mobile TV reception are available in Fig. 5 to Fig. 8. The approximation condition for the QEF reception was previously defined as BER after Viterbi decoding equal to 2.10^{-4} or less. This is the limit at which the subsequent FEC Reed-Solomon decoder still delivers an output BER of 1.10^{-11} or less. This presents one error per hour. There were analyzed results of the OFDM in 2k and 8k mode with GI (Guard Interval) used in large SFN and equal to 1/4.

5 Conclusion

The results are not available in 8k mode and VU30 and MR100 channels, where 2k mode is better to use in case of mobile TV reception. Experimental results were compared with reference results presented in [9] [10]. Theoretical minimal C/N value in 8k mode, code rate 1/2 and non-hierarchical modulated 16-QAM is equal to (13.5, 13.8, 14.5, 14.6) dB in the (PI3, PO3, VU30, MR100) channel profile respectively. Theoretical minimal C/N value in 8k mode, code rate 2/3 and non-hierarchical modulated 16-QAM is equal to (17.4, 17.4, 17.9, 18.0) dB in the (PI3, PO3, VU30, MR100) channel profile respectively. These results were achieved using Nokia reference receiver and these theoretical results are not available for the 2k mode.

Presented results supplement existing results of measurements in portable and mobile TV environment [10] – [13]. It can be used for DVB-T/H transmission distortions analysis and evaluation of the non-hierarchical and hierarchical modulation on portable and mobile reception of digital TV services.

Acknowledgments

This paper was supported by the Research program of Brno University of Technology no. MSM0021630513, "Electronic Communication Systems and New Generation Technology (ELKOM)" and the research project of the Czech Science Foundation no. 102/08/P295, "Analysis and Simulation of the Transmission Distortions of the Digital Television DVB-T/H".

References

1. DVB Fact Sheet (2008, November). Digital Terrestrial Television. The world's most flexible and most successful DTT standard, http://www.dvb.org/technology/
2. ETSI EN 300 744 V1.5.1 (2004-11). Digital Video Broadcasting (DVB); Framing structure, channel coding and modulation for digital terrestrial television. ETSI (2004)
3. DVB Fact Sheet (2008, August). Broadcasting to Handhelds. The Global Technology Standard for Mobile Television, http://www.dvb.org/technology/fact_sheets/
4. ETSI EN 302 304 V1.1.1 (2004-11). Digital Video Broadcasting (DVB); Transmission system for handheld terminals. ETSI (2004)
5. Fisher, W.: Digital Video and Audio Broadcasting Technology, 2nd edn. A Practical Engineering Guide. Springer, Berlin (2008)
6. Reimers, U.: Digital Video Broadcasting, The family of international standards for digital television, 2nd edn. Springer, Berlin (2004)
7. ETSI TR 101 290 V1.2.1 (2001-05). Digital Video Broadcasting (DVB); Measurement guidelines for DVB systems. ETSI (2001)
8. ETSI TR 102 377 V1.3.1 (2009-03). Digital Video Broadcasting (DVB); Implementation guidelines for DVB handheld services. ETSI (2009)
9. Celtic Wing TV project report (2006, December). Services to Wireless, Integrated, Nomadic, GPRS-UMTS & TV handheld terminals. Hierarchical Modulation Issues. D4 - Laboratory test results. Celtic Wing TV (2006), http://projects.celtic-initiative.org/WING-TV/deliverables/
10. Kratochvíl, T., Štukavec, R.: DVB-T Digital Terrestrial Television Transmission over Fading Channels. Radioengineering 17(4), 96–102 (2008)
11. Kratochvíl, T., Štukavec, R.: Portable and Mobile TV Transmission over Fading Channels. In: Proceedings of the PIMRC 2008 Conference (CD-ROM). Also online available in IEEE Xplore, pp. 1–6. IEEE France Section, SEE, Cannes (2008)
12. Kratochvíl, T., Štukavec, R.: Hierarchical Modulation in DVB-T/H mobile TV Transmission over Fading Channels. In: Proceedings of the 2008 International Symposium ISITA 2008 (CD-ROM), pp. 1–6. Society of Information Theory and its Applications (SITA), Auckland (2008)
13. Kratochvíl, T.: Hierarchical Modulation in DVB-T/H Mobile TV Transmission. In: Plass, S., Dammann, A., Kaiser, S., Fazel, K. (eds.) MC-SS 2009. Proceedings from the 7th International Workshop on Multi-Carrier Systems & Solutions, May 2009. LNEE, vol. 41, pp. 333–341. Springer, Heidelberg (2009)

Localization to Enhance Security and Services in Wi-Fi Networks under Privacy Constraints

Gareth Ayres[1], Rashid Mehmood[1], Keith Mitchell[2], and Nicholas J.P. Race[2]

[1] Civil and Computational Engineering Centre, Swasea University, Swansea SA2 8PP, UK
[2] Computing Department, InfoLab21, Lancaster University, Lancaster, LA1 4WA
{g.j.ayres,r.mehmood}@Swansea.ac.uk,
{k.mitchell,n.race}@lancaster.ac.uk

Abstract. Developments of seamless mobile services are faced with two broad challenges, systems security and user privacy - access to wireless systems is highly insecure due to the lack of physical boundaries and, secondly, location based services (LBS) could be used to extract highly sensitive user information. In this paper, we describe our work on developing systems which exploit location information to enhance security and services under privacy constraints. We describe two complimentary methods which we have developed to track node location information within production University Campus Networks comprising of large numbers of users. The location data is used to enhance security and services. Specifically, we describe a method for creating geographic firewalls which allows us to restrict and enhance services to individual users within a specific containment area regardless of physical association. We also report our work on LBS development to provide visualization of spatio-temporal node distribution under privacy considerations.

Keywords: Location-Awareness, Security, Privacy, Visualisation, Wireless Networks.

1 Introduction

Mobile services are increasingly pervasive due to the recent developments in localization, context-aware, and mobile technologies. In today's modern society, users are expecting location based and context-aware services to aid them in their daily lives. The increased popularity and usage of location-aware and pervasive mobile systems have brought two broad challenges. Firstly, access to wireless systems is highly insecure due to the lack of physical boundaries. Secondly, the inherent mobile nature of users within wireless networks provides an opportunity to offer location or context based services, however, it does render the users vulnerable since highly sensitive information about them can be extracted from location based systems. First problem can be addressed by developing security systems which exploit node location and contextual information. Security could be considered a service too and hence systems to provide both security and services can be designed and developed on a generic level such that system security is ingrained into location based services and is used as an inherent tool to protect user privacy.

R. Mehmood et al. (Eds.): EuropeComm 2009, LNICST 16, pp. 175–188, 2009.

In this paper, we present our ongoing work on developing systems which exploit node location information to enhance security and services under privacy constraints. The work is based on the initial results of two complimentary methods developed to track node location within large production (or live) University networks comprising of large numbers of both fixed and mobile clients. Lancaster University has mainly focussed on (finer-grained) indoor tracking while Swansea's focus has been on (course-grained, building level) outdoor localisation. An aim is to investigate whether useful contextual information can be extracted from a production wireless network in order to offer value added services.

Specifically, we describe a method for creating geographic firewalls based on user location enabling the restriction and/or enhancement of services to users within a pre-defined 'containment area'. Crucially, we are able to prevent access to mobile users whom are connected through the same Access Point as other users in neighbouring rooms without degrading the service provided to legitimate users. The motivation for this stems from a number of institutional requirements such as being able to disable wireless access to specific rooms or lecture halls on campus during exam periods without affecting neighbouring rooms. Furthermore, we present our work on developing location based services using visualisation technologies for campus network at node activity level. Such location based services (LBS) could be used, for example, by the network operators to find and predict usage patterns, congestion points, traffic and network growth. This strand of work uses open source solutions including Google API to provide visualization of spatio-temporal distribution of network nodes. We describe our work to date and the careful considerations made to user privacy, and show how we are able to extract useful information about nodes activities including mobility across campus without affecting user privacy.

In the process of describing location based firewall, visualisation and other LBS which we mentioned in the paragraph above, we give a discussion on the design and architectural choices for systems that provide location based security and services. The rest of the paper is organised as follows. Section 2 gives a brief literature review of location based security and services. Section 3 describes the network architecture for Swansea and Lancaster University. Section 4 describes the design of location based systems providing security and services. Section 5 presents and discusses results: results on location based security and visualisation services are discussed in Section 5.1, while Section 5.2 gives a brief literature review and discussion on Privacy in the context of Swansea's work on network visualisation. Section 6 concludes the paper. This work is part of the Janet UK Location Awareness Trials [1] which aims to explore the possible applications of location awareness in a wireless context within the education sector.

2 Location Based Security and Services

Wireless and mobile technologies have progressed to a point where the use of wireless networks is common place in most businesses, academic institutions and homes in modern societies. The move from wired to wireless communication systems has brought about many challenges as well as opportunities. Location Based Services (LBS) are one such opportunity. LBS apply to wide range of applications that exploit the physical location of the user through GPS or other technologies to facilitate user-specific and personalized services. On the other hand, users are no longer bound to physical locations and are free to roam wherever there is sufficient wireless coverage. This ability of users to roam and become 'mobile' has brought about lots of new hurdles and problems with respect to security and access control. It is no longer sufficient to rely on the assumption that users who connect to the network are users who are already physically located inside the institution. Wireless networks penetrate physical boundaries and have therefore required a new approach to security.

The problem of securing the traffic over the wireless medium has been addressed with varying success over the years with encryption protocols such as WEP, WPA and WPA2. These are now addressed by the IEEE 802.11i standard. IEEE 802.1x allows for enterprise level authentication over wireless networks and its use combined with IEEE 802.11i currently provides a secure and accountable solution to wireless network security. This solution, however does not address the problem of providing different levels of network access control and security according to the location of the user. To achieve location based security it is important to be able to accurately obtain the location of the user. The problem of localization of wireless nodes has been tackled using a number of wireless technologies. A fundamental paper in this field is [2] which identifies a number of techniques for locating and tracking wireless nodes using RF signal measurements. Outdoor location discovery is usually solved with GPS, but this approach will not work indoors. A number of technologies have been explored to help with indoor location discovery. The Active Bat [3] system uses ultrasonic RF measurements to locate nodes, while the Active Badges [4] system uses infra-red. The Cricket [5] system uses a combination of ultrasound and RF beacons. These technologies are surveyed and compared well in [6, 7]. See also our earlier work for a brief review of LBS applications and methods, and UWB (Ultra WideBand) based localisation in indoor environments [8].

Although the technologies mentioned work well they are aimed at specific problems and require significant hardware and/or software investment. The more specific problem of the localization of IEEE 802.11 nodes has also been addressed by a number of researchers. Nearly all localization techniques are based around the RF signal measurement techniques originated from [2] and make use of the received signal strength indicator RSSI value. The initial problems identified with Wi-Fi network localization are that it is not very accurate (up to 1-2 meters accuracy at best) and requires an understanding of the physical layout of the wireless environment. The problem of improving accuracy from RSSI values has been worked on by [9-12] and a number of algorithms have been proposed with varying results. The problem of the wireless physical environment is one that has been 'passed-off' by a number of commercial applications which put the burden of calibration on network administrators. This approach is time consuming and tedious, and is often not desirable to network administrators and as a results does not get done correctly or even at all. A number of solution to this have been proposed, one of the first being [13] which work towards a easy self calibration of a wireless environment with limited user input. There are localization techniques not based on signal strength values but on data obtained through RADIUS packets and SNMP data. These were first described by [14]. There are also a number of attack vectors possible based on location information, these are described well in [15].

Once the location of a node has been determined, it is then possible to build location based security into the system. There are a number of ways to achieve this which are either client (node/user) side, server (network infrastructure) side or a combination of both. A client side example based on user intervention is [16], it relies on users selecting their location via a GUI once they have associated to a wireless network. This work was the precursor for the location selection option seen today in Microsoft Vista once user first connects to a wireless network. A server side example is [17] which has a server that monitors RSSI values of clients and then modifies firewall rules accordingly. The approach adopted by a lot of commercial products generally involves a similar server side approach, making use of RSSI values and similar location discovery techniques as described in [2]. Most products then augment the location data with user inputted maps and floor plans to provide LBS such as asset tracking and usage visualization. Privacy is an increasingly important and sensitive topic today, which we discuss in Section 5.2, in context of location based services.

3 Wireless Infrastructure

The Lancaster University campus is set in 250 acres of parkland and lies approximately 3.5 miles south of the City of Lancaster. The University operates a wireless network both on campus and within areas of the city of Lancaster. Overall, approximately 400 Access Points have been deployed with the aim of providing coverage across all academic departments and service·buildings (i.e. libraries) as well as social and public spaces. Wireless network coverage is not provided to student residences since access within student rooms is provided through a separate 100Mbps wired network infrastructure known as RESNET. The hardware infrastructure deployed at Lancaster is based on Cisco's Wireless Location Appliance (LA). The overall solution comprises of the Cisco LA which is used in conjunction with the Cisco Wireless Control System (WCS), Cisco wireless LAN controllers, and Cisco Aironet lightweight access points (LWAP). The APs are essentially used to record sightings of wireless clients which is stored in the LA database. The WCS provides a web front end for information visualization and management of the overall system. Additionally, the location information is also available to third party applications through a Web Services (SOAP/XML) interface (API) on the appliance and it is through this interface which we extract mobile node information.

Swansea University is largely a single campus oriented university based on the Swansea sea front consisting of 43 Buildings surrounded by Singleton Park. There are also two areas off campus used for halls of residence. Swansea University provides an IEEE 802.11g wireless internet service to students and staff within all of its campus buildings, halls of residence on campus, Student Village off campus and Beck House residence. The wireless network is primarily composed of 760 Cisco 1100/1200 Aironet Access Points in Light Weight mode, 4 Cisco Wireless Service Module (WiSM) blades and a Cisco Wireless Control Server (WCS).

4 Location Based Security and Services – Design and Architecture

As mentioned earlier, wireless networks cannot be secured using physical bounds alone since any device within range of a wireless signal is able to listen or attempt to connect to the network. Also, in certain environments, such as a university lecture theatre, it may be necessary to restrict certain network traffic types to users confined by the physical bounds of the lecture theatre, while still allowing users outside the theatre to connect through the same wireless network access point. Location based security approaches can help solve these problems. Security in this context can be considered a service, leading to the development of generic system architectures to provide both security and services based on location or context. This section presents and discusses the design and architecture of our systems providing locations based security and services. Section 4.1 discusses the system design in the context of location based firewall (security) being developed at Lancaster. Section 4.2 briefly presents the work on location based services and visualisation at Swansea University. From a system design perspective, most of the architectural details of the two strands of work at Swansea and Lancaster are similar.

4.1 Toward a Location Based Firewall at Lancaster

There are two distinct challenges to providing location based security (or service). The first is how you ensure you receive timely updates regarding user location in order to rapidly resume or restrict network access (or to provide another service). The second relates to the method of controlling (i.e. restricting/resuming) network access in real time for production environments in situations where mobile devices are highly mobile. Therefore, in order to effectively deploy a location based firewall solution within an existing wireless infrastructure, the development of additional services are required, namely: *Location Data Gathering* to collect and manage sighting pertaining to digital assets (tags, mobile devices, etc); *Location Based Security Policies* in order to accurately link geographic location with authentication, authorization and accounting; *Access Control* in order to implement and enforce the chosen security policies. These are discussed in the following three subsections.

4.1.1 Location Data Gathering

In this section, we introduce the method adopted for obtaining and determining user location within our production wireless network. We (at Lancaster) have developed third party software which communicates with the Cisco Location Appliance (LA) through a Web Services (SOAP/XML) interface (API) on the appliance. This interface exposes details relating to all aspects of the wireless infrastructure (maps, clients, statuses, etc) and these sources of information are used to extract mobile node information in a timely fashion. There are two basic approaches to collecting this information. Polling: Here, a third party application polls the location engine via SOAP/XML and gathers a list of clients and their current location. Notifications: Using this method, the location engine is pre-configured in order to generate SNMP traps or push XML to a configured IP address when pre-determined events occur, such as a client moving into a defined region.

The software developed at Lancaster for the Location Awareness trials has been written in C#.NET and makes use of the Cisco Location Service API (via XML Web Services) in order to enable third party applications to access the location information stored within the location appliance (LA). Our initial implementation consists of two components, the first manages the communication to/from the location server and gathers the relevant location information and the second is responsible for managing the access control. For the purposes of application described below, we poll the location appliance in response to specific user requests rather than having a series of pre-defined notifications. Once data of interest has been retrieved from the LA, this is processed by the access control component which makes explicit requests to the location based firewall, which in turn controls access to the wireless medium.

The data gathering engine consists of a dedicated process which communicates with the Cisco Location Appliance server using SOAP/XML over HTTP or HTTPS. This communication protocol consists of 3 basic message types: *Request:* Sent from a client to the server to set or get information stored in the LA. *Response:* Sent from the location server to a client in response to a particular request. *Notification:* Sent from the server to a client asynchronously upon a particular server event occurring. A client application may first register for notifications based on a set of criteria the client application defined in the request for notification. With the exception of the initial login request all subsequent SOAP request messages consist of a *request name* to identify the method being called on the server, *a unique session id* (the server rejects all calls not containing a valid session if), a list of *objects* that act as the parameters to the method request and an optional list of *attachments* (for example images). All server response messages are indicated by a response flag, followed by a list of objects for the client to process, which contain the results of the request.

4.1.2 Implementing Location Based Security

The application we have developed as part of this paper has been designed to allow lecturers or speakers to restrict wireless access within rooms for a specific time period. This stems from a series of institutional requirements such as being able to disable wireless access to specific rooms or lecture halls on campus during exam periods without affecting neighbouring rooms. In practice, this can also be applied to restricting access during lectures and conferences on campus. In essence, our aim is to link geographical location with authentication, authorization and accounting (AAA). At present corporations like Cisco do not link these two elements and it is here where some of our efforts have been focused in order to bridge between them.

The prototype client application we have developed resides on each of the lecture room PC's (each lecture hall on campus has dedicated data projector and networked PC). An authenticated user logged into the PC (i.e. members of staff only) is able to navigate to a simple web page which, based on their location, provides a list of rooms available in that building and on that floor. From this page the user is able to select a room and a time window before selecting the disable button. Initiating the request to disable access initiates a call to the third party location and tracking service (LocoTrak). The LocoTrak service acts as a proxy service and handles all requests targeted for the Location Appliance (LA). Upon receiving a request, LocoTrak queries the LA for a list of all mobile devices stored within the database located at that location at that time. The LA returns a list of *AesMobileStationLocation* objects filtered by the specified room id. The result is a list of MAC addresses recorded for that location and, by default, the location appliance returns the list of devices sighted within the past 24 hours. This list is then filtered by LocoTrak so that only those recorded in the past 2 minutes are stored. This MAC address list is then forwarded to the GeoFirewall server, which is responsible for granting/denying access to the network.

The LocoTrak service provides a response to the user's web browser and indicates the number of initial devices found. Further, the service spawns a new process which runs for the duration of the specified time period, for example, a 50 min lecture. During this time, the thread periodically (5 min intervals) queries the LA the list of all mobile devices stored within the database located at that location. New devices discovered are forwarded to the GeoFirewall to deny access temporarily; similarly, devices who appear to have left the area (after not been discovered after 3 continuous scans) have their access restrictions lifted.

4.1.3 Access Control

The process of access control is non-trivial and within a production environment we need to have a reliable way of receiving and processing location updates. The first step is to determine whether any restrictions are necessary based on the individual users' current locality or whether they are allowed access to the network. We believe that there are four different approaches to dynamically restricting access to network services and we are currently investigating each in order to evaluate the most effective and reliable solution.

a) Preventing clients from connecting to the wireless network by setting up MAC filters on the Wireless LAN Controller and by sending de-authentication requests to clients: From a conceptual point of view this appears to be the most trivial method and would appear to offer the most efficient and fast method overall because mobile clients would become de-authenticated and lose network connectivity immediately. However, the main challenge is that on its own it is not effective enough as it could be bypassed by changing the MAC address on the mobile client device. A further drawback of significant concern within a live production environment is that this method would provide a distinct lack of feedback to the end user which would detail the reason why they have lost network connectivity. For this reason, we have not pursued this avenue further.

b) Use our existing role based firewall and captive portal hardware from BlueSocket: We use a BlueSocket BSC-2100 to restrict access to network services and to limit bandwidth usage. This is done based on roles that the BlueSocket assigns to users during the authorization phase. Roles are based on faculty membership and on user status, such as undergraduate, postgraduate or staff. The BlueSocket also supports the ability to quarantine individual users based on their MAC address and, further, provides a SOAP interface which makes it flexible enough to allow third party applications to access its features. However, during the course of our initial trials we have discovered that although the quarantine function when applied does accurately block clients immediately, the re-establishment process is extremely cumbersome. More specifically, once a mobile client (e.g Windows XP, Vista, Linux) has their quarantine restriction lifted, they do not automatically gain access to the wireless medium as one might expect. To re-gain access, a client has to re-authenticate with the wireless network explicitly and to best achieve this, the wireless interface ideally needs to be disabled and then re-enabled in order to initiate the re-authentication process. As with the previous option, this means that behaviour is likely to be inconsistent and unexplained from the end user point of view making this approach unsuitable for production services. Additionally, since the quarantine is again based on MAC address only, one could easily bypass it.

c) Dynamically configure a traditional firewall: An alternative approach we are investigating is the use of IPTables on a dedicated Linux based server in order to restrict access. This approach can be based on client IP address or physical MAC address, which although could both be manually changed by users and therefore bypassed, has other advantages. Other issues which we seek to explore fully are, whether this method is able to block established streams effectively (e.g. a client already streaming a video prior to being blocked) and, how well this approach would scale given a situation where hundreds or thousands of clients are connected. The biggest advantage of this approach is that the inclusion of another entity means that we can redirect web (HTTP) traffic to a well known web page which can be used to provide clear feedback as to why a user has been blocked as well as support instructions.

d) Null route clients at Layer 3: A final involves null routing each discovered IP address at the border of the network and we do not currently have the required hardware in order to test this approach fully.

4.2 Location Based Services

We now briefly describe the work being carried out at Swansea on developing Location Based Services using open source software and technologies; referred to here as the Locaware System. The Locaware system is composed of two servers and applications written in Java and PHP. The first server 'locaware' acts as a listener to collect all the location data sent to it by the Cisco WiSM's. Once it receives this data - in the form of SNMP Traps - it records the data to a database. PHP scripts running on the web server can then be called via a 'HTTP GET' API call to analyse the data in the database and provide location information. This can be seen in Figure 1. PHP was used to define groups of access points, and then perform localisations calculations based on the data contained in the location database. In the example in figure 4 each group represents a building. Node1 makes a request for a LBS embedded in a web page. The web service will use an API provided by the Locaware system to request the location of Node 1 using the IP address from the HTTP headers. This IP address is then looked up in the DHCP server for the corresponding MAC address, and hash code is generated. This hash code is then used to look up current location of the node from the location database.

This system will allow for the easy adoption of the use of location based services by Swansea University web service developers. The number of possible location based services feasible is considerable, but current developed are: Location aware wireless statistics and reporting allowing users to make informed decisions on where is the least congested place to access the wireless network and enhanced wireless problem reporting that allows technicians to provide better support. In particular, we are developing network visualisation technologies, as a location based service, to aid us in traffic and network monitoring, prediction of congestion points, future traffic and network growth. The need for such tools arises because wireless network deployments are now a fundamental service provided by universities and large institutions alike, and a more detailed understanding of the usage patterns of users is vital in order to provide an acceptable level of service. With the growing trend of wireless deployments performing a uniform distribution, or 'blanket installation', of wireless coverage across a campus, emerges the inherent problem of congestion. As users do not spread themselves geographical uniformly, but tend to group together in locations such as eating areas and lecture rooms, a blanket installation may require the addition of extra wireless coverage in areas of high congestion. Some Preliminary visualisation results are discussed in the next section.

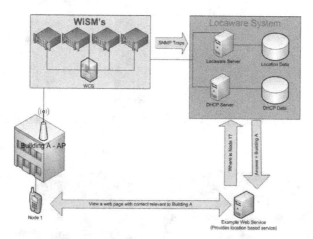

Fig. 1. Location Data Gathering

5 Results and Discussion

5.1 Network and Node Activity Visualisation

We now present and discuss some selected results, first for Lancaster and then for Swansea. Figure 2 shows the mobile node activity across the campus for a 24-hour period on 30th March 2009, which reflects a typical day. We have not yet carried out individual measurements per location on campus but know that the most heavily used areas on campus are the Library and the Management School, since these have the greatest density of APs, meeting rooms and work spaces available. Figure 3 shows a heat map for one of the floors within a building on campus, InfoLab21. This map shows the location of the APs and the coverage area supported by that AP, all associated clients and their IP addresses and finally the regions (or containers) defined in relation to that floor.

The key results from Lancaster's perspective relate to the quality and accuracy obtained from the Cisco Location Appliance, specifically: **Incompleteness**: The current version of the Cisco LA SOAP API does not provide data consistent with similar queries entered via the WCS. Data appears to be inconsistent internally when querying for the same object using both the web interface and the XML based API. **Scale**: Location values (x, y coordinates) mismatch. **Determining and Managing location**: The Cisco Location Appliance does accurately present the third party developers with location information which can be related to the granularities of buildings, rooms and containment areas. Associated with each response for a location is a confidence factor which can be used to determine the reliability of the response. A large confidence (say 75) factor implies that the system has calculated with 95% accuracy that a node is located within a 75m^2 region. Further, these results can be filtered according to a number of factors such as SSID associated and specified time periods.

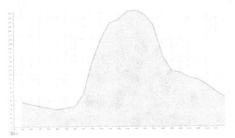

Fig. 2. Node Activity across campus

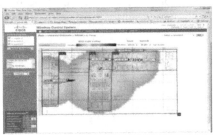

Fig. 3. Heat map for a floor (InfoLab21)

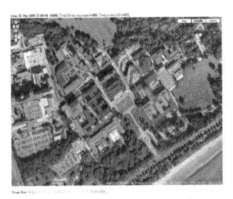

Fig. 4. Wireless Usage at 14:00

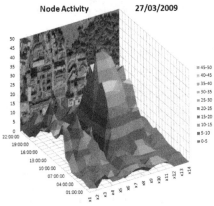

Fig. 5. Wireless Node Actvity

In general, we found evidence to support the general guidelines (provided by Cisco) that each mobile device or asset needs to be heard at better than -75 dBm by at least three access points or monitoring stations in order to provide a useful and accurate location. Although it is clear that the more APs/Monitors that hear a device the better, this obviously depends on the deployment environment and building layout(s). Optimal AP/Monitor density is approximately one every 25 meters depending on the environment and WLAN requirements and in general, placing APs towards the perimeter of rooms and coverage areas provides the best overall coverage and location fidelity. Additionally, for providing coverage within corridors or walkways, the best results are obtained when the APs are staggered along alternating walls rather than placing the APs on the ceiling along the centre line of the corridor. Despite this, we have also found that a large number of deployed access points do not guarantee the correct density needed for effective location awareness. Specifically, the placement of access points for the provision of a wireless network service doesn't mean that this automatically achieves good location fidelity and location awareness possibilities.

We now discuss visualisation of wireless nodes activity for Swansea. Figure 4 shows the wireless usage for a day and time chosen randomly (Monday 2 June 2008 at 2pm). The figure shows a total of 480 node associations with users spread around most of campus, and still heavily at the halls of residence. The Google API was used to display a Google Maps visualization of Swansea University campus using satellite imagery. The usage data was then used to create an overlay of the Google Map showing semi-transparent polygons for each grouping of usage data, colorized according to a predefined scale. The colour of each polygon indicates the level of wireless usage in that grouping, in this case 'building'. The figures are colour dependant and the scale range consists of nine values in descending RGB intensity.

Figure 4 depicted the node activity at a fixed point of time. In Figure 5 we plot the node location activity for a 24-hour period on 27 March 2009 (randomly selected). The campus 2D plane is converted into a 1D plan by aggregating all the campus node activity usage for a certain number of 1D chunks, in this case 14 chunks. The reminaing 2 dimensions in Figure 5 show the number of associations and time (24 hours). These visualisations could be used, for example, by the network operators to look at the wireless network usage around the year and hence to find and predict usage patterns, congestion points, traffic and network growth. Note that it is possible for us to plot mobility patterns of each individual node or group of nodes across campus. It is also possible for us, for example, to find and plot relationships between individual nodes or group of nodes based on their activity patterns in time and space. Activity patterns may include mobility and presence in groups. However, collection, analysis and visualisation of such data may transgress on individuals privacy. We have looked at the analysis and visualisation of node location data with the aim to develop policies for the storage, usage, and release of node location data. The results presented in this section, for example, do not disclose any personal data of nodes, however these results are of limited use for network operators and could not be used to provide rich LBS's. Further discussion of the privacy issues and solutions is given in the next section.

5.2 Location Data and User Privacy – Swansea Considerations

One of the first criticisms of a Location Based Service (LBS) by its users is the perceived privacy implication of using a system where tracking user's movement is a fundamental principle of the technology. It is this alarming realisation that leads users to contemplate the possible effects that this data could have on their privacy, and in some cases causes an immediate rejection of the technology.

This reaction is understandable in a world where the terms *Big-Brother* and an *Orwellian State* are branded daily by the press, combined with headlines of governments on one hand wanting to create *Super Databases* [18] while with the other are losing personal data on buses and in the post [19]. Most users of networks in large institutions such as Universities are happy to use computers to browse the internet and communicate with friends and colleagues without considering how private that activity is. They are likely unaware that their internet browsing activity is being logged and the chat communications is being sent unencrypted and open to interception by network administrators or other agencies or hackers. It is only the fact that LBS immediately cause users to become consciously aware of the fact that their location data is what drives the service and that data is being controlled by a computer somewhere that causes the kneejerk reaction. Privacy is considered a fundamental human right by the Universal Declaration of Human Rights and most democracies around the world [20]. Therefore the issue of location data and privacy must be taken seriously, and there has been substantial work to help provide privacy while also maintain the usefulness of LBS's.

One of the first considerations is the granularity of the location data. The granularity of meters could provide more information about a user than the granularity of kilometres [6]. The level of granularity in Swansea's LBS is per building, which removes a significant amount of detail from location data while still provide enough to offer a valuable LBS. Granularity alone does not provide any real privacy, and is vulnerable to correlation attacks as well as inference and assumptions based on historical data. One of the concerns of location data is how it is stored, and if the stored data could be abused by anyone who gains access, whether legitimately or not, to that data. One solution proposed to solve this is to annonymise the data using pseudonyms. Pseudonymity provides anonymity to location data while maintaining a relationship between the data that is used to help the LBS function. Recording a pseudonym and location as a location data record allows for the movement of a node to be tracked while removing any identifiable data from the record [21]. This adds a level of privacy to the system that would protect a user if the data was stolen or misused, however it does not offer complete privacy as a user's identity could still be inferred from the history of a nodes movement in some cases. One solution to this problem is the addition of dummy nodes that add a level of 'noise' to the LBS that does not affect the quality of the service but helps remove the ability of a possible attacker to infer the identity of a node based on the history of a nodes movements [22]. Another possible addition to add privacy is the use of mix zones which provide a trusted middleware that facilitates distribution of anonymised location information to third-party applications by defining spatiotemporal zones [23]. This does not directly fit into the system design at Swansea, but should be considered for the future.

The importance of privacy is fully understood by the research community and this is reflected in the amount of research undertaken in this area. But it has been suggested that the public put less significance on the importance and value of privacy and more on the short term benefits of the technology [24]. Regardless of the perceived value and importance of location privacy by the public it is vital that their privacy is maintained to the highest level, while still providing a valued service, in order to protect them from future and current threats to their human right of privacy.

6 Conclusions and Future Work

Systems security and user privacy have been major hurdles in the mass uptake of seamless mobile services. Location and context based approaches could provide additional network intelligence in securing networks. Privacy will have to be traded off for mobility and convenience; however, system designers could work to bring the trade-off equation more in the favour of privacy. We will continue to improve our work in these directions.

Acknowledgment. This work has been carried out partly through the JANET Location Awareness programme funds, whose support we acknowledge here.

References

1. Location Awareness Trial, Janet UK
2. Bahl, P., Padmanabhan, V.N.: RADAR: an in-building RF-based user location and tracking system (2000)
3. Harter, A., et al.: The Anatomy of a Context-Aware Application. In: Proc. 5th Annual ACM/IEEE Int. Conf. on Mobile Computing and Networking (1999)
4. Want, R., et al.: The Active Badge Location System. ACM Transaction on Information Systems, 1992 (10), 91–102 (1992)
5. Priyantha, N.B., Chakraborty, A., Balakrishnan, H.: The Cricket location-support system. In: Proceedings of the 6th annual international conference on Mobile computing and networking. ACM, Boston (2000)
6. Grlach, A., Heinemann, A., Terpstra, W.W.: Survey on location privacy in pervasive computing, in Privacy, Security and Trust within the Context of Pervasive Computing. The Kluwer International Series in Engineering and Computer Science. Kluwer Academic Publishers, Dordrecht (2004)
7. Hightower, J., Borriello, G.: A Survey and Taxonomy of Location Systems for Ubiquitous Computing, pp. 57–66 (2001)
8. González, M.C., Mehmood, R.: Experiences in Designing a UWB-based Indoor Localisation System. In: Eighth IASTED international conferences on Wireless and Optical Communications (WOC) 2008, Montreal, Canada. ACTA Press (2008)
9. Castro, P., et al.: A Probabilistic Room Location Service for Wireless Networked Environments. In: Proceedings of the 3rd international conference on Ubiquitous Computing. Springer, Atlanta (2001)
10. Jason Small, A.S., Seiwiorek, D.P.: Determining user location for context aware computing through the use of a wireless LAN infrastructure. ACM Mobile Networks and Applications 6 (2001)
11. Haeberlen, A., et al.: Practical robust localization over large-scale 802.11 wireless networks. In: Proceedings of the 10th annual international conference on Mobile computing and networking. ACM, Philadelphia (2004)
12. Youngjune, G., Jain, R., Kawahara, T.: Robust indoor location estimation of stationary and mobile users. In: INFOCOM 2004. Twenty-third Annual Joint Conference of the IEEE Computer and Communications Societies (2004)
13. John Krumm, J.C.P.: Minimizing Calibration Effort for an Indoor 802.11 Device Location Measurement System. Microsoft Research, MSR-TR-2003-82 (2003)
14. Koo, S.G.M., et al.: Location Discovery in Enterprise-based Wireless Networks: Implementation and Applications. In: Proceedings of the 2nd IEEE Workshop on Applications and Services in Wireless Networks (ASWN 2002), pp. 3–5 (2002)
15. Ferreres, A.I.G.T., Alvarez, B.R., Garnacho, A.R.: Guaranteeing the Authenticity of Location Information. IEEE Pervasive Computing 7(3), 72–80 (2008)
16. Aura, T., Roe, M., Murdoch, S.J.: Securing network location awareness with authenticated DHCP. In: Security and Privacy in Communications Networks and the Workshops. SecureComm. (2007)
17. Garg, S., Kappes, M., Mani, M.: Wireless access server for quality of service and location based access control in 802.11 networks. In: Proceedings of Seventh International Symposium on Computers and Communications. ISCC 2002 (2002)
18. Anderson, R., Brown, I., Dowty, T., Inglesant, P., Heath, W., Sasse, A.: Database State. Joseph Rowntree Reform Trust (2009)
19. Gauardian, 25 Million Peoples Data Lost (2007)
20. Nations, U., Universal Declaration of Human Rights, General Assembly Resolution 217 A (III) (1948)

21. Chaum, D.: Untraceable electronic mail, return addresses, and digital pseudonyms. Communications of the ACM (24), 84–88 (1981)
22. Gruteser, M., Grunwald, D.: Anonymous Usage of Location-Based Services Through Spatial and Temporal Cloaking. In: Proceedings of the 1st international conference on Mobile systems, applications and services. ACM, San Francisco (2003)
23. Beresford, A.R., Frank Stajano, U.o.C.: Location Privacy in Pervasive Computing. IEEE Pervasive Computing, 10 (2003)
24. Acquisti, A., Grossklags, J.: Privacy and rationality in individual decision making. IEEE Security & Privacy 3(1), 26–33 (2005)

A Proportional Fairness with Bandwidth-Borrowing Scheme for a Two-Tier NEMO System

Bing-Chi Kuo and Tsang-Ling Sheu

Department of Electrical Engineering
National Sun Yat-Sen University
Kaohsiung, Taiwan
sheu@ee.nsysu.edu.tw

Abstract. In this paper, we present a proportional fairness with bandwidth-borrowing (PFBB) scheme for a two-tier NEMO system. When traffic load is light, free-slot borrowing is employed to maximize system utilization. On the other hand, when traffic load is heavy and session arrival rates in different tiers are not proportional to their distributed areas, busy-slot borrowing is used to achieve proportional fairness. A mathematical model is built to analyze the performance in terms of the system utilization, blocking probabilities, and fairness index. Analytical results show that fairness index can be affected significantly, when session arrival rates in different tiers are varied.

Keywords: Proportional fairness, Traffic distributtion, Bandwidth borrowing, Makov chains, and NEMO.

1 Introduction

NEtwork MObility (NEMO) proposed by IETF is an integrated approach to maintain the connectivity of a mobile network so that internal mobile devices can perform seamless roaming between different Internet attachment points. Hierarchical NEMO architecture [1] plays an important role in improving the coverage of wireless communications, since it can effectively support large number of mobile devices roaming in different geographical areas. Hierarchical mobile networks were proposed in [2-3], where a mobile node (MN) attaches to an access router (AR) or a mobile router (MR), depending on the geographical area where it resides. In other words, an MN may set up a multimedia (video/audio/data) session to an AR if it is located in the service area of AR, and it may have to communicate indirectly with AR via a neighboring MR, if it is outside the service range of AR. Due to limited resources of a wireless NEMO system, it is important to provide an adequate bandwidth allocation strategy especially when there are insufficient network resources. As shown in [4-5], Channel-borrowing schemes were mainly focused on wireless cellular networks and they did not consider channel allocations in a multi-tier hierarchical NEMO system. By taking into account the effect of queuing times for different traffics, a Markov model proposed by Salih *et al.* [6] evaluated the performance of a two-tier cellular network. However, their works did not investigate how to apply fairness criterion to a multi-tier hierarchical

R. Mehmood et al. (Eds.): EuropeComm 2009, LNICST 16, pp. 189–199, 2009.

NEMO system. Thus, many studies have dealt with different kinds of fairness, e.g., max-min fairness in [7] and proportional fairness in [8].

In this paper, the proposed proportional fairness with bandwidth-borrowing (PFBB) scheme endeavors to achieve balance between the fairness of bandwidth sharing and the improvement of system utilization. The ratio of session arrival rates between direct- (Tier-0) and indirect-link (Tier-1) in a two-tier NEMO system is assumed to be proportional to the ratio of MN distributed areas between Tier-0 and Tier-1. In light traffic, PFBB employs free-slot borrowing to maximize system utilization. On the other hand, when traffic load is heavy and the ratio of data-session arrival rates between Tier-0 and Tier-1 is not proportional to the MN distributed areas, busy-slot borrowing scheme is employed to achieve proportional fairness. A mathematical model with 6-D Markov chains is built to evaluate the PFBB performance in terms of the system utilization, blocking probability, and fairness index.

The rest of this paper is organized as follows. In Section 2, we describe the traffic model and the proposed PFBB scheme in a two-tier hierarchical NEMO system. In Section 3, we introduce the 6-D Markov model to analytically derive the performance metrics, such as system utilization, proportional fairness index, and session blocking probability. Numerical results and discussions are presented in Section 4. Finally, Section 5 contains our concluding remarks.

2 System Models

For a NEMO network, assuming each MN maintains only one session at a time and each AR has a capacity of C slots allocated for serving the session requests of MNs. A logical view of the NEMO scheme, shown in Fig. 1, an MN can establish a direct-link (Tier-0) session to an AR if it is located within the service area of the AR. In addition, the MN also can establish an indirect-link (Tier-1) session via the intermediate MR to the adjacent AR. Session 1 and Session 3 are Tier-0 connections of high-speed and low-speed levels, respectively. Similarly, Session 2 and Session 4 are Tier-1 connections of high-speed and low-speed levels, respectively. Therefore, four kinds of traffic types in Fig. 1, Session 1, Session 2, Session 3, and Session 4, are expressed in terms of *Type-H0*, *Type-H1*, *Type-L0*, and *Type-L1*, respectively.

In our previous works [9], a NEMO network is assumed to be homogeneous such that session generations are uniformly distributed in the service area of AR. In fact, unfair sharing of wireless bandwidth is occurred while the unequal traffic distribution in the service area, i.e., session generations of different traffic types are non-proportional to their distributed areas. Therefore, impact of fairness on the sharing wireless bandwidth between Tier-0 and Tier-1 is our major concern.

A logical view of distributed areas of Tier-0 and Tier-1 can be depicted in Fig. 2. For simplicity, the service areas of AR and MR are assumed to circles and the radii of AR and MR are denoted as R and r, respectively. The distributed area of Tier-0 (A_0) can be covered within the whole service area of AR because any generated Tier-0 session is lived only if the associated MN is located within the service area of AR. When the MN moves across the border of service area of AR (MN_N), it can send a session request of Tier-1 to AR via an intermediate MR that can communicate with AR and MN at the same time. As the MN moves across the border of service area of

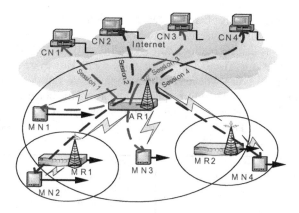

Fig. 1. A two-tier hierarchical NEMO system

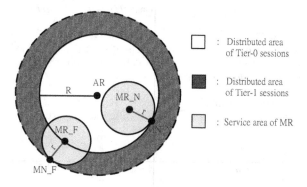

Fig. 2. Distributed areas in Tier-0 and Tier-1

MR (MN_F) and the MR also moves across the border of service area of AR (MR_F), the associated Tier-1 session would become invalid since the intermediate MR no longer communicates with AR and MN simultaneously. Therefore, the shaded region in Fig. 2 can represent the distributed area of Tier-1 (A_1). Thus, the distributed-area ratio of A_0 to A_1 (r_D) can be expressed as in Eq. (1).

$$r_D = \frac{R^2}{(R+r)^2 - R^2}.$$ (1)

Considering a single AR model in a two-tier NEMO network, total number of C slots can be divided into two partitions: Tier-0 slots with the capacity of C_0 and Tier-1 slots with the capacity of C_1. To achieve fair sharing of wireless bandwidth between Tier-0 and Tier-1, the capacity ratio of C_0 to C_1 is compatible with the distributed-area ratio of A_0 to A_1 (r_D), i.e., $C_0 / C_1 = r_D$. A bandwidth borrowing is active when the ratio of slot occupancies between Tier-0 and Tier-1 is incompatible with r_D. A borrowing limit (B), with the range from 0 to the minimum of C_0 and C_1, explicitly implies the maximum slots for each traffic type involved in bandwidth borrowing. If B is equal to 0, it can be viewed as the original scheme without performing borrowing.

Two kinds of borrowing mechanisms can be explained as below. A free-slot borrowing is employed for increasing system utilization under the light traffic load. Any free Tier-0/Tier-1 slots can be reallocated to Tier-1/Tier-0 sessions on their arrival if the original capacities for Tier-0/Tier-1 are fully used. However, reallocating free slots of different traffic types will lead to non-proportional ratio of slot occupancies between Tier-0 and Tier-1. Therefore, performing free-slot borrowing by *Type-H0* and *Type-H1* sessions is more appropriate than that by *Type-L0* and *Type-L1*. Under heavy traffic load, busy Tier-1 slots can be reallocated to Tier-0 sessions on their

```
// When a session arrives
Case 'H0':  // a Type-H0 session arrives
   If (S₀<C₀ and S <C)
      i=i+1;
   Else if (S₀ ≥ C₀ and S₀<C₀+B)
      If (S<C) // performing free-slot borrowing
         i= i+1;
      Else   // S=C
         Reject it;
   Else if (S₀<C₀ and S=C)
      If (w>0) // perform busy-slot borrowing
         i=i+1, w=w–1, y=y+1;
      Else   // perform busy-slot borrowing
         i=i+1, x=x–1, z=z+1;
Case 'L0':  // a Type-L0 session arrives
   If (S₀<C₀ and S<C)
      j=j+1;
```

```
   Else if (S₀ ≥ C₀ and S₀< C₀+B)
      Reject it;
   Else if (S₀<C₀ and S=C)
      If (x>0)  // perform busy-slot borrowing
         j=j+1, x=x–1, z=z+1;
      Else   // perform busy-slot borrowing
         j=j+1, w=w–1, y=y+1;
Case 'H1':  // a Type-H1 session arrives
   If (S₁<C₁ and S<C)
      w=w+1;
   Else if (S₁ ≥ C₁ and S₁<C₁+B)
      If (S<C)  // perform free-slot borrowing
         w=w+1;
      Else  // S=C
         Reject it;
   Else if (S₁<C₁ and S=C)
         y=y+1;
```

```
Case 'L1':  // a Type-L1 session arrives
   If (S₁<C₁ and S<C)
      x=x+1;
   Else if (S₁ ≥ C₁ and S₁<C₁+B)
      Reject it;
   Else if (S₁<C₁ and S=C)
      z=z+1;
// When a served session leaves
Case 'H0':  //a served Type-H0 session leaves
   If (y ≠ 0)
      i=i-1, w=w+1, y=y-1;
   Else if (z ≠ 0)
      i=i-1, x=x+1, z=z-1;
   Else
      i=i–1;
Case 'L0':  //a served Type-L0 session leaves
   If (z ≠ 0)
      j=j-1, x=x+1, z=z-1;
   Else if (y ≠ 0)
      j=j-1, w=w+1, y=y-1;
   Else
      i=i–1;
```

```
Case 'H1':  //a served Type-H1 session leaves
   If (y ≠ 0)
      y=y–1;
   Else if (z ≠ 0)
      w=w-1, x=x+1, z=z-1;
   Else
      w=w–1;
Case 'L1':  //a served Type-L1 session leaves
   If (z ≠ 0)
      z=z-1;
   Else if (y ≠ 0)
      x=x-1, w=w+1, y=y-1;
   Else
      x=x–1;
// When a queued session leaves
Case 'H1':  //a queued Type-H1 session leaves
      y=y–1;
Case 'L1':  //a queued Type-L1 session leaves
x=x–1;
```

Fig. 3. Slot allocation algorithms in PFBB

arrival when the ratio of slot occupancies between Tier-0 and Tier-1 is incompatible with the distributed-area ratio of A_0 to A_1 (r_D). If the ratio of slot occupancies between Tier-0 and Tier-1 becomes larger than r_D, it would perform busy-slot barrowing mechanism from the served Tier-1 sessions to the arriving Tier-0 ones in balance of the slot occupancies of both traffic types.

Nine parameters, $i, j, w, x, y, z, S_0, S_1$, and S are used to show the status of the employed sessions when performing bandwidth borrowing. First, i, j, w, and x are the numbers of *Type-H0*, *Type-L0*, *Type-H1*, *Type-L1* sessions allocated in the slots, respectively. Then, y and z are the numbers of *Type-H1* and *Type-L1* sessions queued in the buffer, respectively. S_0 is the sum of the number of *Type-H0* and *Type-L0* sessions allocated. S_1 is the sum of the number of *Type-H1* and *Type-L1* sessions allocated. Finally, S is the sum of the number of all sessions allocated. The value ranges of these discrete parameters are $i \in [0, C_0 + B]$, $j \in [0, C_0]$, $w \in [0, C_1 + B]$,

$x \in [0, C_1]$, $y \in [0, B]$, $z \in [0, B]$, $S_0 \in [0, C_0 + B]$, $S_1 \in [0, C_1 + B]$, and $S \in [0, C]$.

Pseudo-code of the proposed PFBB is shown in Fig. 3. Any arriving Tier-0/Tier-1 sessions are allocated with their original capacities if free Tier-0/Tier-1 slots exist. When S_0 (S_1) is reached C_0 (C_1), an arriving *Type-L0* (*Type-L1*) session is rejected while a *Type-H0* (*Type-H1*) session on its arrival is reallocated a free Tier-1 (Tier-0) slot by free-slot borrowing. When S equals C and S_0 is smaller than C_0, after performing busy-slot borrowing, next arriving Tier-0 session is reallocated with the busy Tier-1 slots and the original occupied Tier-1 sessions will be interrupted and queued in their corresponding MRs. On the other hand, Tier-1 sessions on their arrival will be queued to wait for the next free slots if S_1 is smaller than C_1.

3 Mathematical Analysis

3.1 Markov Model

An analytical model of the proposed PFBB is built with 6-D Markov chains, where each state (i, j, w, x, y, z) exists as long as the following four constraints are met.

1. $\forall i, j, \quad i + j \leq C_0 + B$.
2. $\forall w, x, \quad w + x \leq C_1 + B$.
3. $\forall i, j, w, x, y, z, \quad i + j + w + x + y + z \leq C + B$.
4. If $i + j + w + x < C$, $\quad y + z = 0$.

Furthermore, the following assumptions are also made in the traffic model: The data-session arrival rates of Tier-0 and Tier-1 are independent Poisson processes with mean λ_0 and λ_1, respectively. The mean speed of MNs in the NEMO system is assumed to be constant, v, and the speed ratio between high- and low-mobility MNs is also assumed to be constant, R_v. The mean speeds of high- and low-mobility MNs (v_H, v_L) can be calculated as $2vR_v/(R_v+1)$ and $2v/(R_v+1)$, respectively. The ratio of data-session arrival rates between high- and low-speed MNs is assumed to be constant, R_λ. The duration time of each session (T_d) is exponentially distributed with a mean $1/\mu$. The residence times of Tier-0 and Tier-1 sessions ($1/\tau_0$, $1/\tau_1$) can be simply derived by $\pi R/2v$ and $\pi r/2v$, respectively, where R and r are the radii of AR's and MR's service area. The residence times of *Type-H0*, *Type-L0*, *Type-H1*, and *Type-L1* sessions $(1/\tau_{H0}, 1/\tau_{L0}, 1/\tau_{H1}, 1/\tau_{L1})$ are obtained by $\pi R/2v_H$, $\pi R/2v_L$, $\pi r/2v_H$, and $\pi r/2v_L$, respectively. The data-session service times (T_s) are also exponentially distributed with means $1/(\mu + \tau')$, where τ' is defined as

$$\tau' = \begin{cases} \tau_{H0}, & \text{for a } \textit{Type-H0} \text{ session.} \\ \tau_{L0}, & \text{for a } \textit{Type-L0} \text{ session.} \\ \tau_{H1}, & \text{for a } \textit{Type-H1} \text{ session.} \\ \tau_{L1}, & \text{for a } \textit{Type-L1} \text{ session.} \end{cases} \tag{2}$$

The queuing times of *Type-H1*, and *Type-L1* sessions $(1/\tau_{QH}, 1/\tau_{QL})$ is also assumed exponentially distributed with means τ_{QH} and τ_{QL}, respectively, and can be denoted as:

$$\tau_{QH} = \frac{(2\lambda_{H1} + \lambda_{H0} + \lambda_{L0})\tau_{H1}}{2(\lambda_{H1} + \lambda_{H0} + \lambda_{L0})}. \tag{3}$$

$$\tau_{QL} = \frac{(2\lambda_{L1} + \lambda_{H0} + \lambda_{L0})\tau_{L1}}{2(\lambda_{L1} + \lambda_{H0} + \lambda_{L0})}. \tag{4}$$

Here, the borrowing probability of *Type-H1* session is assumed to be equal to the borrowing probability of *Type-L1* session and the mean queueing time of *Type-H1* (*Type-L1*) session can be simply expressed by the products of the data-session service time of *Type-H1* (*Type-L1*) and the ratio of data-session arrival rates among *Type-H1* (*Type-L1*), *Type-H0*, and *Type-L0*.

3.2 Balance Equations

Let $P(\mathbf{n})$ be the steady-state probability of state (i, j, w, x, y, z), where $\mathbf{n} \equiv [i, j, w, x, y, z]$. To facilitate the expression of balance equations, two indicator functions are used.

$$I_0(a,b) = \begin{cases} 1 & a \neq b \\ 0 & a = b \end{cases}. \tag{5}$$

$$I_1(a,b) = \begin{cases} 1 & a = b \\ 0 & a \neq b \end{cases}. \tag{6}$$

The steady-state balance equations can be divided into the following six cases.

1. E_1 ($0 \leq i + j < C_0$, $0 \leq w + x < C_1$, and $y + z = 0$): the arriving Tier-0 and Tier-1 sessions will be allocated to their free slots in original capacities.
2. E_2 ($C_0 \leq i + j \leq C_0 + B$, $i + j + w + x < C$, and $y + z = 0$): only *Type-H0* and Tier-1 sessions can be allocated to the free Tier-1 slots due to Tier-0 slots have been fully occupied.
3. E_3 ($C_1 \leq w + x \leq C_1 + B$, $i + j + w + x < C$, and $y + z = 0$): Tier-1 slots have been fully used and only *Type-H1* and Tier-0 sessions can be allocated to the free Tier-0 slots.

4. E_4 ($C_0 \leq i+j < C_0 + B$, $i+j+w+x = C$, and $0 \leq y+z < B$): the arriving Tier-1 sessions will be queued in corresponding MRs to wait for the next released slots.

5. E_5 ($C_1 \leq w+x < C_1 + B$, $i+j+w+x = C$, and $0 \leq y+z < B$): Tier-0 sessions on their arrival can be reallocated to the busy Tier-1 slots.

6. E_6 ($i+j+w+x = C$, and $y+z = B$): all the arriving Tier-0 and Tier-1 sessions will be rejected.

We can obtain the steady-state probabilities by solving the steady-state balanced equations with the following initial condition.

$$\sum_{k=1}^{6} P(\mathbf{n} \mid \mathbf{n} \in E_k) = 1. \tag{7}$$

3.3 Performance Metrics

To evaluate the proposed PFBB, three performance metrics, system utilization, proportional fairness index, and session blocking probabilities are derived. System utilization (U) in Eq. (8) is defined as the normalized throughput.

$$U = \frac{1}{C} \sum_{k=1}^{6} \left[(i+j+w+x) P(\mathbf{n} \mid \mathbf{n} \in E_k) \right]. \tag{8}$$

Proportional fairness index (*PFI*) in Eq. (9) is defined to determine how fair the system model is. It can be estimated by the ratio of two terms, the ratio of slot occupancies between Tier-0 and Tier-1 and the distributed-area ratio of Tier-0 to Tier-1. For the fairest case, *PFI* = 1, As *PFI* is larger than 1, the ratio of slot occupation between Tier-0 and Tier-1 is not proportional to their distributed areas. If *PFI* is smaller than one, Tier-1 sessions gets more bandwidth than they are expected.

$$PFI = \frac{\sum_{k=1}^{6} \left[(i+j) P(\mathbf{n} \mid \mathbf{n} \in E_k) \right]}{r_D \sum_{k=1}^{6} \left[(w+x) P(\mathbf{n} \mid \mathbf{n} \in E_k) \right]}. \tag{9}$$

In the proposed PFBB, any Tier-0 session will be blocked on its arrival if total number of associated slot occupancy is greater than or equal to ($C_0 + B$). Furthermore, we can distinguish between the probabilities of *Type-H0* and *Type-L0* with the condition of *E2*. Similarly, Tier-1 sessions will be blocked if total number of associated slot occupancy is greater than or equal to ($C_1 + B$). Session blocking probabilities of *Type-H0*, *Type-L0*, *Type-H1*, and *Type-L1* are represented as

$$P_{b\_H0} = \left[\sum P(\mathbf{n} \mid \mathbf{n} \in E_{2,1}) + \sum P(\mathbf{n} \mid \mathbf{n} \in E_4) + \sum P(\mathbf{n} \mid \mathbf{n} \in E_6) \right] \tag{10}$$

$$P_{b\_L0} = \left[\sum P(\mathbf{n}\,|\,\mathbf{n}\in E_{2,2}) + \sum P(\mathbf{n}\,|\,\mathbf{n}\in E_4) + \sum P(\mathbf{n}\,|\,\mathbf{n}\in E_6) \right]$$

$$P_{b\_H1} = \left[\sum P(\mathbf{n}\,|\,\mathbf{n}\in E_{3,1}) + \sum P(\mathbf{n}\,|\,\mathbf{n}\in E_5) + \sum P(\mathbf{n}\,|\,\mathbf{n}\in E_6) \right]$$

$$P_{b\_L1} = \left[\sum P(\mathbf{n}\,|\,\mathbf{n}\in E_{3,2}) + \sum P(\mathbf{n}\,|\,\mathbf{n}\in E_5) + \sum P(\mathbf{n}\,|\,\mathbf{n}\in E_6) \right],$$

where $E_{2,1} = \left\{ \mathbf{n} \,\middle|\, \sum_{E_2} i + j = C_0 + B \right\}$, $E_{2,2} = \left\{ \mathbf{n} \,\middle|\, \sum_{E_2} i + j \geq C_0 \right\}$, $E_{3,1} = \left\{ \mathbf{n} \,\middle|\, \sum_{E_3} w + x = C_1 + B \right\}$, and

$$E_{3,2} = \left\{ \mathbf{n} \,\middle|\, \sum_{E_3} w + x \geq C_1 \right\}.$$

Then, session blocking probability of Tier-0 ($P_{b\text{-}0}$) can be introduced to the union of the blocking probabilities of *Type-H0* and *Type-L0*. Similarly, session blocking probability of Tier-1 session ($P_{b\text{-}1}$) can be viewed as the union of the blocking probabilities of *Type-H1* and *Type-L1*. They are shown as follows.

$$P_{b\_0} = \left[\frac{\lambda_{H0}}{\lambda_0} \sum P(\mathbf{n}\,|\,\mathbf{n}\in E_{2,1}) + \frac{\lambda_{L0}}{\lambda_0} \sum P(\mathbf{n}\,|\,\mathbf{n}\in E_{2,2}) + \sum P(\mathbf{n}\,|\,\mathbf{n}\in E_4) + \sum P(\mathbf{n}\,|\,\mathbf{n}\in E_6) \right]$$

$$P_{b\_1} = \left[\frac{\lambda_{H1}}{\lambda_1} \sum P(\mathbf{n}\,|\,\mathbf{n}\in E_{3,1}) + \frac{\lambda_{L1}}{\lambda_1} \sum P(\mathbf{n}\,|\,\mathbf{n}\in E_{3,2}) + \sum P(\mathbf{n}\,|\,\mathbf{n}\in E_5) + \sum P(\mathbf{n}\,|\,\mathbf{n}\in E_6) \right].$$

$$(11)$$

4 Performance Evaluation

By running on the MATLAB tool, we give a numerical example. System parameters used in the example are listed in Table 1.

Table 1. Parameters used in the numerical analysis

Parameters	Values	Parameters	Values
C	10	λ_0	0.25 (1/s)
B	5	λ_1	0.25 (1/s)
R	5000 (m)	R_λ	1
R	2000 (m)	v	20 (m/s)
T_d	1/180 (s)	R_v	1.5

The results of system utilization under different area ratios of A_0 to $(A_0 + A_1)$ are plotted in Fig. 4. When the area ratio of A_0 to $(A_0 + A_1)$ is increased, the system utilization (U) in PFBB declines as the ratio of session arrival rates between Tier-0 and Tier-1 is decreased from 1/3 to 1/6. It is a trade-off between achieving the proportional fairness and maximizing the system utilization when traffic load is heavy. Proportional fairness indexes (*PFI*) under different data-session arrival rates and different ratios of session arrival rates is shown in Fig. 5. As can be observed, both schemes, if in smaller ratio of data-session arrival rate ($\lambda = 0.01$), cannot reach the target fairness index since the system is under loaded. Higher ratio of data-session arrival rate ($\lambda_0/\lambda_1 = 3$) has benefit in increasing the slot occupancies of Tier-1. As the session arrival rate increases, however, the *PFI* in PFBB is close to the target no matter the ratio of data-session arrival rates is higher or lower.

Referring to Equation (11), Fig. 6 and Fig. 7, respectively, show the blocking probabilities of Tier-0 and Tier-1 sessions. P_{b-0} and the P_{b-1} monotonically increase with respect to the increase of session arrival rate ($\lambda_0 + \lambda_1$). P_{b-0} in PFBB is always higher than that in original scheme when the ratio of session arrival rates is high ($\lambda_0/\lambda_1 = 3$). On the contrary, Tier-0 sessions in PFBB get more bandwidth than that in the original scheme when the ratio of session arrival rate is low ($\lambda_0/\lambda_1 = 1/3$).

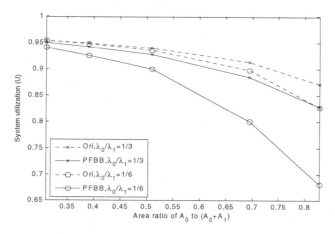

Fig. 4. System utilization vs area ratio (Tier-0)

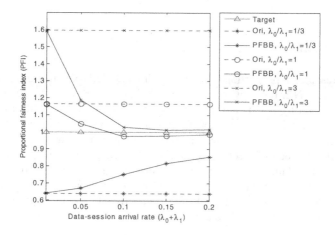

Fig. 5. Proportional fairness index

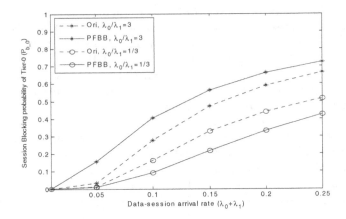

Fig. 6. Session blocking probability of Tier-0

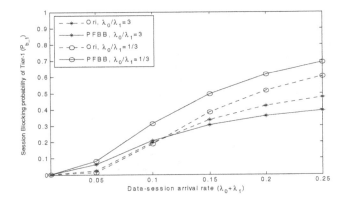

Fig. 7. Session blocking probability of Tier-1

5 Conclusions

We have presented a proportional fairness with bandwidth-borrowing scheme in two-tier hierarchical NEMO networks. A free-slot borrowing is employed to maximize system utilization by borrowing available slots when the traffic load is light. In our design, a busy Tier-1 slot can be borrowed to an arriving Tier-0 session if the ratio of slot occupancies between Tier-0 and Tier-1 is smaller than their distributed-area ratio while the NEMO network becomes congested. For the purpose of validation, an analytical model was built to compare the performance between our proposed scheme and the original scheme. From the analytical results, we have demonstrated that the proposed model can achieve the goal of fairly bandwidth sharing between Tier-0 and Tier-1 according to their distributed-area ratio.

References

1. Kuo, G.S., Ji, K.: NXG04-6: Novel Hierarchical Network Mobility Support Protocol with Bidirectional End-to-end Route Optimization Solution for Nested Mobile Networks. In: Proc. of GLOBECOM, San Francisco, pp. 1–6 (2006)
2. Soliman, C.H.C., Malki, K.E., Bellier, L.: Hierarchical Mobile IPv6 Mobility Management (HMIPv6). IETF RFC 4140 (2005)
3. Yoo, S.J., Choi, S.J., Su, D.: Analysis of Fast Handover Mechanisms for Hierarchical Mobile IPv6 Network Mobility. Wireless Pers. Comm. 48(2), 215–238 (2009)
4. Kadi, E., Olariu, S., Wahab, A.: A Rate-Based Borrowing Scheme for QoS Provisioning in Multimedia Wireless Networks. IEEE T. Parallel Distr. 13(2), 156–166 (2002)
5. Yuen, J., Chan, E., Lam, Y.: A Buffered-Bandwidth Approach for Supporting Real-Time Video Streaming over Cellular Networks. Multimed. Tools Appl. 28(1), 141–155 (2006)
6. Salih, T., Fidanboylu, K.M.: Modeling and Analysis of Queuing Handoff Calls in Single and Two-Tier Cellular Networks. Computer Communication 29(17), 3580–3590 (2006)
7. Bejerano, Y., Han, S.J., Li, L.: Fairness and Load Balancing in Wireless LANs Using Association Control. IEEE Trans. Netw. 15(3), 560–573 (2007)
8. Jiang, L.B., Liew, S.C.: Proportional Fairness in Wireless LANs and Ad Hoc Networks. In: Proc. of WCNC, New Orleans, pp. 436–440 (2005)
9. Sheu, T.L., Kuo, B.C.: An Analytical Model of Two-Tier Handoff Mechanisms for a Hierarchical NEMO System. Wireless Networks 14(6), 795–802 (2008)

Intelligent Healthcare Systems (IHS)

Healthcare Information Systems –
Requirements and Vision

John G. Williams

Professor of Health Services Research, Swansea University, UK
Director of Health Informatics Unit, Royal College of Physicians, UK Swansea University

Abstract. The introduction of sophisticated information, communications and technology into health care is not a simple task, as demonstrated by the difficulties encountered by the Department of Health's multi-billion programme for the NHS. This programme has successfully implemented much of the infrastructure needed to support the activities of the NHS, but has made less progress with electronic patient records. The case for health records that are focused on the individual patient will be outlined, and the need for these to be underpinned by professionally agreed standards for structure and content. Some of the challenges will be discussed, and the benefits to health care and clinical research will be explored.

R. Mehmood et al. (Eds.): EuropeComm 2009, LNICST 16, p. 203, 2009.

The Impact of eHealth on the Quality
and Safety of Healthcare

Azeem Majeed[*], Ashly Black, Josip Car, Chantelle Anandan, Kathrin Cresswell,
Brian McKinstry, Claudia Pagliari, Rob Procter, and Aziz Sheikh

[*] Imperial College London, London, UK
University of Edinburgh, Edinburgh, UK

Abstract. There is considerable interest in using information technology (IT) to
enhance the quality and safety of healthcare. We undertook a systematic literature review to assess the impact of eHealth applications on the quality and
safety of healthcare. We retrieved 46,349 potentially relevant publications, from
which we selected 67 relevant systematic reviews for inclusion. The literature
was found to be poorly collated and of variable quality in its methodology, reporting and utility. We categorised eHealth applications into three main areas:
i). storing, managing and transmission of data; ii). supporting clinical decision-
making; and iii). facilitating care from a distance. We found that relative to the
potential benefits noted within the literature, little empirical evidence exists in
support of these applications. Of the few studies revealing the clearest evidence
of benefits, many are from academic clinical centres where developers of new
applications have also been directly associated with their evaluation. It is therefore unclear how effective these applications would be if deployed outside the
environment in which they were developed. Our review of the impact of
eHealth applications on quality and safety of healthcare demonstrated a vast gap
between the postulated and empirically demonstrated benefits. In addition, there
is a lack of robust research on risks and costs. Consequently, the cost-
effectiveness of these interventions has yet to be demonstrated.

R. Mehmood et al. (Eds.): EuropeComm 2009, LNICST 16, p. 204, 2009.
© Institute for Computer Science, Social-Informatics and Telecommunications Engineering 2009

e-Labs and Work Objects:
Towards Digital Health Economies

John D. Ainsworth* and Iain E. Buchan

School of Community Based Medicine,
University of Manchester,
Manchester Academic Health Science Centre,
Manchester, M13 9PL, United Kingdom
{john.ainsworth,iain.buchan}@manchester.ac.uk

Abstract. The optimal provision of healthcare and public health services requires the synthesis of evidence from multiple disciplines. It is necessary to understand the genetic, environmental, behavioural and social determinants of disease and health-related states; to balance the effectiveness of interventions with their costs; to ensure the maximum safety and acceptability of interventions; and to provide fair access to care services for given populations. Ever expanding databases of knowledge and local health information, and the ability to employ computationally expensive methods, promises much for decisions to be both supported by best evidence and locally relevant. This promise will, however, not be realised without providing health professionals with the tools to make sense of this information rich environment and to collaborate across disciplines. We propose, as a solution to this problem, the e-Lab and Work Objects model as a sense-making platform for digital health economies - bringing together data, methods and people for timely health intelligence.

Keywords: Health Intelligence, Collaboration, Work Objects, e-Lab, Digital Economy, Health Economy, Analysis Workbench.

1 Introduction

In the 1970s Archie Cochrane and colleagues alerted the medical profession to the need to weed out subjectivity and anecdote from clinical practice [1]. At the same time there was a move to improve the safety of medicines. Since then the evidence-based care movement has grown and is now accepted by most healthcare professionals to be best practice. However, there are serious problems with the evidence on which healthcare and public health practice is based: it is expensive to produce; it takes a long time to produce; it takes a long time to influence professional practice; it is crude, relating to the average participant and simple treatment definitions under ideal conditions – in other words, it gives a low-resolution picture of how a patient might respond to treatment or a how a sub-group of the community might respond to a public health intervention. There is

---

* Corresponding author.

R. Mehmood et al. (Eds.): EuropeComm 2009, LNICST 16, pp. 205–216, 2009.
© Institute for Computer Science, Social-Informatics and Telecommunications Engineering 2009

also a lack of public benefit from investments in science and public services, due to fragmentation of communities, data and analytical methods. In other words; silos of research that could be more effective and efficient if the researchers had easy ways to find and share resources when they need them. The divisions are common between disciplines, for example social vs. biomedical science investigations of obesity. But they also exist within disciplines, for example between biomedical scientists investigating nutritional vs. physical activity components of obesity. Most of the health informatics literature on electronic health records and putting evidence into practice is about weaving the existing evidence-base into healthcare decision-making. The role of clinical information systems in improving the evidence-base, however, has been neglected, but they are essential to providing a timely and more flexible evidence base for future healthcare. This future could be called *high resolution healthcare*; it would enable personalised medicine, efficient and opportunistic clinical trials, complex (including genomic) epidemiology, and tactical development of local services based on local environmental factors and outcomes at the population level. High-resolution care and research requires information systems to link relevant data, methods and people in a clear and timely fashion.

The history of public health intelligence shows rapid advancement in the discipline through the application of information technology [2], [3] and [4]. Increasingly complex analysis methods requiring High Performance Computing (HPC) resources are being used. Simultaneously, there has been a rapid increase in the range of data sources available to the public health practitioner, encompassing electronic health records, research databases, geographical information systems and socio-demographic profiles. Ubiquitous connectivity and middleware enables HPC resources to be shared, and data collections to be accessed from anywhere. However the applications used to make sense of these electronic resources themselves tend to be very specific to the problem being addressed resulting in isolation of outputs and duplication of effort when the same problem is solved for each discipline [5].

2   Related Work

Over the course of the past decade, we have witnessed the growth of e-Science [6] and much progress in developing the middleware required for sharing resources, both computational and data. The plethora of Grid frameworks [7] and grid deployments represents the main thrust of these efforts, but it has not become the universal infrastructure envisioned by its pioneers [8]. In fact the most successful Grid deployments are actually as part of a complete vertical application such as the CERN Large Hadron Collider Grid. Service Oriented Architectures (SOA), usually realised through Web Services, offer an alternative approach to sharing, typically by providing a workflow tool for orchestration [9]. The e-Science movement has also spawned numerous Virtual Research Environments [10] drawing on the collaboratory concept [11], but no generic, reusable, electronic equivalent of the laboratory workbench or lab notebook has emerged. The Open Provenance

Model [12] provides a standard way of capturing the history of the production of digital objects, with the goal of providing repeatability of *in-silico* experiments. myExperiment [13] draws on the social networking paradigm to provide a platform for curating and sharing scientific workflows. myExperiment also contains an aggregation mechanism known as a "pack", which enables user to bind related artefacts together. This capability is further developed as Research Objects in [13]. The Open Archives Initiative (OAI) have developed a standard for aggregating web-based resources through the Object Reuse and Exchange protocol [14], which is being widely adopted within the digital repositories community. The concept of Boundary Objects, as a means of cross-discipline communication, was first identified by Star and Griesemer [15] two decades previously.

3 Motivating Use Cases

The use cases presented below serve to illustrate the need for an electronic laboratory for health.

3.1 Obesity Investigations

The obesity epidemic [16] and its potential to break financial models of healthcare has raised the urgency of understanding the epidemiology of obesity and the effectiveness of large-scale measures to tackle it. However, identifying the determinants of obesity, which are very complex, requires understanding social and behavioural as well as biomedical mechanisms [17]. Obesity-relevant information is contained in a number of large surveys, such as Health Surveys for England and the British Household Panel Survey. However, these surveys are difficult to navigate, and are under-used in obesity research. The difficulty arises from the number of variables measured in each survey, and subtle differences in measurement techniques and variable names, which can only be resolved by digging through supporting documentation. Researchers fail to learn from one another about finding, extracting and analysing relevant data. Furthermore, individual researchers may be unable to reproduce an analysis, based on a complex survey after they have forgotten the steps they took. The statistical analysis is usually encapsulated in scripts, but this is not usually chained to the data extraction. Surveys that are repeated on a regular basis, for example the annual Health Survey for England, may have differences in measurement, sampling, or simply labelling of variables, which makes analysis across surveys difficult. It is unsurprising therefore that social and health scientists asking similar questions using HSE would usually in isolation from one another. Social researchers don't usually know where or how to get at the full range of data relevant to obesity research, for example data collected by healthcare services or schools. And for obesity research in the public health service, there is often a lack of analytical capacity, for example to resolve spatial or temporospatial patterns of obesity from geocoded data sets.

3.2   Genetic Epidemiology

Understanding the genetic basis for disease, and how genetic factors interact with environments and behaviours is a grand challenge for science. Biotechnologies are providing vast amounts of genetic and gemonic data. For example, out of the three million or so genetic factors that vary between people, half a million factors can now be measured on a blood sample for around two hundred dollars. These points of variation, or Single Nucleotide Polymorphisms (SNPs), are usually studied for their relation to disease states by running statistical analyses over tens of thousands of study subjects, hundreds of thousands of genetic factors and a handful of other factors such as age. This is a computationally expensive task [18], even with the crudest types of analysis. Ideally more relaistically complex analyses, such as seeking clusters of interacting genetic factors, would be commonplace, but this is restricted by statistical and computational limits at present. The development and/or application machine learning methods may make the more compelx analyses tractable. Validation of the causal relationship between a genetic variation and a disease state, must take into account environmental exposures of individuals as these may contribute significantly. This information can be acquired through a clinical study of the cases or from medical records. The successful interpretation of genotype and phenotype data requires a specialist understanding of the disease. The ideal genomic research information system would enable collaboration between methodologists (bioinformaticians, biostatisticians and biomathematicians), domain experts (clinicians, epidemiologists and biologists) and computer scientists. The system would provide a timely thinking space for teams of experts to co-develop insights into the genetic basis of disease from a combination of perspectives.

3.3   Pharmacovigilance

Post-marketing surveillance of medicines (also known as Phase IV of clinical trials) is required to assess the safety, and to some extent the effectiveness, of newly licensed medicines 'in the wild', oustide the artificial environments of clinical trials. Phase III clinical trials do not usually include all of the types of patient, for example women of child bearing age or patients with other dieases taking other medicines, who might be eligible for treatment with the drug after it is licensed. Therefore the evidence from clinical trials does nto provide a full picture of the public health implications of the drug. Regarding saftety: a system of Adverse Event Reporting (AER) is employed, which relies on clinicians identifying, and reporting harmful affects to a central authority. It may be the case that adverse reactions are not identified as being caused by a particular medicine and so not reported. Important signals about the safety and effectiveness of newly licensed medicines could be extracted from electronic health records. For example, if patient A has the same indication for new medicine X as patient B, but patient A's physician is not yet prescribing X, then a natural experiment takes place - the challenge is to identify appropriate natural control patients like A and make careful statistical analyses to compare X with existing treatment 'in the wild'. However, there is no central database that can be analysed; the data is held within multiple systems that not only cover a subset of the population but it further fragmented by the type of care being provided, typically primary and secondary care. The difficulty of combining the relevant data is further compounded by the need to preserve patient privacy and to comply with the information governance requirements of each organisation that holds a part of the patient's overall the health record. An ideal system would enable analysts to extract anonymised data across a federation of electronic health record databases, effectively treating it as a single virtual population data set. Effective analysis requires a combination of statistical method expertise and clinical expertise to interpret the findings [19].

3.4   Modelling Healthcare for Populations

Long-term conditions, such as Coronary Heart Disease (CHD), consume the largest proportion of healthcare budgets, and are a major focus of public health initiatives. Moving interventions 'up stream' to earlier stages of disease would reduce the amount of suffering over the average lifetime and save money. Health policy makers and those planning and managing local health services are poorly served by over-simple estimates of the potential public health impacts of making changes to the pathways of care or taking preventive public health measures. These estimates are often unreliable [20], because the models do not represent the complexity of the disease, population or care over time. It is possible to construct graphical models [21] and to use Discrete Event Simulation to model a disease in a population [22]. Such a simulation would enable the user to test various different scenarios, with the ability to modify both clinical and public health interventions, and measure both the effectiveness based on clinical outcomes and costs. Larger simulations, in terms of the population size, results in better accuracy but require greater computational resources. Discrete event simulations are amenable to parallelisation, and so there is a benefit to employing HPC resources. The construction of models requires collaboration between health economists, epidemiologists, biostatisticians and typical decision-makers/leaders (public health professionals, healthcare managers, and clinicians). The execution of simulation scenarios is of interest to public health professionals, clinicians and service commissioners and the results of simulations are used to inform policy decisions. The ideal system would enable user to construct and share models around 'what if scenarios' easily; to execute individual simulations quickly; and to share simulations and their results.

3.5   Use Case Summary

From these domain specific use cases, we can identify a set of common requirements. The electronic laboratory must:

1. Provide a mechanism for organising work, such that it can be shared, repeated, audited, reused and reviewed.
2. Provide easy access to resources such as data sets and computational resources.

3. Provide support for the scientific method such that investigations can be planned, constructed, executed recorded and repeated.
4. Provide support for collaboration through the formation of ad-hoc communities of interest, both within and between disciplines.

Our goal is to support both the reuse of content and the reuse of software. The curation and discovery of content via Work Objects within an e-Lab can serve to act as an organisational memory, as training materials, as an accelerant to the discovery process, and as means to reduce duplication. Within health services we envisage a key benefit of the e-Lab/Work Object paradigm to be analytical capacity building among the workforce. The reuse of content between e-Labs will require a standard interexchange format for Work Objects to be developed. The e-Lab software architecture must foster the reuse of functionality and interoperability, but allow specialisation for domain specific tasks.

4   The e-Lab

An e-Lab is an information system for bringing together people, data and analytical methods at the point of investigation or decision-making. It provides a secure environment for managing, exploring and analysing data from anonymised, integrated health records. The functional architecture of the e-Lab is shown in Figure 1. The e-Lab provides access to three different types of workspace for each user: personal space that is private to the user; group collaboration spaces that are visible only to members of the group; and public space that is visible to all e-Lab users. Collaboration facilities – such as people search and messaging – are provided, as is the capability to organise communities of interest around Work Objects. Syndication is available for users to track the development of Work Objects. The e-Lab enables access to computational and data resources. Computational resources may range from private compute clusters, required for secure processing of medical records, genomic data and images, to national and international Grids. The e-Lab embeds anonymised clinical data and enforces information governance policies. The e-Lab provides the capability to link across data sources, to perform statistical analysis and visualise the results. Users may upload their own data sets – retaining full control over access rights – and the e-Lab will add it to the data resource catalogue so that it can be used in the same way as the embedded data resources. We distinguish between 'expert users' and 'routine users'. Expert users are able to create and publish methods to support the knowledge discovery process into the e-Lab as Work Objects. These Work Objects can then be re-used by routine users to accelerate their own knowledge discovery. The e-Lab is secured through both technical and operational governance procedures. Maintaining privacy and confidentiality of individuals whose anonymised medical records are stored in the e-Lab is paramount. Privacy preserving data linkage [23] and statistical disclosure control [24] is used. Furthermore, users are only permitted to access data for which they have the approval of the governance board and full audit trails of all activity in the e-Lab are maintained. The e-Lab employs a Service Oriented Architecture (SOA), which

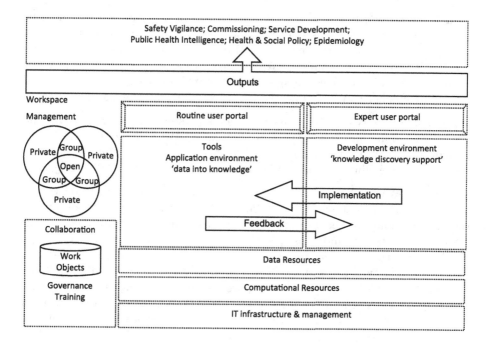

Fig. 1. The e-Lab functional architecture

enables both reuse of software and reuse of operational services between e-Lab deployments. We define the core set of e-Lab services to be a Work Object repository, data set repository, metadata catalogue, statistical analysis, visualisation, governance, and access control.

5   Work Objects

Work Objects are central to the e-Lab, providing the capability to curate and share information, which in turn builds analytical capacity and organisational memory. Work Objects are collections of digital content assembled to support a specific work task or a series of work tasks – for example to provide a persistent record of an investigation, to publish to a community of interest a statistical method for reuse, or to group together training examples for a tutorial.

Repeatability. A useful analogy can be drawn between a Work Object and a scientific paper. In theory, the paper should give the community all the information necessary to reproduce the results of the research, however there is rarely sufficient information in the paper for another scientist exactly to recreate the investigation. A Work Object representing an investigation can capture all the information necessary to reproduce the results, by recording each step in the process, the data sources used, any transformations applied, the analysis methods and models used, and the commentary underpinning the interpretation of results.

Reuse. Furthering the analogy with scientific papers, a Work Object must be able to reference other Work Objects, in a similar fashion to citations in papers and these references must be navigable. However the Work Object concept goes further. It is possible to embed a Work Object inside another Work Object. For example a Work Object containing a method of statistical analysis could be used inside any number of Work Objects each representing an investigation.

Permanence. A Work Object must provide a persistent record of activity and the associated findings. The process of publishing a Work Object into the public domain must cause a permanent record to be made. A Work Object contains metadata that enables searches to be made over a collection of Work Objects.

Typing. A Work Object must provide a mechanism that enables constraints to be place on its contents, to define application specific content types, and to describe relationships between the content items. This mechanism enables Work Objects to be typed, and consequently systems that are aware of the type of Work Object that they are producing or consuming can provide a richer user experience. The typing of a Work Object requires the specification of the allowed content items, their format and the required number of each; it requires specification of the precedence of content items, for example "data set A and method B must be populated before results C"; it requires specification of production relationship between contents items, for example "executing query I on data source J produces data set K". This specification defines a Work Object's lifecyle that compliant systems will enforce. As an example a Research Object must contain a definition of a research question; the design of the investigation; the ethical approval; the measurements; a record of the steps used to transform the data into results; the results; finished documents about the results. The typing mechanism is extensible, allowing for new types of Work Object to be created as and when required by a community of users.

Graceful degradation of understanding. All systems producing and consuming Work Objects must implement the Work Object as a container; it is not necessary to understand any specific Work Object type. We term these systems Work Object Compliant. An example of this type is a Work Object Repository that is able to store Work Objects, and provides the capability to search for specific Work Objects by querying the metadata. Systems that produce/consume Work Objects and understand one or more types are application specific but are able to reuse components that are Work Object Compliant . Furthermore, Work Objects inherit from OAI ORE [14], and so any system that it Work Object Compliant is also ORE compliant as shown in Figure 2.

Content Items contained in a Work Object maybe embedded directly or indirectly referenced by URI. There are pros and cons associated with either approach. Embedded Content Items can be guaranteed to be immutable and are always accessible. There can be no such guarantees with Reference Content Items, although it may be possible to enforce this through service level agreements with the content provider. It is impractical to embed some content items because of their size, for example genomic data sets, and impossible for others

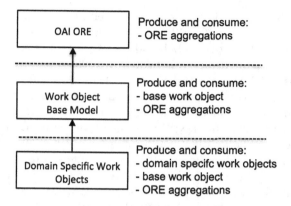

Fig. 2. Levels of Work Object Compliance and Understanding

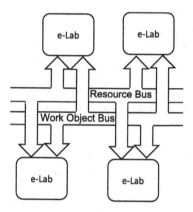

Fig. 3. e-Lab Federation

where they are subject to copyright. A published Work Object is considered to be in the public domain, however it is possible to restrict access to Content Items. Any Content Item may be encrypted so that it is not visible without prior arrangement with the author. This applies to both embedded content items and the URI of a referenced content item. Furthermore, although the URI of a Referenced Content Item may be visible, the content provider may apply access control.

6   Discussion and Future Work

The e-Lab and the Work Object work together to provide a solution to the problems of resource access, collaboration, reuse and organisation of work. We expect that it will be used in the UK NHS to build analytical capacity and accessible organisational memory. The e-Lab model will be fully developed in the North

West e-Health (NWeH) project, a collaborative effort between the University of Manchester, Salford Primary Care Trust and Salford Royal Foundation Hospital Trust. NWeH is developing the e-Lab and the Work Object software. The first operational e-Lab will be deployed in Salford in 2009, with further deployments following across the North West of England. These community e-Labs will be federated creating a virtual e-Lab for large-scale population-based research containing data on over 2 million people across the North West of England, and Work Objects contributed from NHS personnel from all members of the federation – tapping into the existing culture of sharing across the NHS. The core e-Lab software will be further developed across a range of projects in the Northwest Institute for Bio-Health Informatics (http://www.nibhi.org.uk) including the Shared Genomics Project [18], the Obesity e-Lab [25] and the Manchester Collaboration for Leadership in Applied Health Research and Care (Systems Research Theme, which is producing new methods for care pathway modelling and simulation).

We have presented e-Labs, and their enclosed Work Object repositories. This model can be extend to enable sharing of resources and sharing or Work Objects between communities centred around an e-Lab. We introduce the Resource Bus and the Work Object Bus as a means of federating e-Labs (Figure 3). If a community wishes to trust another community it can export a Work Object, which could be used by the receiving community to accelerate service provision or research and ensure that it is consistent across communities. A published Work Object is considered to be in the public domain, however it is possible to restrict access to it contents. Any content item may be encrypted so that it is not visible without prior arrangement with the author or if the content item is indirectly referenced, the content provider may apply additional access control. The Resource Bus enables the sharing of data and computational resources between Health Economies. The Resource Bus enables users to discover the resources that are available to them from other e-Labs, contingent on the trust relationships that exist between any two e-Labs. These resources can then be used as part of an investigation. For example, e-Labs can expose their embedded health data resources, derived from integrated electronic health records, onto the Resource Bus, creating a single virtual database of the entire population from the participating health economies. The virtual population database can then by accessed in the same way as any embedded e-Lab data resources. This model of distributed collaboration ensures that access control and governance arrangements of each e-Lab are maintained at a local level, which is not possible with traditional approaches that utilise a central data warehouse.

The e-Lab Technical Architecture Group at the University of Manchester was established to bring together projects from disciplines outside of health such as bioinformatics and chemistry. The goal of this group is to standardise Work Objects and define a common, reusable e-Lab infrastructure.

Acknowledgments. We would like to thank the members of the Obesity e-Lab (funded by the UK Environmental and Social Research Council), Shared Genomics (funded by Microsoft), the Manchester Collaboration for Leadership in

Applied Health Research and Care (funded by UK National Institute for Health Research), and North West e-Health (funded by the UK Northwest Development Agency) projects for their input and the e-Lab Technical Architecture Group at the University of Manchester for many insightful discussions.

References

1. Cochrane, A.L.: Effectiveness and Efficiency. Random Reections on Health Services. Nuffield Provincial Hospitals Trust, London (1972)
2. Hersh, W.: Medical informatics improving health care through information. Journal of the American Medical Association 288(16), 1955–1958 (2002)
3. AbouZahr, C., Boerma, T.: Health information systems: the foundations of public health. Bulletin of the World Health Organization 83, 578–583 (2005)
4. Hersh, W.: Health care information technology progress and barriers. Journal of the American Medical Association 292(18), 2273–2274 (2004)
5. O'Carroll, P., Yasnoff, W., Ward, E., Ripp, L., Martin, E.: Public Health Informatics and Information Systems. Springer, New York (2003)
6. Hey, T., Trefethen, A.: The UK e-science core programme and the grid. Future Generation Computer Systems 18(8), 1017–1031 (2002)
7. Stockinger, H.: Dening the grid: a snapshot on the current view. The Journal of Supercomputing 42(1), 3–17 (2007)
8. Foster, I., Kesselman, C.: The Grid: Blueprint for a New Computing Infrastructure. Morgan Kaufmann, San Francisco (1999)
9. Stevens, R., Robinson, A., Goble, C.: myGrid: personalised bioinformatics on the information grid. Bioinformatics 19(90001), 302–304 (2003)
10. Fraser, M.: Virtual research environments: overview and activity. Ariadne (2005)
11. Chin Jr., G., Lansing, C.: Capturing and supporting contexts for scientic data sharing via the biological sciences collaboratory. In: Proceedings of the 2004 ACM conference on Computer supported cooperative work, pp. 409–418. ACM, New York (2004)
12. Moreau, L., Freire, J., Futrelle, J., McGrath, R., Myers, J., Paulson, P.: The open provenance model. Technical Report, University of Southampton (2007)
13. De Roure, D., Goble, C., Aleksejevs, S., Bechhofer, S., Bhagat, J., Cruickshank, D., Fisher, P., Hull, D., Michaelides, D., Newman, D., et al.: Towards Open Science: The myExperiment approach. Concurrency and Computation: Practice and Experience (in press, 2009)
14. Lagoze, C., Van de Sompel, H., Johnston, P., Nelson, M., Sanderson, R., Warner, S.: Open Archives Initative Object Reuse and Exchange (OAI-ORE). Technical report, Open Archives Initative (2007), http://www.openarchives.org/ore/0.1/toc
15. Star, S., Griesemer, J.: Institutional ecology, translations and boundary objects: Amateurs and professionals in Berkeleys Museum of Vertebrate Zoology, 1907-39. Social studies of science, 387–420 (1989)
16. James, P., Leach, R., Kalamara, E., Shayeghi, M.: The worldwide obesity epidemic. Obesity 9(11s), 228S–233S (2001)
17. Canoy, D., Buchan, I.: Challenges in obesity epidemiology. Obesity Reviews 8(s1), 1–11 (2007)
18. Deldereld, M., Kitching, L., Smith, G., Hoyle, D., Buchan, I.: Shared Genomics: Accessible High Performance Computing for Genomic Medical Research. In: IEEE Fourth International Conference on eScience, 2008. eScience 2008, pp. 404–405 (2008)

19. Bates, D., Gawande, A.: Improving safety with information technology. New England Journal of Medicine 348(25), 2526–2534 (2003)
20. Morabia, A. (ed.): A History of Epidemiologic Methods and Concepts. Birkhauser Verlag, Basel (2004)
21. Bishop, C.: Pattern recognition and machine learning. Springer, New York (2006)
22. Unal, B., Critchley, J., Capewell, S., Liverpool, U.: IMPACT, a validated, comprehensive coronary heart disease model. Technical Report, University of Liverpool, United Kingdom (2006),
    http://www.liv.ac.uk/PublicHealth/sc/bua/IMPACT-Model-Appendices.pdf
23. O'Keefe, C., Yung, M., Gu, L., Baxter, R.: Privacy-preserving data linkage protocols. In: Proceedings of the 2004 ACM workshop on Privacy in the electronic society, pp. 94–102. ACM, New York (2004)
24. Elliot, M., Purdam, K., Smith, D.: Patient record data: Statistical disclosure control for grid based data access. In: Proceedings of the second international conference on e-Social Science (2006)
25. Obesity e-Lab, http://www.obesityelab.org.uk

Mandatory and Location-Aware Access Control for Relational Databases

Michael Decker

Institute AIFB, University of Karlsruhe (TH)
Kaiserstr. 89, 76 128 Karlsruhe, Germany
decker@aifb.uni-karlsruhe.de

Abstract. Access control is concerned with determining which operations a particular user is allowed to perform on a particular electronic resource. For example, an access control decision could say that user *Alice* is allowed to perform the operation *read* (but not *write*) on the resource *research report*. With conventional access control this decision is based on the user's identity whereas the basic idea of Location-Aware Access Control (LAAC) is to evaluate also a user's current location when making the decision if a particular request should be granted or denied. LAAC is an interesting approach for mobile information systems because these systems are exposed to specific security threads like the loss of a device. Some data models for LAAC can be found in literature, but almost all of them are based on RBAC and none of them is designed especially for Database Management Systems (DBMS). In this paper we therefore propose a LAAC-approach for DMBS and describe a prototypical implementation of that approach that is based on database triggers.

Keywords: Location-based Services, Database Management Systems (DBMS), Mandatory Access Control (MAC), Mobile Computing, Security Models.

1 Introduction

Location-based Services (LBS) [14] are services for mobile computers (e.g. PDA, smartphones) that evaluate the user's location to provide the service. A standard example for a LBS is that of a Point-of-Interest-Finder service which guides a user to a facility of a particular category (e.g. restaurant, monument, pharmacy) in his nearer surrounding. The realization of LBS is enabled by the availability of techniques to determine a mobile computer's location. Examples for such locating systems are the satellite-based *Global Positioning System (GPS)* or special systems for indoor locating based on infrared light or ultrasound waves. A good overview concerning various locating technologies can be found in [14]. Our work concentrates on a special kind of LBS called *Location-Aware Access Control* (LAAC). Access control in the domain of computer systems means to determine if a user is allowed to perform a particular operation on a particular resource or not [11]. For example, the access control component of a computer

R. Mehmood et al. (Eds.): EuropeComm 2009, LNICST 16, pp. 217–228, 2009.
© Institute for Computer Science, Social-Informatics and Telecommunications Engineering 2009

system could prohibit that user Alice performs the operation *read* on the resource *payroll file*. The special idea of LAAC is that for an access control decision also (or even only) the current location of the user is considered [8]. Using LAAC we could enforce the policy that a user is only allowed to access a file with confidential business data while he stays at the premises of the company.

To implement access control a special data model is needed to manage the rules in a way that can be understood by human administrators as well as the computer system; such a model is called *Access Control Model* (ACM). A simple form of an ACM is the *Access Control Matrix* where each row represents one user and each column one resource [11]. Each element in the matrix then lists operations the respective user is allowed to perform on that resource.

In this article we introduce a novel ACM for Database Management Systems (DBMS) that is location-aware and follows the principle of Mandatory Access Control (MAC). In MAC-based systems users and data objects have security labels. The system then allows or forbids operations a user wants to perform on a particular resource depending on rules that evaluate the label of both resource and user. While there are several papers proposing location-aware ACM (LAACM) that are extensions of RBAC, there are almost no publications dealing with LAACM that implement the MAC or DAC concept. Further there is considerable work concerning ACM for DBMS (e.g. [10,16]), but none of them is location-aware.

The remainder of the article is organized as follows: In the next section 2 we discuss some basics concerning access control and relational database management systems. For the description of a LAACM we need a location model that is introduced in section 3. The main contribution of our article is a location-ware ACM for DBMS in section 4. Section 5 is devoted to a description of a prototypical implementation of the model. Related work is covered in section 6 before we conclude in section 7.

2   Basics

2.1   Mandatory Access Control

In the pertinent literature like [11] usually three groups of ACM are distinguished: Discretionary Access Control (DAC), Mandatory Access Control (MAC) and Role-Based Access Control (RBAC). Since the novel ACM proposed in this paper is a MAC model we give only a superficial discussion of DAC and RBAC before MAC is introduced in more detail.

DAC is the approach implemented by most conventional file systems (e.g. those of MS Windows and Linux): The creator/owner of a resource has all permissions for a resource and it is on his *discretion* to give permissions on this resource to other users (and maybe revoke them later). For example, if *Alice* created a file she could grant the permission for the operation *read* to her colleague *Bob*. The *Access Control Matrix* mentioned above is an ACM for DAC.

The basic idea of RBAC is that job descriptions within an organization rarely change but the assignment of jobs to people changes quite often, e.g. employee hired, fired or promoted [11]. So there are *roles* as mediators between users and permissions: roles are created according to job descriptions (e.g. role "secretary", role "manager") and are assigned to the set of permissions that is necessary to fulfil that job. Then users are assigned to roles; however, it is forbidden to assign users directly to permissions. Contemporary variants of RBAC also support *Role Hierarchies* and *Separation of Duties (SoD)*, i.e. sets of roles can be defined that are mutually exclusive at administration time (static SoD) or at runtime (dynamic SoD).

The "mandatory" in "MAC" means that access control rules are imposed by the system without the demand that end users have to (or even can) configure permissions on resources. To implement MAC we need security labels that are assigned to users and resources. If a user wants to perform an operation on a resource the MAC-system will make its decision based on a consideration of both the user's and the resource's labels. To exemplify this we assume the following ordered set of security labels: $Top\ Secret \succ Secret \succ Confidential \succ Public$. If a resource (say an electronic document) is classified as *Secret* then a user with clearance *Secret* or even *Top Secret* would be allowed to read that document; however, a user with lower clearance like *Confidential* or just *Public* wouldn't get read access.

This read rule is called *no-read-up* and actually enforced by the most prominent MAC model, namely the Bell-LaPadula-model [11]. The model has also a rule for write operations which seems to be counterintuitive at the first glance: a user is only allowed to write to a resource if the resource's security label is higher than the user's security clearance. The reason behind this *no-write-down* rule is that it should be prevented that a user (or a Trojan Horse working with the user's permissions) reads data and writes them to resources with lower security level so that users with a lower clearance than that of the original data could gain access. The security labels for the Bell-LaPadula model have not only the above mentioned hierarchical component, but also a non-hierarchical component. This non-hierarchical component is an unordered set of thematic categories like *finance, chemistry* or *nuclear*. If we have two security labels $X = (A, B)$ and $Y = (A', B')$ where A and A' are elements of the hierarchical component and B and B' is from the non-hierarchical component then X dominates Y iff: $Y \preceq X \iff (A' \preceq A \wedge B' \subseteq B)$.

While the Bell-LaPadula-Model is a MAC-model to ensure the secrecy of data there are also models that were developed for the purpose of enforcing the integrity of the managed data. The most prominent model for integrity is the Biba-model [2]: one of its rule is called *no-write-up*, i.e. a user is not allowed to write into an object with a higher integrity level. The rationale for this is that it should be prevented that a user at a low integrity level "pollutes" a data object at a higher integrity level with inferior data.

MAC is usually combined with DAC to absorb configuration mistakes in the DAC configuration. For many years MAC was only applied to secure information systems used by organizations like military and intelligence service. However, nowadays there are MAC implementation for "ordinary" computer systems available, e.g. Security-Enhanced Linux (SE-Linux). In section 6 presenting "Related Work" we will also mention a few database systems that support MAC.

2.2 Basics of DBMS

A DBMS is a special software system designed to store and manage a large amount of structured data records in an efficient way [10]. The management aspect includes especially the capability for the retrieval of data records that meet dynamically specified conditions. Further, a modern DBMS should be able to handle concurrent requests by many users. Nowadays the prevalent paradigm for DBMS is the relational model: the basic idea of this concept is that data is stored in tables; a database can be considered as a collection of tables (also called *relations*). Each table defines columns of a specified data type and stores the data records as rows. It is further possible that one record of a table references a row in another table (foreign key relationship).

More formally, the tables and their actual rows are considered as relations of a particular relation schema $R(A_1, A_2, \ldots, A_n)$. Each attribute A_i is the name of one column that contains values of a particular domain denoted by $dom(A_i)$. Such a domain could be the set of all unsigned 32-bit-integer numbers or of all character strings with a maximum length of nine characters. For a relation schema R the function $r()$ returns the relation or the current state of a table, i.e. all the tuples or rows t_i: $r(R) = \{t_1, t_2, \ldots, t_m\}$. To refer to the value of attribute A_j of tuple t_i we write $t_i.A_j$. The set of all relation schemas is denoted by $\mathbb{R}$, i.e. $\mathbb{R} = \{R_1, R_2, \ldots, R_k\}$.

Today most DBMS support the Structured Query Language (SQL), a declarative command-language to manage the database's structure (e.g. to set up new tables), to insert, update and query the data and for administrative commands like granting permissions on database objects to users. DBMS usually have also some kind of access control that follows the DAC approach: The creator of a database object (e.g. a table) as owner of that object can grant permissions on that object to other users. For a table for example one usually can grant permissions for individual operations like viewing (selecting), updating, inserting or deleting data rows. This is supported by special SQL commands, namely GRANT and REVOKE.

3 Location-Model

For our work so far the following simple location model is sufficient (figure 1): The geometric locations of the model describe a polygon that is a non-empty subset of the reference space called *universe*. Since with a polygon each spatial extent can be approximated as precise as demanded the restriction to use only polygons is a weak one. A polygon together with a name like *London* or *England* is called *location instance* or *location* for short. Locations are grouped in *location classes*: each location instance belongs to exactly one location class. This principle can be also found in the geographic markup language (GML) where each feature (object with spatial dimension) belongs to a feature type [15]. Also many systems that provide support to visually work with geographical data like maps (e.g. Geographic Information Systems (GIS)) support the concept of several layers that can be switched on and off individually; each of these layers usually contains

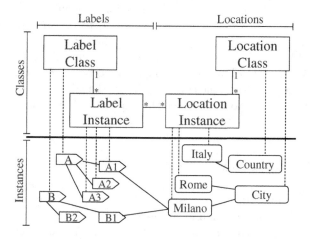

Fig. 1. Location model

the spatial objects of one type (or location class), e.g. there is one layer for the streets and another one for forest areas. From the perspective of object-oriented software design this is also a natural principle.

Formally, L is the set of all location classes and l the set of all location instances. The function $\lambda()$ maps a location class to the set of all its instances. With $\mathbb{P}(l)$ as the power set of all locations instances (i.e. the set of a all possible subsets of l including the empty set $\emptyset$) this can be written as follows: $\lambda : L \rightarrow \mathbb{P}(l)$.

To exemplify the model we consider the following set of location classes: $L = \{universeclass, cities, countries\}$ For location class *cities* we have two instances $\lambda(cities) = \{London, Milano\}$ and for location class *countries* there are also two instances: $\lambda(countries) = \{U.K., Italy\}$. For all the location instances of a given location class two properties have to hold: (1) Two location instances do not overlap spatially; (2) The union of all location instances covers the universe completely. These two properties guarantee that for a given location class and a given point we always can determine exactly one location instance belonging to that class which covers this point.

We further need different classes of security labels which in turn have instances. A security label class corresponds approximately to the compartments (component with unordered labels) found in the Bell-LaPadula-model [1]. Using the security label instances of one security class we can classify documents and locations under the view of a particular topic or domain. The number of different labels for each class may vary and is defined in the security class whereas the strictest label has always the value "1"; the remaining classes have the following natural number $2, 3, \ldots, n \in \mathbb{N}$. As example we consider a company operating plants in all European countries that produces two types of main products A and B. In some countries the company has to fear espionage because there are local companies that are also active in the market for these product. The company therefore defines two classes of labels: $S = \{A, B\}$. To obtain the subset of label instances from the set of all labels s for a given class from S there is function: $\sigma : S \rightarrow \mathbb{P}(s) \setminus \emptyset$. Label class A is used to classify data records and location instances according to product A and has $|\sigma(A)| = 3$ labels, namely $\sigma(A) = \{A1, A2, A3\}$. Countries were no espionage has to be feared will get a clearance of $A1$; if a mild level of espionage has to be feared because of a small competitor in a country then the country will get the label $A2$; however, if strong espionage activities have to be assumed the label $A3$ will be assigned as clearance to the country.

4   LAACM for DBMS

The novel ACM for DBMS proposed in the article at hand supplements the basic DAC by allowing to assign location-constraints (LC) to individual rows in a table. A row with such a location-constraint can only be accessed when the user currently stays at a location which is in accordance with that LC. Because we are following the MAC approach these LC are created automatically by the runtime system when the respective data row is created and inserted into a table. Further it is not possible to alter or remove such a location-constraint by an usual administrative operation. Our MAC models supports *direct* and *indirect* LC so far:

Direct LC (DLC): For this case each individual row of a table obtains a LC that restricts the access to that row to users who currently stay within a particular location-instance. To activate the creation of DLC for a table $R \in \mathbb{R}$, the table has to point to one location class: $\rho_1 : R \rightarrow L \cup \emptyset$. When a user inserts a new row into this table the instance $l \in \lambda(L)$ that covers the current location of that user is looked up and assigned to this row as location constraint.

Indirect LC (ILC): For this case security labels can be attached to each individual row of a table. To activate the creation of ILC the table R has to point to at least one security label class: $\rho_2 : R \rightarrow \mathbb{P}(S)$. When a user inserts a new row to a table the runtime system determines all location instances that cover the user's current position. Since it is demanded that two location instances of the same location class don't overlap each other, this implies that we'll get not more than one instance of each location class. Afterwards it is evaluated if security labels belonging to one of the security classes returned by $\rho_2(R)$ are assigned to the location instances. If such labels are found they will be attachted to the newly inserted row. Access to this row will then only be granted when the user stays in a location whose security labels are at least as high as those assigned to the row.

To obtain a list of of all LC assigned to a given row of a table we introduce the functions τ_1 and τ_2. The first function is for DLC and returns DLC the locations where access to that row is allowed: $\tau_1 : t \rightarrow \mathbb{P}(l)$. If no DLC is assigned to that row the empty set will be returned. This means that the respective row can be accessed at all locations. The second function τ_2 returns a possible empty set of all security labels assigned to a row: $\tau_2 : t \rightarrow \mathbb{P}(s)$.

5   Implementation

For the prototypical implementation we chose PostgreSQL[1] (PG) for several reasons: PG is known as the most powerful open source DBMS and provides a good implementation of the pertinent standards. Its PostGIS-plugin[2] offers an excellent implementation of the OGC's *Simple Features Specification* [15], which is an extension for SQL to work with spatial data.

We developed an implementation of the proposed ACM using PG's support for procedural programming, namely the PL/pgSQL language to write so called *Stored Procedures*. Stored procedures not only encapsulate sequences of conventional SQL commands, they also provide the common features of modern high-level programming languages like loops, variables and if-then-else-decisions. The implementation and the source code fragments presented in this section will only work with PG, but it should be easy to transfer the basic principle to most other modern DBMS.

Our implementation (figure 2) relies heavily on database triggers: triggers allow the definition of stored procedures that are invoked when particular events occur. For our work the events of interest are insertion-, update- und delete-operations on tables. In the body of a trigger procedure there are variables to query the name of the table that raised the event or to access old or new data rows. Using trigger procedures we can prevent the execution of an operation on a database table. This is of interest for update and delete operations on a table row that should be inhibited according to our MAC because the mobile user doesn't stay at the right location. A trigger for insert operations can be employed to set up the location restriction upon creation of a new row in a location-aware table. To prevent read-operations of table rows we would need to set up a triggers on select. However, neither the SQL standard nor PG support select-triggers. As workaround for this problem we resort to *views*. A view presents the result of a SQL-statement like a real table. In this way subsets or combinations of data rows stored in tables can be offered to the user. The command to create a view named v_table1 which hides the rows from the user according to our model is:

```
CREATE OR REPLACE VIEW v_table1 AS
    SELECT * FROM table1 WHERE is_access_allowed (oid, tableoid);
```

This view returns all the columns of *table1*, but may hide rows when the function is_access_allowed() returns *false*. The system parameters oid and tableoid are passed to this function: oid is a row number that is assigned for each row in a table. However, it is not guaranteed that oid is unique over all tables. That's why we also consider tableoid, which is an unique id for each table so a pair of this two id-numbers uniquely identifies a table row in a PG database. We use tableoid as column in a system table named table2locclass that implements the mapping ρ_1 that can assign a location class to a table to activate DLC. An DLC for a table row is stored as row in table named DLC with a pair (oid,tableoid) and a reference to a location instance.

---

[1] http://www.postgresql.org
[2] http://postgis.refractions.net

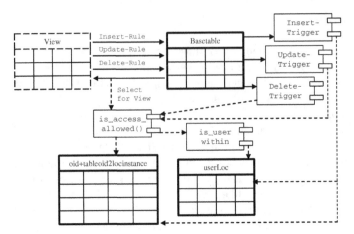

Fig. 2. Main components of the implementation

However, the user should be able not only to query data from a view but also to alter the data of a view respective the basetable behind the view. To enable this PG's rules-feature can be used to redirect insert, update and delete commands performed on the view to the respective basetable. For example, the rule for the insert command looks like this:

```
CREATE OR REPLACE RULE "ins2tab1rule"
    AS ON INSERT TO table1 DO INSTEAD
    INSERT INTO table1 (id ,name) values (NEW.ID ,NEW.name)
```

To work with spatial data we employ PG's PostGIS-plugin which provides an implementation of the OGC's SQL extension for spatial data. As example we take the table `locinstance` which is used to store the location instances (set l according to our formalization): We first create the table using the SQL's conventional **CREATE**-command and then add a column named `polygon` for storing the location instances with the following function call:

```
SELECT AddGeometryColumn (
    'locinstance', 'polygon', −1,'POLYGON', 2);
```

The parameters have the following meanings (in that order): (1) name of the target table, (2) name of the column to create, (3) numeric code (SRID) specifying the employed coordinate system, (4) data type of the new column and (5) dimension of the employed data type. To insert a row into this table we use the following statement:

```
INSERT INTO locinstance values (1, 'District1', 4,
    GeometryFromText( 'POLYGON((0  0, 5  0, 5  10, 0  10, 0  0))'));
```

The elements in the values-expression specify the following things: (1) ID of the location instance, (2) name of the location instance, (3) integer specifying the location class (foreign key reference to table `locclass`), (4) definition of the polygon using a string expression following the *Well-Known Text (WKT)* representation by enumerating the points that span the polygon. The user's current position is stored in a table called `userloc` where each tuple contains amongst other attributes a user name and a point. We assume that the employed locating system (e.g. GPS) updates this value when appropriate. With the **&&**-operator we can test if two geometries overlap. As example we show the statement that lists for each combination of location class and user the location instance that covers the user's current location.

```
select * from userloc , locclass , locinstance
    where locinstance.locclass=locclass.id and
    locinstance.polygon && userloc.location
```

Another approach for the implementation of the model would be to use PGACE (PostgreSQL Access Control Extension), an interface offered by PG to implement custom access control. This interface was introduced for the implementation of SE-PG, the MAC extension of PG (see next section). However, using this interface requires programming in C/C++ which is more prone to errors and doesn't allow the comfortable usage of PostGIS. Also PGACE is a PG-specific interface so that a MAC system implemented with PGACE cannot be transferred to other DBMS implementations.

6   Related Work

Gallagher [12] developed an extension for SQL's DAC that allows to specify location constraints when granting and revoking permissions to users. Using this extension a grant-command can have an *inside*-clause to restrict the permission assigned to a user to a particular region, e.g. GRANT SELECT ON TAB1 TO ALICE INSIDE AREA1. The meaning of this command is to allow user alice to perform the select-command on table `tab1` when she is inside the location referred by `area1`. To the best of our knowledge Gallagher's work is the only approach for LAAC especially for DBMS so far.

In a paper by Casati et al. [3] a DBMS with triggers is employed to implement autorization constraints in workflows by using triggers to enforce workflow-specific access rules like "separation of duties": if a user performed a step of a workflow instance he is not allowed to perform a particular other step for the same workflow instance, e.g. for the handling of the order the company's policy could demand that the user who performed "prepare shipment" mustn't perform "check shipment" for the same workflow instance because a shipment should always be seen by two different employees before it is dispatched. So if a user performs a task that implies a "separation of duties" rule a trigger inserts a row into a table that records which users for which workflow instances are not allowed to perform particular activities.

In [17] the only proposal of a LAACM following the MAC-approach which we are aware of can be found; however, this model wasn't designed with DBMS as special focus. In this model, security levels are assigned to users, electronic resources and locations. If a location lies within another one the inner location needs to have at least the security level of the outer location, e.g. if a building is classified as "Secret" an room within that building cannot be classified below, e.g. as "Confidential". Further, the model assumes that resources are classified manually and prohibits that a resource is stored at a location that has a lower security level than the resource itself.

The most prominent example for a DBMS with MAC is *Seaview* [16]. This model considers secrecy and integrity, however, for the sake of simplicity we only discuss secrecy here. To each row and each single attribute instance a security label is assigned. Depending on his security label a user may not be able to see all rows in a table or all attributes in a row. However, if he wants to insert a row into a table that has the same primary key as a row invisible to him this operation cannot be rejected because in this case the user could infer that there is a hidden row. This means that the row has to be inserted regardless of the fact that this leads to multiple rows with the same primary key (but with different security labels). The term for this phenomenon is *polyinstantiation*. Polyinstantiation can also occur when rows are updated. Further, it is demanded that if a user is able to see any of the elements of a row he is also able to see the primary key elements of that row, i.e. every non-key attribute in a row has to dominate the primary key attributes. Some other MAC models for DBMS can be found in [4].

There are some research contributions that propose location-aware extensions of ACM. Almost all of these works cover RBAC-extensions, e.g. GEO-RBAC, SRBAC, LoT-RBAC or STRBAC. GEO-RBAC [6] allows to switch roles on and off depending on the mobile user's current location. However, in SRBAC the assignment between individual roles and permissions is enabled/disabled according to the user's current location [13]. A survey providing on these models can be found in [8]; this paper also discusses some scenarios for LAAC. However, none of these models provides special support for DBMS.

SE-PostgreSQL is a variant of PG that provides MAC but it runs only on SE-Linux. The strict coupling between DBMS and OS enables to keep the security context of users and data objects between the OS and the DBMS. For example, if a user reads a classified file from the filesystem of SE-Linux and stores it into a database table the classification of this file isn't lost. But there is also another lightweight MAC-implementation for PG called *Veil*[3] that doesn't require that the PG installation runs on SE-Linux. SE PG doesn't provide location-aware MAC. For the other popular Open-Source DBMS, namely MySQL, no MAC-support was implemented at all. MAC is available for the two most popular commercial DBMS, namely *IBM DB2* and *Oracle*, but these MAC implementations do not support location-awareness, too. MAC was introduced as *Label Based Access Control* in Version 9 of *IBM DB2*. The other popular commercial DBMS, Oracle, also offers MAC and calls it *Fine Grained Access Control (FGAC)*. These MAC implementations offer several types of security labels, e.g. as unordered or ordered lists and as hierarchical components. But neither DB2 nor Oracle support location-aware MAC.

Implementing access control based on the determination of a user's location raises the question how resistant a locating system is with regard to manipulation attempts. Deliberate manipulation attempts to forge a mobile user's location are

---

[3] http://veil.projects.postgresql.org

called *location spoofing*. One method to prevent this kind of spoofing is to demand that the mobile device sends some kind of information to the backend system that can only be received at the alleged location, e.g. signals emitted by beacons, e.g. [5]. Another method is to measure the time needed by a mobile device to send back a response that is based on a request that cannot be predicted, e.g. [18]. These *request-response-protocols* are especially interesting if radio waves are employed, because currently no technique is know to send data at a higher speed. An overview on different approaches to harden locating systems against spoofing attacks can be found in [9].

If a mobile user is constantly located for the purpose of LAAC by his employer's information system this raises concerns regarding data protection. In [7] we therefore survey several approaches to tackle this *location privacy* problem.

7   Conclusion: Summary and Outlook

We motivated the need location-aware access control and introduced a novel Access Control Model (ACM) for database management systems. The ACM is a mandatory access control model, i.e. its works "behind the scenes" and doesn't require manual configuration by the user. It allows to restrict the access to individual rows stored in database tables to particular locations.

Ideas for further work include rules distinguishing different operations or assigning different location restrictions to different user groups, e.g. a service technician is only allowed to edit the document in the building where it was created while an executive manager can do this as long as he is in the same country. Our model so far only supports positive restrictions, i.e. it makes a statement where something is allowed. But it is also thinkable to have additional negative restrictions, i.e. restrictions that state where something is forbidden. However, when positive and negative restrictions can be used together contradictions may occur that have to be handled.

References

1. Bell, D.E., LaPadula, L.J.: Secure Computer System: Unified Exposition and Multics Interpretation. Technical Report MTR-2997, The MITRE Corporation (1976)
2. Biba, K.J.: Integrity Considerations for Secure Computer Systems. Technical Report MTR-3153, The MITRE Corporation (1976)
3. Casati, F., Castano, S., Fugini, M.G.: Managing Workflow Authorization Constraints through Active Database Technology. Information Systems Frontiers 3(3), 319–338 (2001)
4. Castano, S., Fugini, M., Martella, G., Samarati, P.: Database Security. Addison-Wesley, Wokingham (1994)
5. Cho, Y., Bao, L., Goodrich, M.T.: LAAC: A Location-Aware Access Control Protocol. In: Third Annual International Conference on Mobile and Ubiquitous Systems: Networking & Services, pp. 1–7 (2006)
6. Damiani, M.L., Bertino, E., Perlasca, P.: Data Security in Location-Aware Applications: An Approach Based on RBAC. International Journal of Information and Computer Security 1(1/2), 5–38 (2007)

7. Decker, M.: Location Privacy – An Overview. In: Proceedings of the International Conference on Mobile Business (ICMB 2008), Barcelona, Spain. IEEE, Los Alamitos (2008)
8. Decker, M.: Location-Aware Access Control: An Overview. In: Proceedings of the Conference on Wireless Applications and Computing (WAC 2009), Carvoeiro, Portugal, pp. 75–82 (2009)
9. Decker, M.: Prevention of Location-Spoofing. A Survey on Different methods to Prevent the Manipulation of Locating-Technologies. In: Proceedings of the International Conference on e-Business (ICE-B), Milano, Italy, pp. 109–114. INSTICC (2009)
10. Elmasri, R., Navathe, S.: Fundamentals of Database Systems, 4th edn. Pearson, Boston (2004)
11. Ferraiolo, D.F., Kuhn, D.R., Chandramouli, R.: Role-Based Access Control, 2nd edn. Artech House, Boston (2007)
12. Gallagher, M.: Location-based authorization. Master's thesis, University of Minnesota (2002)
13. Hansen, F., Oleshchuk, V.: SRBAC: A Spatial Role-Based Access Control Model for Mobile Systems. In: Proceedings of the Nordic Workshop on Secure IT Systems (NORDSEC), Gjovik, Norway, pp. 129–141 (2003)
14. Küpper, A.: Location-based Services – Fundamentals and Operation. John Wiley & Sons, Chichester (Reprint, 2007)
15. Lake, R., Burggraf, D.S., Trninic, M., Rae, L.: GML. Geography Mark-Up Language. Foundation for the Geo-Web. John Wiley & Sons, Chichester (2004)
16. Lunt, T.F., Denning, D.E., Schell, R.R., Heckman, M., Shockley, W.R.: The seaview security model. IEEE Trans. Softw. Eng. 16(6), 593–607 (1990)
17. Ray, I., Kumar, M.: Towards a Location-based Mandatory Access Control Model. Computers & Security 25(1), 36–44 (2006)
18. Sastry, N., Shankar, U., Wagner, D.: Secure Verification of Location Claims. In: Proceedings of the 2nd ACM Workshop on Wireless Security (WiSE 2003), San Diego, California, USA, pp. 1–10 (2003)

The Interaction of Production and Consumption in the News Media Social Space

Gary Graham[1], Finola Kerrigan[2], Rashid Mehmood[3], and Mustafizur Rahman[4]

[1] Manchester Business School, University of Manchester, Manchester M15 6PB, UK
gary.graham@mbs.ac.uk
[2] Department of Management, King's College London, London WC2R 2LS, UK
finola.kerrigan@kcl.ac.uk
[3] School of Engineering, Swansea University, Singleton Park, Swansea SA2 8PP, UK
r.mehmood@swansea.ac.uk
[4] Oxford e-Research Centre, University of Oxford, Keble Road, Oxford, OX1 3QG, UK
mustafizur.rahman@begbroke.ox.ac.uk

Abstract. Newspapers are operating in increasingly competitive and fragmented markets for audiences and advertising revenues, government media policy and changing audience requirements for news and the ways in which it is presented and delivered. A growing army of bloggers and amateur citizen journalists now delivers – but rarely edits – content for all media platforms, while new media technologies, combined with the changing structure of global news industries, are radically changing the ways in which newspapers and media business functions and struggles for profitability. Our research sought to answer the question of how the internet is impacting on producer/consumer value activities in the news media supply chain. To answer this question initial descriptive statistical analysis was performed on 51 newspapers. This was followed by a focus group undertaken with London-based news media organizations and bloggers. The findings showed that in spite of initial fear and rejection, the internet is now firmly embedded in news media supply chain operations. Firms are now using the internet as an operant resource and working proactively with consumers to develop various forms of relationship value. We highlight the role of consumers in the creation of news (editorial) content and consumer-driven moves toward a merged media platform of distribution (including television, online, mobile and printed forms). Regional news media organizations will probably continue to survive if they are able to supply a highly specialized and 'hyper local' community service. This will be in the form of 'hybrid' content: analysis, interpretation and investigative reporting in a print product that appears less than daily combined with constant updating and reader interaction on the web.

Keywords: Emerging Web Applications, News Social Media, Statistical Analysis, Innovation Processes, Digital Economy.

1 Introduction

The sustained decline in circulation, sales and readers for print editions of newspapers, coupled with the more recent challenge to advertising revenues posed by the

R. Mehmood et al. (Eds.): EuropeComm 2009, LNICST 16, pp. 229–239, 2009.
© Institute for Computer Science, Social-Informatics and Telecommunications Engineering 2009

internet, has prompted pundits to speculate about the fortunes of news media suppliers (Currah, 2009; Economist, 2006: 57-59). For instance, a rapid decline in reader numbers has been observed in regional newspapers: sales declined from 2.1 billion in 2000 to 1.7 billion in 2005 (Mintel, 2007). This decline is predicted to continue so that by 2010 sales will have fallen further to 1.4 billion copies. News media firms are changing and adapting their content, style and design, in response to the challenges they confront in an increasingly competitive and fragmented market for consumers and advertisers (Franklin, 2008). Furthermore, it is suggested by Freer (2007) that the biggest challenge facing the news media firm today is the changing means of distribution of news through the new media platforms of the internet and telephony, "... which deliver news, blogs, text alerts, news updates, podcasts and user-generated content (UGC) to 'consumers' at a greater pace; in more accessible formats and when consumers demand them" (ibid.,:101).

Our research therefore sought to investigate the important influence of the internet on the news media supply chain and the producer/consumer intersection. The paper is structured as follows: Section 2 presents the theoretical model and research aims; Section 3 outlines the research design and methodology; Section 4 presents the results of univariate analysis on a random sample of news media organizations while Section 5 provides a number of insights from focus group research; Section 6 concludes by reviewing the findings and assessing the strategic implications of the internet for news media suppliers.

2 Theoretical Model and Research Aims

Figure 1 presents the guiding theoretical model for this work. This model is derived from marketing theory grounded in debates on co-creation (Vargo & Lusch, 2004; Vargo &Lusch, 2006; Sawhney & Prandelli, 2000; Prahalad & Ramaswamy, 2004); operations management (Martinez, 2003; Martinez & Bititchi, 2006), value chains (Porter, 1985; 2001); and newspaper industry research (Hill, 2007; Clemons & Lang, 2003; Lowrey, 2007).

The theoretical model implies that there are a number of different environmental and objective factors impacting on the value creation system for a regional news media supply chain. The size of readership and level of advertising revenues directly impact on the profitability of news media firm supply chain operations. Actors who are participating in supplying raw materials and product distribution include: print manufacturers; ink and paper suppliers; distributors; trade associations and retailers.

There are also a number of external influences: stories are community sourced from the general public, police, courts and local government (though this view has been revised by Picard (2004) to include the increasing amount of local news content sourcing from interest groups and public relations professionals). The thick double headed arrow highlights the potential for value co-creation activities between firm, consumer and blogging community. However, the literature indicates a note of caution regarding the motivation of pro/consumers in their interactions with news organisations and the spaces within which such interaction takes place (Freer, 2007; Ofcom, 2008).

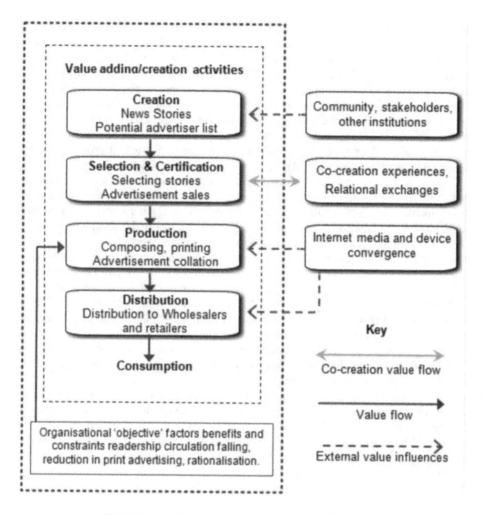

Fig. 1. A theoretical model of the news media value chain

The internet is clearly driving many convergences in media and devices. For instance, newspapers are increasingly being produced and distributed in multi-media formats (including television, online, mobile and printed forms) and this is leading to a relaxing of the rigid structuring of their missions, routines, practices, and relationships (Klinenberg, 2005). In addition, the traditional divide between production and consumption which influenced marketing thought is being eroded and marketing scholars (Prahalad & Ramaswamy, 2004; Vargo & Lusch, 2004; 2006) are now considering issues such as co-creation as central to our understanding of marketing, particularly when considering the online environment (Prahalad & Ramaswamy, 2004; Sawhney et al., 2005).

The aim of this paper is to understand the impact of UGC on the traditional newspaper supply chain; to examine the perception of consumer engagement and value creation within the online environment and to question the manner within which newspapers organisations are engaging with consumers within the online environment. In posing these questions, our research will engage with the new dominant logic of services marketing as initially proposed by Vargo and Lusch (2004) and its further refinement by them (Vargo & Lusch, 2006). Taking the newspaper industry as the research setting, is highly appropriate, as what was once a physical product - the newspaper - has now itself transformed into a service experience (news provision) which is delivered in a variety of ways. Therefore, our paper contributes to marketing theory through exploring the transformation of products into services in the digital economy, rather than a simple increase in the service dimension of products as discussed by Vargo and Lusch (2004).

While their work and those which followed have focused on the goods/service divide, this paper considers moving forward to embrace the notion of goods and services being intertwined. Additionally, Vargo and Lusch (ibid.,:1) introduced the idea that value can only be created and acknowledged by the consumer in the act of consumption. Value cannot be abstractly defined in isolation from the consumption experience, therefore they move from notions of value in exchange (which has underpinned much marketing thought) to value in use. Vargo and Lusch (2006,:44) introduced a refined notion of 'co-production' referring to the customer as 'co-creator of value' rather than the earlier concept of 'co-production' which critics attributed to a more goods dominated approach. Coupled with co-creation of value, they (ibid.,:48) define 'co-production' as "the participation in the creation of the core offering itself".

This provides the ideal theoretical framework within which to examine the changes to the supply chain which are occurring in the news media industry. Firstly, as stated above, news organizations can be viewed as moving from providers of goods, to providers of services. The traditional 'good', the physical newspaper product is being replaced by the mode of distribution of the service. Secondly, the digital economy is placing the consumer as a central figure in the 'co-production' of media products. The notion of the passive consumer of news content no longer holds in the new fragmented media landscape and Vargo and Lusch's conceptualisation of the co-creation of value in use and co-production can shed light on the changes occurring in this industry.

3 Descriptive Statistical Research of the Regional Newspaper Industry

A sample of 51 firms were selected randomly from the Newspaper Society (industry trade association) database of regional newspaper firms operating in the UK. These were then statistically analysed to present general insights into changes in circulation levels (1995 – 2008), the levels of online/offline convergence, website functionality and interactivity. Further comparisons were made between morning and evening editions and also rural to urban-based publications. These initial insights and findings would be explored further in the focus group.

3.1 Description of the Research Method

A focus group was conducted with a dedicated group of professionals from radio, television and newspaper organizations as well as citizen journalists. This was conducted in London in February 2009 and grounded in the theoretical model in order to generate further insights, knowledge and practical advice. It was important to evaluate the level of awareness of virtual consumer behaviour, perceptions of the role of the consumer in the co-creation of value and co-production processes. In addition, we wished to look further into the interaction with suppliers among news media organisations. The expert focus group technique was selected as the most appropriate method of gathering the data for a number of reasons; for example, it is seen to be ideal for obtaining data about feelings and opinions (Basch, 1987).

The 'radio' group - two participants involved in the production and distribution of offline/online content.
The 'television' group – one participant who develops online content to support evening news programmes.
The 'newspaper' group - two participants who are developing online social (community) eco-systems.
The 'blogging' group – two participants who are professional bloggers providing training programmes to news media organisations.

Fig. 2. Focus Group Participants

The focus group followed Krueger and Casey (2000) in design. Three groups of news media suppliers and one group of bloggers took part in the research (see Figure 2). Group discussion was recorded and later transcribed. From the transcripts, key themes were pulled together to allow comparisons to be made.

3.2 Results of the Statistical Analysis

Table 1 reports the changes in the average newspaper sizes for the sample of newspapers from 1995 to 2008. There has been a steady decline from 64,857 (in 1995) to 41,852 (in 2008). This represents a decline in circulation of -35%. Further research of the sample showed that the decline seems to be greater for the evening newspapers such as the Birmingham Mail (which showed the greatest decline among the sample of -62%) compared to the mornings (who had the lowest decline with the Western Morning News (Plymouth) of -12%). This could be because the mornings have a more targeted readership audience than the evenings. Furthermore it is the urban newspapers in the north (Manchester, Liverpool, Leeds, Sheffield) which seem to be having a much steeper decline than rural area publications (Gloucestershire Echo, Daily Post (North Wales) and The Argus, Sussex). To some extent this could reflect the level of internet penetration being much greater in towns and city areas (Ofcom, 2008).

Table 1. Average newspaper sizes

1995	64857	2003	58767
1996	62113	2004	56438
1997	59583	2005	54795
1998	58194	2006	53014
1999	57083	2007	51111
2001	56528	2008	41,852
2002	58356		
% change: - 35%			

Table 2. Newspaper circulation and website users

Newspaper/Website	Circulation (Daily)	Unique Daily Users
Manchester Evening News – MEN.co.uk	153,724	58,826
The Scotsman – Scotsman.co.uk	49,158	67,959
Western Mail – walesonline.co.uk	33,693	24,655
Liverpool Echo – liverpoolecho.co.uk	97,779	18,266
The Herald, Scotland – theherald.co.uk	60,147	16,244
Liverpool Daily Post – liverpooldailypost.co.uk	12,190	13,649
Birmingham Mail – birminghammail.net	61,526	10,192
Lancashire Evening Post – lep.co.uk	28,275	9,954
Evening Chronicle, Newcastle – chroniclelive.co.uk	67,103	9,754
Yorkshire Post – yorkshirepost.co.uk	45,718	9,569
Nottingham Evening Post – thisisnottingham.co.uk	51,526	9,253
Evening Gazette, Teesside – gazettelive.co.uk	46,692	9,117
The Argus, Sussex – theargus.co.uk	30,070	87,444
Derby Evening Telegraph – thisisderbyshire.co.uk	39,152	8,370
Sheffield Star – thestar.co.uk	47,216	8,202
Evening Times, Glasgow – eveningtimes.co.uk	68,422	8,141
Yorkshire Evening Post – yorkshireveningpost.co.uk	49,064	8136
Hull Daily Mail – thisishull.co.uk	51,886	7,906
The Sentinel, Stoke – thisisthesentinel.co.uk	58,049	7,642
Leicester Mercury – thisisleicestershire.co.uk	64,919	7,412
Bristol Evening Post – thisisbristol.co.uk	46,522	7325
Telegraph & Argus, Bradford – thetelegraphandargus.co.uk	34,042	7,043
The Northern Echo, Darlington – thenorthernecho.co.uk	48,783	7,027
Southern Daily Echo, Southampton – dailyecho.co.uk	36,906	6,999
Coventry Telegraph – coventrytelegraph.net	43,594	6,936
The Gazette, Blackpool – blackpoolgazette.co.uk	26,698	15767
Portsmouth News – Portsmouth.co.uk	49,628	6,730
Birmingham Post – birminghampost.net	12,795	6,696
Sunderland Echo – sunderlandecho.co.uk	39,159	6,634
Western Morning News, Plymouth – thisisplymouth.co.uk	37,819	6,506
Gloucestershire Echo, The Citizen – thisisgloucestershire.co.uk	18,850	6,365
Lancashire Telegraph, Blackburn – lancashiretelegraph.co.uk	28,569	6,350
The Journal, Newcastle – journallive.co.uk	32,859	5,763
Sunday Herald, Scotland – sundayherald.com	41,419	5,584
Daily Post, North Wales – dailypost.co.uk	34,601	5,465

Table 2. (*continued*)

Peterborough Evening Telegraph – peterboroughtoday.co.uk	16,428	5,432
South Wales Evening Post – thisissouthwales.co.uk	47,875	5,225
Oxford Mail – oxfordmail.co.uk	22,402	4,969
The Bolton News – theboltonnews.co.uk	27,540	4,618
Cambridge Evening News – cambridge-news.co.uk	25,195	4,578
The Press, York – thepress.co.uk	31,569	4,396
Grimsby Telegraph – thisisgrimsby.co.uk	31,538	4,102
Lincolnshire Echo – thisislincolnshire.co.uk	20,181	4,073
Evening Courier, Halifax – halifaxcourier.co.uk	19,128	3936
Newsshopper – newsshopper.co.uk	113,504	3784
Reading Evening Post – getreading.co.uk	12,879	3661
Swindon Advertiser – swindonadvertiser.co.uk	20,845	2612
Surrey Advertiser – getsurrey.co.uk	27,472	2332
Scunthorpe Telegraph – thisisscunthorpe.co.uk	18,823	2235
Rochdale Observer – rochdaleobserver.co.uk	35,916	1578
Stockport Express – stockportexpress.co.uk	14,611	1361
Average circulation: 41,852		
Average unique users: 11,123		
Convergence: Multiple 10%, Dual 90%		
Offline/online ratio: 0.3		
Website creation: 2008		
Functionality: 80% UGC, 25% Digital editions, 90% RSS		
Interactivity: 45% blogs, 35% forums, 30% journalist email		

Table 2 presents the daily circulations and website users of the sampled newspapers. The average circulation of the sample is 41,852 while the number of daily unique users registered is 11,123. This gives an offline/online ratio of 0.3. In short, daily physical circulations are three times greater than the number of unique daily website users. This might to some extent reflect the struggles of newspapers in dealing with the influence of the internet on their operations and also a need to improve their functionality and interactivity (Franklin, 2008).

The level of multi-platform convergence in respect to distribution is quite low for the sampled newspapers. While 90% have dual distribution platforms – print and online, only 10% of the sample had 'multiple platforms' of distribution (print/online and either television, mobile or radio). All the multiple platforms were for the larger regional newspapers owned by holding companies notably the Manchester Evening News (Guardian Media Group) and the Liverpool Echo (Trinity Mirror). In the case of the Evening News they operate their own television station, Channel M and the Echo, who broadcast through televisions in the back of taxis in the Liverpool area.

The functionality of the sampled websites is developing quickly. Two thirds of the websites have been redeveloped and redesigned in 2008 and now 80% of them are now offering UGC facilities whereby stories, video and photos can be submitted. 90% of them provide RSS feeds. It is only larger sized firms in the sample which provide digital editions of their publications (Bolton News, Cambridge Evening News). In respect to Zheng's (2002) measures of newspaper interactivity levels are still quite low with only 45% of websites having blogs, 35% discussion forums and 30% having personal journalist email contacts directly linked to articles.

3.3 Focus Group Results: London News Media Organizations

Three key questions were posed during the expert focus group. Firstly, we asked participants about the level of disruption evident in media sector as a result of the development of social media/UGC (changing business models, media operations and the manner of interaction). Secondly, we were interested in the potential for wealth/value creation being generated in these networks and finally, we asked about the organizations, control and management of the interactions between the media organizations.

Some clear consensus emerged from the group. Firstly, there was discussion regarding the term 'disruption' being applied to the changes occurring. Bustamante (2004:805) makes a convincing case for rejecting the notion that the digital economy is a revolutionary disruption which is 'rupturing' old media. The focus group respondents also rejected the notion that changes in the creation, distribution and consumption of news and the concurrent intensification of engagement with the consumer was a disruption; but that it should be more appropriately viewed as a development or innovation. Moving away from the concept of disruption could be seen as acceptance of the new dominant logic being proposed by Vargo and Lusch (2004; 2006). News media organizations were providing spaces within which news consumers could engage with each other and with the news provider. In this way, through providing commentary and proposing news stories, consumers could be seen as enacting their consumption of news through the provision of commentary on news stories. Additionally, news organizations are drawing on consumers in order to fact check and to enhance their own news provision, in effect empowering consumers as the producers of news. This follows Pires et al., (2006) conclusions regarding the role of information and communication technologies in empowering the consumer. In this way, news providers are moving beyond what Fellenz and Brady (2008:43) refer to as "transaction focused ICT use in service delivery". However, the news organizations were aware that 'allowing space' for these activities was in a way a spurious act, as the rise in citizen journalism, blogging and provision of news takes place in consumer produced and controlled environments in addition to branded spaces.

In terms of wealth creation, this was an area of much debate. Consensus appeared around the idea of news organisations developing highly specialised commercially valuable 'news' focusing on specific areas such as finance, technology and offering this to consumers for a fee alongside freely available conventional news sources. Finally, the issues of the uncontrollable consumer came to the fore. A consumers' willingness to participate and contribute content is likely to differ throughout the day and the week with most participation occurring at the weekend.

4 Discussion and Concluding Remarks

The research question asked how the internet is impacting on the different producer/consumer value activities within the news media supply chain. The results of the focus group demonstrated that the internet's influence on the newspaper industry supply chain model (presented in Figure 1) is considerable: newspapers are caught in a revenue trap composed of decreasing advertising revenue coupled with declining circulation revenue. The industry is therefore under severe pressure to create value in order to maintain their existing consumer base and to acquire new customers. News media organizations are responding to this pressure by developing a 'multi-tasking' strategy based on media convergence, with the internet seemingly acting as the linking medium.

Our work confirms that of Geyskens et al., (2002) who found that employing both printed and online editions can result in improvements in both. Online editions are attracting more revenue through greater advertising, increased sales, and reader offers; however, at least for the near future, traditional printed newspapers will remain the core offering and revenue source for the three newspaper firms. Although the news media industry is moving towards co-creating value with its consumers through internet mechanisms such as blogs and discussion forums, it is still very much at the customisation stage. Macdonald and Uncles (2007) stress that consumers have different levels of sophistication in engaging with technology, but our study moves beyond existing studies of technology bridging the producer consumer interface in examining how pro/consumers have instigated moving into online modes of distribution, rather than organisations looking to save costs through incorporating information and communication technologies.

The focus group indicates that socio-technical networks and systems are changing the balance of power in news production and distribution. Bloggers and citizen journalists are challenging the traditional power and control of news production systems by creating their own distribution mechanisms. The very idea of news is changing, as bloggers jostle with journalists for 'scoops'. However, our research setting allows us to clearly contribute to the debate around Vargo and Lusch (2004; 2006) new dominant logic for services. Newspaper organisations engagement with consumers has intensified in the digital economy. While many of the 'interactions' which occur can be seen merely as new versions of existing practices (the letters page replaced by opportunities to post comments), pro/consumers are engaging more with both setting the news agenda and contributing to shaping and fact checking news stories. As Busmante (2004:803) notes, the function of old media is to inform society. However, news organizations are finding themselves less relevant as consumers turn to other, non corporate sources for 'news'. This is leading to falling advertising revenues, the cutting down of their market share, and the marginalising of previous sources of firm strength.

However this research indicates that regional news media firms are not a dying breed as predicted by Meyer (2004; 2008), but are evolving from product supplier into a multimedia content service provider. In response to the challenges of the internet they are retaining their community influence - for being trusted sources of locally produced news, analysis and investigative reporting about public affairs. Though there are concerns that news media organizations are moving online into the (virtual) space rather than creating their own space. This raises questions over whether consumers will be willing to interact in these spaces or whether they will wish to create/find their own spaces. Therefore there is a need for more understanding and greater marketing knowledge about the quality of producer/consumer interaction occurring in these spaces, so as to assess the viability to generate future online value chains and business models.

In examining the changes taking place within news media organizations, in the digital economy, this paper contributes to evolving theories of the co-production of value between a producer and consumer, within a reframed notion of the 'service'. In addition to this theoretical contribution, the paper has clear managerial implications. As acknowledged by the respondents, traditionally media organizations may be too large at present to sustain the drop in advertising revenue occurring. However, many of the central functions of news organizations remain. News organizations should seek revenue creating opportunities through specialising in commercially valuable specialist publications and through a focus on 'hyper localised' community news provision. Future research questions posed by this paper should focus on profiling consumer engagement with news media and investigating perceptions of value in the digital age.

Acknowledgement

We would like to acknowledge the contribution of the participants in the focus group workshop and other meetings. These are Zoe Smith (ITN), Anthony Munnelly (Blogger), Sarah Hartley (Manchester Evening News), Kirsten Schlyder (Journalist), Jennifer Tracey (BBC Radio 4, iPM), Chris Vallance (BBC Radio 4, iPM), Graham Holliday (Blogger), Cagri Yalkin (King's College London) and Peter Kawalek (Manchester Business School).

References

1. Basch, C.E.: Focus group interview: an underutilised research technique for improving theory and practice in health education. Health Education Quarterly 14(4), 411–448 (Winter 1987)
2. Bishop, J.: Increasing participation in online communities: A framework for human-computer interaction. Computers in Human Behaviour 23, 1881–1893 (2006)
3. Bustamante, E.: Cultural industries in the digital age. Media, Culture and Society 26(6), 803–820 (2004)
4. Clemons, E.K., Lang, K.R.: The decoupling of value creation from revenues: a strategic analysis of the markets for pure information goods. Information Technology and Management 4(2-3), 259–287 (2003)
5. Currah, A.: What's happening to our news. An investigation into the likely impact of the digital revolution on the economics of news publishing in the UK, RISJ/Joseph Rowntree Reform Trust Report, Reuters Institute of Journalism, University of Oxford, Oxford (2009)
6. De Souza, C.S., Preece, J.: A framework for analyzing and understanding online communities. Interaction with Computers 16, 579–610 (2004)
7. Douglas, S.P., Craig, C.S., Nijssen, E.: Integrating branding strategy across markets: building international brand architecture. Journal of International Marketing 9(2), 97–114 (2001)
8. Economist, Special report: The newspaper industry. More media, lessnews, pp. 57-59 (August 26, 2006)
9. Fellenz, M., Brady, M.: Managing the innovative deployment of information and communication technologies (ICTs) for global service organisations. Journal of Management & Organization 3(1), 39–55 (2006)

10. Franklin, B.: Pulling Newspapers Apart: Analysing Print Journalism. Routledge, London (2008)
11. Freer, J.: UK regional and local newspapers. In: Anderson, P., Wood, G. (eds.) The Future of Journalism in the Advanced Democracies, Ashgate, London, pp. 89–103 (2007)
12. Geyskens, L., Gielens, K., Dekimpe, M.: The market valuation of internet channel additions. Journal of Marketing 66(2), 102–119 (2002)
13. Hill, J.: British newspapers and the internet. Admap, pp. 2–4 (February 2007)
14. Klinenberg, E.: Convergence: news production in a digital age. The ANNALS of the American Academy of Political and Social Science 59(1), 48–64 (2005)
15. Kozinets, R.: E-tribalized marketing?: The strategic implications of virtual communities of consumption. European Management Journal 17(3), 252–264 (1999)
16. Zheng, Q.: From print to online world: examining the predictors that influence the level of interactivity of newspaper's world wide web pages, Unpublished MSc thesis, Graduate Faculty of Louisiana State University, Louisiana (2002)

Optimization of TCP/IP over 802.11 Wireless Networks in Home Environment

Toni Janevski[1] and Ivan Petrov[2]

[1] University "Sv. Kiril i Metodij", Faculty of Electrical Engineering and
Information Technologies, Karpos 2 bb, 1000 Skopje, Macedonia
tonij@feit.ukim.edu.mk
[2] Macedonian Telecom, Key Customers Business Centre, Orce Nikolov bb,
1000 Skopje, Macedonia
ivan.petrov@telekom.mk

Abstract. Internet connectivity today is based mainly on TCP/IP protocol suite. Performance of the Internet transport protocols may significantly degrade when end to end connection includes wireless links where packets delays and losses are caused by mobility handoffs and transmission errors. In this paper we perform analysis of the achievable throughput for different TCP versions, such as TCP Tahoe, TCP Reno, TCP New Reno, TCP Vegas and TCP SACK, in IEEE 802.11 wireless networks. The analysis showed the strong impact of Medium Access Control parameters, such as number of retransmissions and interface queue length in 802.11 networks on the obtained throughput.

Keywords: TCP, Throughput, Transmission Protocols, Wireless Network.

1 Introduction

Rapid increase in number of active wireless hot spots is providing people to be connected in almost every building and every street, in their homes as well as in their offices. Large amount of nomadic users are using the IEEE 802.11a/b/g/n wireless access technology for checking emails, web surfing, video/audio streaming, and P2P file sharing, either in infrastructure mode (when connected to Internet) or in ad-hoc mode (in office, home or personal environment). Mobile users are starting to use the benefit of these applications as well. Also, such wireless scenario will be applicable in the home environment for interconnecting communication electronic devices, entertainment devices, various sensors in the home or in the car etc. In all such applications, most of the traffic will be based on TCP/IP protocol suite, either for data traffic i.e. non-real time traffic, such as www, ftp, email etc., or for real time traffic, such as voice over IP and IPTV.

It is well known that TCP/IP protocol stack is the most widely used one in the today's Internet world. However, its parameters were carefully tuned in order to maximize its performance on wired networks where packet delays and losses are caused by congestion [1-5]. In the wireless networks, delays and losses are mainly caused by mobility handoffs and transmission errors due to bad wireless channel conditions. With the recent developments in mobile wireless networking, the performance of the

R. Mehmood et al. (Eds.): EuropeComm 2009, LNICST 16, pp. 240–251, 2009.
© Institute for Computer Science, Social-Informatics and Telecommunications Engineering 2009

Internet transport protocols in mobile wireless environment is becoming more important. We should mention that the protocols for wireless access have been designed in order to maximize the utilization of the wireless channel for web browsing and file downloading applications in an environment with restricted mobility, which is the main reason why the buffers and the local Medium Access Control (MAC) retransmissions are tuned in a way to maximize the throughput and the reliability for this kind of applications. In this context it is necessary to define and fine tune the technical standards in order to guarantee full interoperability between different digital applications in wireless environment as well as to provide proper wireless/wired interconnection. We focus our attention of the impact of diverse MAC layer and buffer settings of IEEE 802.11g wireless access technology over the Internet native transport protocol suite during the distribution of multimedia applications in realistic outdoor static as well as mobile multimedia scenario.

The paper is organized as follows: Section 2 gives brief overview of the transport protocols, discusses some related work and motivates the need for our approach. It briefly describes the 802.11 MAC protocol. Section 3 describes our simulation scenario and section 4 presents the simulation results. Section 5 concludes the paper.

2 Transport Protocols

Applications can be grouped in two major classes: downloading (using TCP) and real-time (using UDP). The first class is using reliable data transfer while the second class is based on quick delivery of packets. The performances that are measured by booth classes of applications are completely different. The first class is measuring the performance in terms of how much time is required to have the whole file transferred that is different from the second one where the performances are measured in terms of percentage of packets that reach the destination within a certain time interval. We can say that FTP, HTTP, SMTP are applications that belong to the first class and that the interactive on-line games, real-time IPTV, video/audio chatting, represent examples of applications that are part of the second class. So, we can distinguish the downloading and real-time applications by the transport protocol: TCP or UDP. The TCP protocol guarantees the reliable and in order delivery of every packet sent by using the congestion control functionality. Every TCP flow probes the link with higher and higher data rates eventually filling up the channel. We can be sure that the packets will be queued at the buffer associated with the bottleneck of the link until it overflows causing packet losses. In this situation TCP retransmits the lost packets, and halves its sending rate to diminish the congestion level. Finally, the regular increase of the sending rate is reestablished and so forth. This is not the case with the UDP transport protocol which is much simpler then TCP because packets are immediately sent toward the receiver with a data rate decided by the sender. UDP does not guarantee reliable and in order packet delivery, but its small overhead and lack of retransmissions make it less prone to introduce additional delays due to packet retransmissions as TCP does. This is the main reason why the UDP transport protocol is mainly used by real-time applications. The first TCP implementations were using cumulative positive acknowledgements and required a retransmission timer expiration to send a lost data during the transport. They were following the go-back-n model. In order to enable good user throughput and to control network congestion a lot of work has been done in order to improve its characteristics and with time TCP has evolved. Today's TCP implementations contain variety of algorithms that enables to control the network congestion and to maintain good user throughput in the wired network. Several variants of TCP can be found in the today's wired networks. TCP Tahoe, TCP Reno, TCP New Reno, TCP Vegas and TCP Sack are few of them that are going to be used in ours simulation scenarios. The most used variant of TCP in the real world today is TCP New Reno. However, every of these TCP variants have unique congestion and flow control mechanisms. A problem is defined in the coexistence of the TCP and UDP traffic in a given wireless channel, caused by the TCP congestion control functionality. TCP continuously probes for higher transfer rates, eventually queuing packets in the buffer associated with the bottleneck of the connection. The wireless connection can be shared by several devices and applications. In such case it is obvious that the connection level and the queue lengths may increase, thus delaying the packet delivery and hence jeopardizing the requirements of the real-time applications. Such situation is even worse because the wireless medium allows transmission of only one packet at a time and in most of the wireless networks it is not full-duplex as in wired links [6-10]. This means that packets should wait their turns to be transmitted. Interference, errors, fading, and mobility are causing additional packet losses, and the IEEE 802.11 MAC layer reacts through local retransmissions which in turn cause subsequent packets to wait in the queue until the scheduled ones or their retransmissions eventually reach the receiver. The back off mechanism of the IEEE 802.11 introduces an increasing amount of time before attempting again a retransmission. In the recent years there was a lot of research regarding the problems that TCP and UDP encounters in a wireless environment [11-15].

3 Simulation Scenario

The network layout of the simulation scenario that is subject of the conducted analysis in this paper is presented at Fig. 1.

We have used the network simulator NS2 (version ns-2.28) in order to simulate the outdoor environment presented in Fig. 1. We can notice that the network topology is consisting of four wired nodes (A0-A3), two wireless base stations (BS0-BS1) and four wireless nodes (n0-n3).

The wireless stations are configured to work according the IEEE 802.11g Standard. Wired connections are configured as given in Table 1. Maximum achievable bandwidth rate is 20Mbps, instead of the maximal 54Mbps for IEEE 802.11g standard, due to home environment.

The queue size value used in the simulation is calculated by multiplying the longest RTT (Round Trip Time) with the smallest link capacity on the path, which is the 20Mbps throughput effectively available over the wireless link. In Table 2 are presented several applications that are used during the simulation. In the simulation we have used real trace files for video chat and movie traffic. Two VBR H.263 Lecture Room-Cam are used for the Video chat and high quality MPEG4 Star Wars IV trace file is used for the movie [15]. In this simulation the game events have been generated at the client side every 60ms [11].

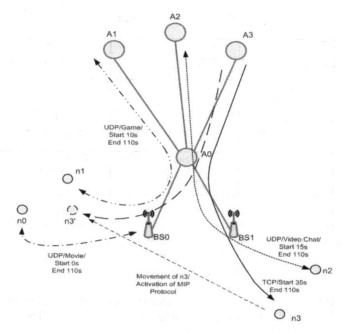

Fig. 1. Simulation Scenario

Table 1. Configuration of wired links simulated at scenario

Node 1	Node 2	Delay	Capacity
A1	A0	10ms	100 Mbps
A2	A0	20ms	100 Mbps
A3	A0	30ms	100 Mbps
A0	BS0	10ms	100 Mbps
A0	BS1	10ms	100 Mbps

Table 2. Types of applications and traffic simulated in the presented scenario

From	To	Type	Transport Protocol	Start	End
BS0	n0	Movie Stream	UDP	0s	110s
A1	n1	Game Traffic	UDP	10s	110s
n1	A1	Game Traffic	UDP	10.1s	110s
A2	N2	Video Chat	UDP	15s	110s
N2	A2	Video Chat	UDP	15.1s	110s
A3	N3	FTP	TCP	35s	110s

Table 3. Simulation parameters

Parameter	Values	Comments
MAC data retransmissions	1,2,3,4	Default value is set at 4
User-BS distance (m)	50,100	Common outdoor environment
MAC queue size (pkts)	25,50,100	Common values
Velocity	static; 4 m/s	Random choice
TCP Transport protocol	TCP Tahoe, TCP Reno, TCP Newreno, TCP Vegas, TCP Sack	Commonly used types of TCP protocols in wired networks.

At the server side updates were transmitted every 50ms toward the client. The payload generated by the client has been set to 42Bytes and the payload generated by the server has been set to 200Bytes. The rest of the packets were set to standard value of 512Bytes for TCP segments. The values for different parameters used in this scenario are listed in Table 3.

For the simulation we have used the shadowing model. The shadowing deviation (σ_{dB}) was set to 4 while the path loss exponent (β) was set to 2.7. These parameters are common for urban environment.

4 Analysis of Transport Protocols

In the following part we observe simulation results from scenario presented in Fig.1, obtained by using the configuration parameters of the links given in Table 1 and applications defined in Table 2. We study the behavior of the UDP/TCP applications and the TCP impact on real time applications in 802.11 wireless networks regarding the throughput as the most important performance metric for non-real-time flows (which use the TCP on transport layer).

The queue size at the MAC layer and the number of MAC layer retransmissions impact the TCP throughput. In Figs. 2 and 3 we show analyses of the throughput of an FTP application as a function of the distance, queue size and the number of MAC layer retransmissions. The results are shown for TCP Tahoe and TCP New Reno.

From the results one may conclude that the queue size of the MAC layer does not impacts the throughput for a given value of the number of MAC layer retransmissions (the curves for different queue sizes and same other parameters are overlapping). Hence, if we increase the number of the MAC layer retransmissions we shall obtain better throughput. The best throughput in this case is obtained when the number of MAC layer retransmissions is set to 4 retransmissions. One may notice that the queue size (i.e. IFQ) at the MAC layer drastically impacts the throughput. It is obvious that if we increase the queue size we will obtain better throughput. It is also obvious that the same throughput is achieved for given values of the MAC layer queue size when the number of the MAC layer retransmissions is set to 3 and 4 retransmissions. The best throughput is achieved when Interface Queue (IFQ) has value of 100 packets.

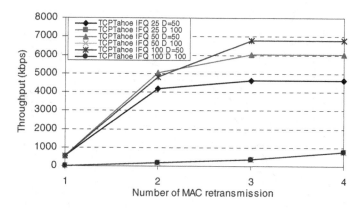

Fig. 2. TCP Tahoe throughput for different access point distances; different MAC queue sizes

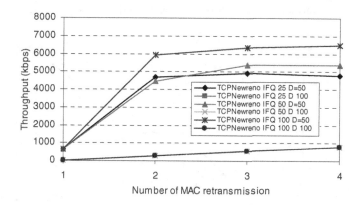

Fig. 3. TCP NewReno throughput for different access point distances; different MAC queue sizes

So far now we are able to conclude that the throughput for all of these transport protocols (i.e. TCP versions) is decreasing as a function of the distance and is increasing as a function of IFQ buffer size and the number of MAC layer retransmission. Drastically lower throughput is achieved at longer distances (i.e. 100m) for all used transport protocols. The queue size at distance of 100m does not impact the throughput as it is a case when the distance is shorter (50m). Highest throughput is achieved for up to four MAC retransmissions. Nearly the same throughput is achieved when MAC retransmissions are set to values of three and four for a given value of MAC queue size (in this scenario the wireless terminal is 50m away from BS).

If we compare the throughput achieved when node is 50m away from the BS for different values of IFQ buffer size and MAC layer retransmissions (Fig. 4) then we can notice that best throughput is achieved for three or higher number of MAC retransmissions. However, the results showed that there is no need for more than 3 retransmission on MAC layer, because there is no significant improvement in average throughput when number of MAC retransmissions is higher than 3 (e.g., 4, 5 etc.).

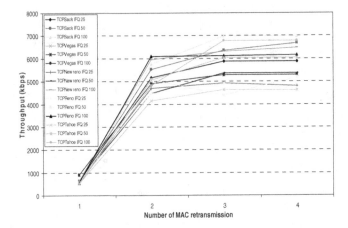

Fig. 4. Throughput of variety TCP protocols for different MAC queue sizes and different number of MAC retransmissions; Distance between n3 and the AP, BS1 is 50m

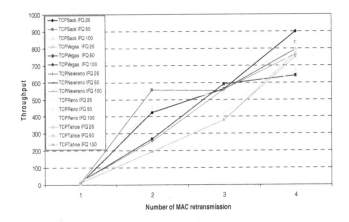

Fig. 5. Throughput of variety TCP protocols for different MAC queue sizes and different number of MAC retransmissions; Distance between n3 and the AP, BS1 is100m

At this point we may fix the number of retransmission to number of 3 at the MAC layer for all TCP versions. Furthermore, the best throughput is achieved with TCP SACK as a transport protocol. TCP Tahoe with larger buffer size (IFQ=100) is the second best case from all TCP versions and all IFQ values. On the other side, TCP Tahoe performs very poor for small IFQ values, i.e. it shows the worst performances for IFQ=25 (the smallest IFQ value in our analysis) when compared with all other cases in Fig. 4. Further, TCP New Reno has slightly better performance than TCP Reno. The overall worst performances are achieved with TCP Vegas excluding the case when the MAC queue size has value of 25 packets (in such case the throughput achieved with TCP Vegas is the second best, after the one achieved when TCP SACK is used as a transport protocol).

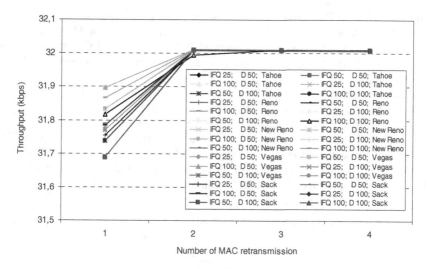

Fig. 6. Comparation of average throughput of the game traffic between the nodes A1-n1 when FTP flow is enabled for different TCP protocols

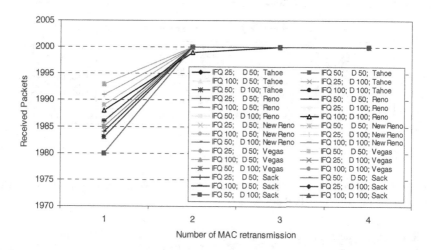

Fig. 7. Received packets of the game traffic between the nodes A1-n1 when FTP flow is enabled for different TCP protocols

In Fig. 5 we present the throughput achieved when the distance between wireless terminal and base stations is 100m. In this scenario, one may conclude that when are needed four MAC retransmission to achieve maximum performances regarding the wireless network and the TCP version. Longer the distance between the BS and the terminals means more MAC retransmissions to achieve the maximum performance in the 802.11 wireless networks. Again, best throughput is achieved with TCP Sack. The second best is achieved with TCP Reno except when the IFQ size is 25 packets (in such case TCP New Reno and TCP Tahoe show better throughput performances). The worst throughput is achieved with TCP Vegas for average of four MAC retransmissions. On the other side, when we use three MAC retransmissions the best throughput is achieved with TCP Vegas, while in such case the worst performance is achieved with TCP Tahoe.

In the following part of this section we provide analysis of the UDP traffic (generated by game application) in presence of background TCP traffic (generated by an FTP flow). If we analyze the results presented in Fig. 6 we will notice that the average throughput of the game traffic between the nodes A1-n1, when FTP flow is enabled, has constant value for different TCP versions when the number of the MAC layer retransmissions is bigger then two, for all possible scenarios. The same note is also valid for the number of received packets, which is presented in Fig. 7.

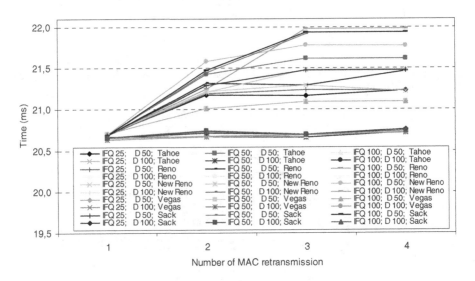

Fig. 8. Comparation of average delay of the game traffic between the nodes A1-n1 when FTP flow is enabled for different TCP protocols

Table 4. Average delay of the game traffic (A1-n1) in (ms) when the MAC retransmissions are set at value of three and the node n3 is 50m away from BS1

L=3	IFQ (pkts)	25	50	100
	TCP Tahoe	21.1711	21.6210	21.9826
	TCP Reno	21.2408	21.2902	21.9826
D=50m	TCP NewReno	21.2953	21.4861	21.7785
	TCP Vegas	21.0952	21.0952	21.0952
	TCP Sack	21.4726	21.9197	21.9386

The results of the average packet delay for game traffic (UDP traffic) when different TCP versions are used for the background TCP traffic (i.e. the FTP flow) are shown in Fig. 8. Numerical results for the packet delay of game traffic are given in Table 4. Lower delays are obtained for larger IFQ buffers and vice versa. The optimal number of MAC retransmissions for smaller IFQ buffers regarding all TCP versions is three, while two retransmissions are good choice for larger buffers, which is similar to conclusions regarding the throughput of the UDP game flow (Figs. 6 and 7). Hence, for UDP game traffic, the optimal number of MAC retransmission is two, which is independent from the distance (i.e. the same results are obtained for different distances between the wireless node and the AP).

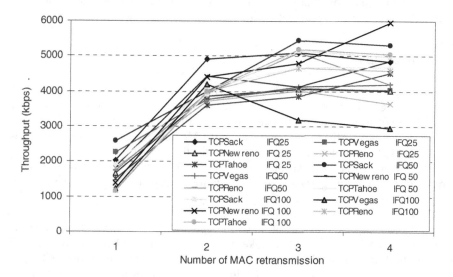

Fig. 9. Average Throughput of the FTP traffic when the node n3 is moving toward BS0 with speed V=4m/s

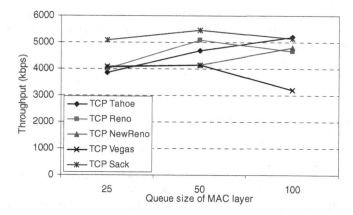

Fig. 10. Average Throughput of the FTP traffic when the node n3 is moving toward BS0 with speed V=4m/s, Number of MAC retransmissions are set at value three

After we have finished the simulations when the node has static position we have conducted the same analysis of the traffic when the node n3 is mobile. As given in Table 3 the mobile node n3 is moving with three different velocities. We have observed scenario when n3 is moving with velocity of 4 m/s (home environment). In Fig. 9 we present the average throughput of the TCP traffic. As one may expect, increasing the number of MAC retransmissions leads to increasing of the average throughput. According to the results optimum value for MAC retransmissions is three retransmissions.

The dependence of the average throughput upon the number of MAC retransmission in 802.11 wireless networks with user mobility in home environment is shown in Fig. 10. The results show that best performances can be achieved when one is using TCP SACK as a transport protocol. Worst results are obtained with TCP Vegas.

5 Conclusions

In this paper we have performed detailed traffic analyses regarding the performances of different TCP versions in 802.11 wireless networks. We have compared different transport protocols by using the throughput as a merit.

The results showed the high importance of the Medium Access Control (MAC) parameters in 802.11 wireless networks regarding the throughput.

The simulations have shown that the best setup in 802.11 wireless networks regarding to the TCP traffic (where TCP counts for most of the traffic in the Internet today): the optimal number of 802.11 MAC layer retransmissions is three, and the MAC queue size is 50 packets for most cases.

If the node becomes mobile the best throughput for TCP-based applications is obtained by using TCP Sack. If we take into consideration the behavior of the TCP traffic in the simulations, the best performance are obtained by using the TCP Sack transport protocol in 802.11 wireless environment. This leads to possibility to create an open transport protocol layer, especially for the case of ad-hoc networks in the home or in the office, when there is no direct communication with other hosts on the global Internet.

Future work is targeted to solutions for open transport layer protocols in future wireless terminals, which is a target for wireless local networks, but it is not limited to them in the wireless world.

References

1. Jacobson, V.: Congestion Avoidance and Control. In: SIGCOMM Symposium on Communications Architectures and Protocols, pp. 314–329 (1988)
2. Floyd, S.: SACK TCP: The sender's congestion control algorithms for the Implementation. Technical report, IETF, March 7 (1996)
3. Fall, K., Floyd, S.: Simulation Based Comparison of Tahoe, Reno and SACK TCP. Lawrence Berkeley National Laboratory One Cyclotron Road, Berkeley (1996)
4. Moraru, B., Copaciu, F., Lazar, G., Dobrota, V.: Practical Analysis of TCP Implementations: Tahoe, Reno, NewReno. In: 2nd RoEduNet International Conference (2003)

5. Mo, J., La, R.J., Anantharam, V., Walrand, J.: Analysis and comparison of TCP Reno and Vegas. In: Proceedings of Eighteenth Annual Joint Conference of the IEEE Computer and Communications Societies. INFOCOM 1999. IEEE, Los Alamitos (1999)
6. Boyden, S., Mahanti, A., Williamson, C.: TCP Vegas Performance with Streaming Media. In: Performance, Computing, and Communications Conference. IPCCC 2007, Dept. of Comput. Sci., Calgary Univ., Alta (2007)
7. Nikitin, P.V., Celebioglu, O., Kukrer, V.(USA): TCP performance in mobile wireless environment: channel modelling and network simulation. In: SCI 2002 (2002)
8. Chiasserini, C.F., Garetto, M., Meo, M.: Improving TCP over wireless by selectively protecting packet transmissions. In: 4th International Workshop on Mobile and Wireless Communications Network, Bombay, India (2002)
9. Singh, A.K., Iyer, S.: ATCP: Improving TCP performance over mobile wireless environments. In: 4th International Workshop on Mobile and Wireless Communications Network, Bombay, India (2002)
10. Palazzi, C.E.: Residual Capacity Estimator for TCP on Wired/Wireless Links. In: WCC 2004 Student Forum IFIP World Computer Congress 2004, Toulouse, France (August 2004)
11. Palazzi, C.E., Pau, G., Roccetti, M., Ferretti, S., Gerla, M.: Wireless Home Entertainment Center: Reducing Last Hop Delays for Real-time Applications. In: ACM International Conference Proceeding Series, vol. 266 (2006)
12. Le Albayrak, S.L., Elkotob, M., Toker, A.C.: Improving TCP Goodput in 802.11 Access Networks. In: ICC 2007, IEEE International Conference on Communications (2007)
13. Lau, C.K.: Improving Mobile IP Handover Latency on End to End TCP in UMTS/WCDMA Networks, Thesis submitted at School of Electrical Engineering and Telecomunications, The University of New South Wales (March 2006)
14. Palazzi, C.E., Chin, B., Ray, P., Pau, G., Gerla, M., Roccetti, M.: High Mobility in a Realistic Wireless Environment: a Mobile IP Handoff Model for NS-2. In: Testbeds and Research Infrastructure for the Development of Networks and Communities, TridentCom 2007 (May 2007)
15. Movie trace files, http://www-tkn.ee.tu-berlin.de/research/trace/ltvt.html (Last accessed, January 2009)

Analysis of the Contextual Behaviour of Mobile Subscribers

Hannu Verkasalo and Borja Jimenez Salmeron

Helsinki University of Technology
hannu.verkasalo@tkk.fi

Abstract. In this paper, contextual behavior of mobile subscribers is studied with data collected straight from smartphones. The paper develops an approach to study how people use mobile devices in different contexts, by proposing an algorithm that works with device-based sensor data. This approach consists of context detection and data analysis. The context detection algorithm analyses cellular network radio logs in modeling the location of people. This paper then analyses usage patterns over different contexts. Demonstration of the contextual modeling with a sample of Finnish smartphone users proves that the applications of the approach are numerous.

Keywords: context modeling; context detection; mobile phone usage.

1 Motivation

The programmability of smartphones has facilitated new research topics, such as the modeling of contextual behavior of people [1]. The issue how people use their mobile phones in different situations is a new topic in market research.

Earlier mobile end-user research (see [14] and [15]) has focused on the analysis of application usage patterns or data service adoption, for example. However, the utilization of handset-based research data facilitates additional dimensions of end-user research. More specifically, analysis of service usage can be conducted over contexts, and locations. This essentially means that in addition to time stamps, also location data is used in the analysis. This gears end-user research towards more context-specific directions. This is a natural evolution path of mobile end-user research, as mobile services themselves are supposed to deliver context-specific value to end-users [16].

The scope of this paper is the analysis of context-specific data collected from mobile handsets, and analysis of that data from perspective of end-user research. The research problem of the paper is: "*What kinds of end-user research approaches are being facilitated by the automatic collection and processing of contextual data from mobile phones?*"

2 Background

Several studies related to context and context-aware systems conclude that a definition of context varies depending on the particular situation and the aim of the study.

R. Mehmood et al. (Eds.): EuropeComm 2009, LNICST 16, pp. 252–266, 2009.

Context-aware systems are used for different purposes such as sensors-based context-awareness for PDA interfaces, adaptive mobile phone application or mobile context-aware tour applications (see [2], [3], [4]). On the other hand, smartphones facilitate contextual computing easier than earlier, with programmable software platforms. Although attempts to create a standardized definition of use-context have been made, context is an abstract concept generally adapted to every specific application that models it [5]. Based on earlier research, context can be understood as something related to all situational factors around the user in a particular use case, a group of variables, parameters and characteristics that specifies the situation of an entity in its current environment where time and location are key aspects for its classification (see e.g. [6], [19], [20]).

Rule induction and machine learning are both valuable data mining techniques transforming data on cell-id transitions to information of location and context. The application of this discipline in the use of algorithms that automatically process huge amounts of cell-id location data has been proven as an accurate method to model end-user context. Once the detection of different contexts, automation of data processing or the visualization of results are solved research questions, the interest focuses on the analysis of these data and the extraction of results. [6]

Context modeling can be applied to social sciences as well in matters such as group behaviour (families, friends, etc) through application usage (study of the likings and the connections among people by listing their music preferences) [7]. The analysis of contextual behaviour of mobile subscribers also covers relevant aspects related to marketing like user segmentation. This paper focuses on how to utilize the data outputs of a context detection algorithm in order to deliver results and interpret them (intensity analysis based on propensity to use is presented as a method to extract reliable conclusions).

Most of the earlier research tends to use location and context as synonyms, understanding the process of context detection as geographical positioning. Vast majority of the applications and tools developed are like sensors that provide additional support rather than noticing the current location (e.g. context phone applications informing about friends in close locations), although some attempts to identify present location and predict future movements have been carried out in the last years (e.g. [8], [9]). But context is much more than mere location and the translation of contexts into geographical locations becomes a secondary objective from the academic point of view.

Previous research on context-aware applications and services pinpoints the difficulty of modeling and identifying context. However, the user's necessity to know contextual information of the person they want to contact to has been presented in several papers (e.g. [10], [11], [12]). Privacy matters regarding to the personal data used for the new tools, methods and experiments in social and context-aware systems must be taken into account as well [13].

The present paper introduces an algorithm to detect end-user context through transitional cell-id logs. With the results obtained of applying this algorithm to real data from the Finnish market, the paper analyses the contextual behaviour of mobile subscribers and explores possible applications in different studies where the contextual perspective can provide with additional and valuable information (e.g. propensity to use mobile services, visualization of movements and service usage distribution). Conclusions are presented last, with special focus on the future research.

3 Context Detection Algorithm

Figure 1 illustrates the context detection process of the algorithm used for modeling contexts [6]. The goal of this algorithm is to extract contextual information of mobile subscribers from data logs of their cell-id transitions and classify every cell visited for every user into abroad, home, office or on the move context. The logic of the algorithm can be divided in three main steps: pre-processing of the input data, cluster extraction and context detection. Finally, the algorithm generates several output files about the context of the user at every moment during the panel. The unique part of the algorithm is that it is developed specifically for smartphone-based sensor data, and it can be used easily to study other phenomena like how people use devices, in a post-analysis mode.

The algorithm has been developed as a main supportive aspect in the modeling of mobile end-user context and it has been applied in several studies regarding the "Modeling of Mobile Internet Usage and Business" project (e.g. [6], [17], [18]).

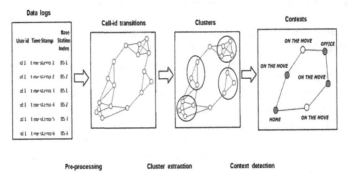

Fig. 1. Context modeling process

3.1 Pre-processing

The preparation of the data logs used as input for the algorithm and time-based calculus are the main parts of this stage. The handset-based end-user research method applied not only measures the usage frequencies, durations and volumes of all terminal features and applications, but also stores transitional information regarding base station connections. The algorithm cleans these logs from missing variables, wrong data or duplicated cases and prepares a file containing the map of every user's movements. This log file is a sequence of timestamps and cell-ids. Every time a user changes the position, a new connection to the base station covering the present cell takes place and this transition is stored in the data logs mentioned. At the end of the day, all the movements are mapped in these logs.

Once the algorithm has pre-processed the data, new variables reflecting the time spent at every cell are calculated. These variables store not only total time spent for a user on every cell id, but also time spent during weekends, at nights or during working hours (night and working hours are defined in the context detection section). The time-based calculus is the key for context detection and it is used in the process of cluster extraction as well.

3.2 Extraction of Clusters

The objective of the cluster extraction process is to group all the cells that are physically close to each other into clusters, utilizing specialized clustering heuristics developed for this purpose and appropriate for the nature of cell-id logs. The coverage of base stations generally overlaps in their limits because the zones without network coverage have to be minimized in order to provide service at every place. Power looses, interferences or movements inside households placed in these overlapping zones that force the handsets to connect to a different base station for a short period of time produce long sequences of transitions among close cells.

The data log used contains many sequences of changes between particular cells, changes that are very short in time mostly. Thus, it can be observed a significant number of cases where a handset connected to a base station changes to a new base station in the following case and presents another transition to the first one afterwards (it can be seen as a "*sandwich*"). These transitions between base stations usually appear many times in the file, what means they are not just a bug because of a dead battery, interference or a power loose of one of the base stations involved. A repeated sequence of cells like that is relevant in the way that it permits the extraction of user behaviour and contextual information.

The algorithm searches for this kind of situations in the file, detecting the exact number of repetitions of these transitions between every pair of cells. If the number of transitions is higher than a pre-determined threshold, both cells are grouped into one renaming their cell-ids into the same. At the end, all the cells are grouped into clusters. These clusters will consist of a non determinate number of cells or, in some cases, the clusters will be formed by a single cell (generally for most of cells detected as on the move context since users do not stay on them for long periods of time what minimizes transitions among them).

3.3 Classification of Cell-Id Clusters

The cluster extraction is the first step in the context classification since the context detection algorithm works with groups of cells. In this step, every cluster is classified into abroad, home, office or on the move context. The algorithm follows a set of rules in order to identify to which group of contexts every cluster belongs to as described in the decision tree on Figure 2.

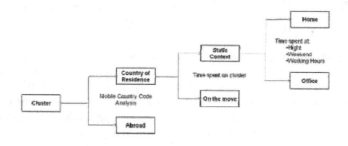

Fig. 2. Decision tree for the context detection process

Abroad context detection is carried out by examination of the mobile country code present in every report. After the identification of the country of residence for every user (the most frequent country code visited), the algorithm searches and marks every visit abroad.

For the rest of the contexts, time-based heuristics are required. First, the algorithm classifies between static and on the move contexts by comparing the amount of time spent at every cluster to a pre-established threshold. If the context is a static one, the next step sets the cluster under analysis as home or office checking and comparing the amount of time spent at nights, weekends and working hours to every corresponding threshold.

The decision of the thresholds as well as the definition of working and night hour is not free of subjectivity. In spite of this, a rigorous sensitivity analysis has been carried out to determine the thresholds that optimize the results [6].

4 Analysis

The context detection algorithm described above generates several output files storing contextual information of mobile subscribers. The analysis section focuses on how to interpret these outputs in order to provide valuable results that can be applied to several fields such as marketing (user segmentation), social sciences (behavioral analysis) or adoption of new technologies and services (technology and service usage analysis) among others [21].

4.1 Dataset

The data used in this paper comes from the context detection algorithm's output files commented in section 3. This algorithm transforms cell-id transitions contained in handset-based data logs of mobile subscribers into contextual information as already described [6, 14, 22].

All the data utilized comes from a Finnish panel provided by Nokia. It can be considered a representative sample of the Finnish market composed of 576 users. From those, 211 users with home and office context properly detected were finally indentified (for this purpose, questionnaires regarding context/location and demographic information were used) [6]. Figures illustrating following sections have been carried out using information from these 211 users.

4.2 Modeling of Movements

The context detection algorithm presented in the previous section is able not only to identify end-user contexts but also to generate a result file storing the physical movements of every user analyzed. These movements can be easily translated into a network plot. Despite the conversion of base stations into geographical locations is not possible because of privacy issues, these visualizations can help in the context detection by giving a new type of information. The advantage of a graph is that it offers the possibility to understand a big mass of data at first sight using nodes, arrows, sizes and colours. The nodes are clusters of network cells, the arrows represent the transitions between these clusters (movements of the user), the size of the nodes symbolize the importance of the clusters in terms of time (total amount of time spent for the user in a cluster) and the code of colours for the nodes informs about the most frequent hours of the day in which the user spends his time in the cluster represented by that node.

Although the result is not a geographical map, it provides information about movements (these visualization show all the "paths" that a user follows over the time of the study), relevant context environments (groups of connected clusters) and the most visited locations (represented with the biggest nodes). Besides, these figures can be used to test the process of context detection (e.g. the environment of a cell classified as office should be, generally, green and orange because these are the colours assigned to the block of the day when people usually work at office; office context should not appear in the weekends visualizations; the node representing home context should be the biggest, etc).

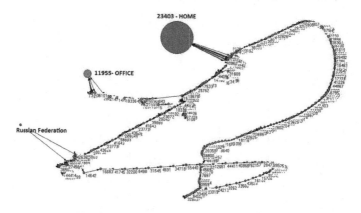

Fig. 3. Movement's network for a single user

The analysis of the average number of different cells visited per hour shows how during weekdays there are two peaks in the number of different cells visited at 7 a.m. and 4 p.m. corresponding to the hours where users typically go to work. There is a noticeable fall between these two peaks corresponding to the standard working hours. Weekend's analysis presents, however, a different curve closer to a Gaussian with its peak of movement at 3 p.m. and a bigger number of movements per hour in average.

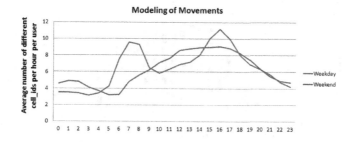

Fig. 4. Average number of different cells visited per hour

4.3 Time Distribution

Additional conclusions can be inferred through the visualization of the proportion of time spent on context. First, there is a logical increase at office context presence during standard working hours (i.e. from 7 a.m. to 4 p.m.) corresponding to a consequent fall at home. Next, the presence at office context during night time does not reach absolute 0% because of the big number of users analyzed (not every one of these users e.g. has to have a day shift) and the algorithm's restrictions (the conditions used in the context detection process tend to be flexible rather than strongly restrictive in order to identify all the possible office contexts) [6]. Last, on the move context presence reaches a peak from 4 p.m. to 7 p.m. corresponding to the time when most of the working users leave office. Curiously, there is no similar peak in the morning when users are supposed to go to work. It can be explained by the randomly chosen plans and paths coming up at the end of a working day.

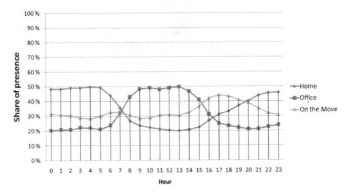

Fig. 5. Proportion of time spent on context

4.4 Distribution of Application Usage

The time distribution of application usage (in launches per hour) gives another perspective of the mobile subscriber behavior. Wide use of voice calls and messaging along the day (excluding night time) with a peak of usage at 3 p.m., the increase in the

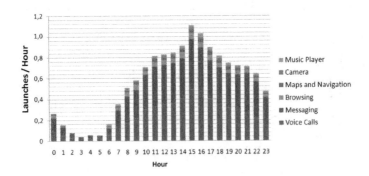

Fig. 6. Distribution of launches per hour between applications and hours of weekdays

usage of maps and navigation applications at hours when users are supposed to go to office or come back home from there, and the similar usage at any time of the rest of the applications (excluding again night time from 0 p.m. to 7 a.m.) are some initial conclusions extracted from figure 6. The comparison of weekday's and weekend's usage (Figure 12 in Appendix A) shows that from 10 a.m. to 11 p.m. there is less variation at weekends although general usage decreases when comparing it to weekdays.

4.5 Propensity to Use Mobile Services

Basic service usage analysis under contextual perspective have shown how deceptive the results can be when considering absolute usage times or relative rates normalized using the total amount of time spent for the user under analysis [6].

The classification of the context into home, office and on the move suggests the use of different variables to analyze results since the time spent at home is, for obvious reasons, bigger than the time spent at the other two contexts although this fact does not imply that the service usage is more intense at home. On the contrary, graphical results have shown that the intensity of usage is bigger on the move and at office contexts rather than at home in all of the services and applications analyzed.

Analysis of the propensity to use of mobile services and applications considers time spent on every context individually what makes it a better measurement of user activity giving a more realistic perspective and a more accurate result. The following descriptive figures regarding propensity to use certain applications consider the time spent on every application at every specific context and hour of the day.

Individual studies of applications over contexts at weekdays show that voice is the most used application at home and on the move, closely followed by SMS. However, SMS is preferred to voice at office context where substitutes such as land lines or meetings probably explain the fall in voice call usage. The figures describing propensity to use camera, music player or browsing show that although usage is much lower compared to voice or SMS services, the propensity to use these applications at on the move and office is considerably higher than at home (see Figures 7, 8 and Appendix B). Results are logical considering that camera and music player are basically on the move applications and that alternative ways to access the Internet at home and office makes browsing another clear on the move application.

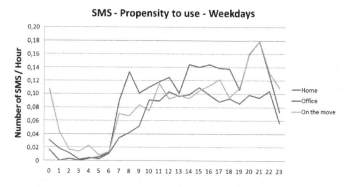

Fig. 7. Propensity to use "SMS" applications during weekdays (number of SMS sent/Hour)

Propensity to use maps and navigation tools at weekdays illustrates that this is again a clear on the move application reaching two peaks at 11 a.m. and 5 p.m. (see Figure 8). First one can be explained by movements related to job during working hours and the second illustrates the time when most users go back home.

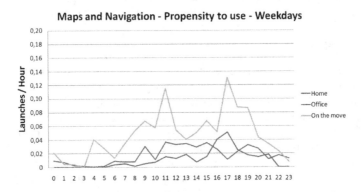

Fig. 8. Propensity to use "Maps and Navigations" applications during weekdays

Further analysis over maps and navigation, voice and music player applications has been carried out. Figures 17, 18 and 19 in Appendix C compare weekdays and weekends usage at home and on the move contexts. For all applications, usage at on the move is higher than at home what proves that this context is the most active considering the time spent on it (here lies the relevance of the propensity to use parameter). Focusing at on the move context, usage at weekdays tends to be higher than at weekends in all applications but in maps and navigation. As it is obvious, needs regarding this application during weekends becomes bigger as Figure 4 indicated in section 4.1 (the number of different cells visited per hour at weekends is higher than at weekdays what means that the users move more frequently at these moments and, consequently, the use of maps and navigation applications increase).

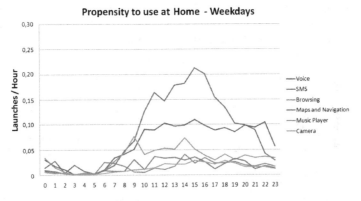

Fig. 9. Propensity to use applications at home context during weekdays

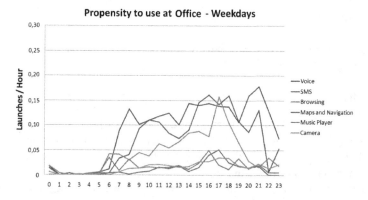

Fig. 10. Propensity to use applications at office context during weekdays

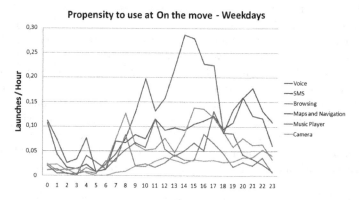

Fig. 11. Propensity to use applications at on the move context during weekdays

Figures 9, 10 and 11 compare the propensity to use all the applications analyzed at every specific context during weekdays. Figure 9 illustrates how the usage of voice and SMS imposes on the rest at home context. As commented before, alternative access to the Internet, substitute leisure devices and the lack of movement explain the fall at home of browsing, music player or camera and maps and navigation applications, respectively.

Figure 10 shows how usage of voice and SMS at office context decreases probably motivated for land lines and e-mail as replacement of SMS for communicating. The rest of applications present low rates of usage similar as the ones at home context.

In Figure 11, propensity to use applications on the move is illustrated. General usage of all the studied applications increases at every hour while on the move. Interesting conclusions can be drawn from the peaks reached at specific hours for certain applications. For example, maps and navigation presents an important peak at 5 p.m. when most users go back home. On the other hand, music player reaches two peaks at 8 a.m. and at 4 p.m., times when most of users are on the way to their offices.

5 Conclusion

This conclusion summarizes the main results, and proposes an agenda for further work in this area.

5.1 Results

This paper is focused on the application of the results of the context detection algorithm presented in section 3. The algorithm provides with a new dimension: context (e.g. [18], {21]). How to use the contextual dimension in standard service usage analysis among others is the matter of study.

The combination of the modeling of mobile subscriber movements, time distribution over contexts and time distribution of application usage lead to the use of a new variable for the analysis of the context-specific behavior of mobile subscribers: the propensity to use. This parameter has been proven as a suitable method to interpret results where context has to be considered. Propensity refers to the intensity to use mobile applications at specific contexts. Graphical plots have demonstrated how on the move context is the most active or, in other words, how the propensity to use every one of the applications analyzed is higher at on the move. The figures show also that propensity to use at weekdays is higher than at weekends in all applications but maps and navigations (the needs of location information increase during weekends when users move more frequently). Visualizations comparing propensity to use all services at different contexts illustrates the dominance of voice and messaging applications over the rest at any hour of the day in every context analyzed. On the other hand, general usage of all applications decreases at office context, particularly voice and SMS.

Although results prove that mobile subscribers use applications more actively on the move, home can be considered as the most important context considering total time of use. Despite this, the variable propensity to use applications has a big value in service usage analysis for academia and industry (e.g. adoption of new services or matters related to segmentation).

5.2 Future Research

The addition of contextual information improves classic service usage analysis helping in the understanding of mobile-subscribers behavior. Thus, a more detailed context analysis (e.g. regarding the number of sub-contexts detected) is an interesting line of research as far as wireless network traffic amounts continue increasing and intelligence of wirelessly connected devices evolves. If the importance of indoor areas increases, a deeper classification of contexts becomes relevant.

The integration of the context identification service in handsets that leads to the adaptation of devices to the current context is an important topic for future research. But before this, improvement on the accuracy of the context detection algorithm and the measurement client used to collect data can be done.

As it has been demonstrated along this paper, contextual information can be used in studies regarding adoption of new technologies. Propensity to use applications provides valuable support to network operators informing about where, when and how much their mobile subscribers use the applications and services installed on their devices. But the context detection process does not only cover service usage analysis neither is a supportive tool just for academia. The interest for industry is increasing for obvious reasons. Context detection can be applied to different fields such -as targeted marketing or user segmentation. The usage of contextual information to support person-situation segmentation and the search of killer applications under a contextual perspective are some examples of possible applications [18].

References

[1] Verkasalo, H., Hämmäinen, H.: Handset-Based Monitoring of Mobile Subscribers. Department of Electrical and Telecommunications Engineering. Helsinki Mobility Roundtable. Helsinki School of Economics (2006)
[2] Schmidt, A., Beigl, M., Gellersen, H.-W.: There is more to Context than Location. In: Proceedings of Workshop on Interactive Applications of Mobile Computing, Rostock, Germany (November 1998)
[3] Esbjörnsson, M., Weilenmann, A.: Mobile Phone Talk in Context. In: Dey, A.K., Kokinov, B., Leake, D.B., Turner, R. (eds.) CONTEXT 2005. LNCS (LNAI), vol. 3554, pp. 140–154. Springer, Heidelberg (2005)
[4] Long, S., Aust, D., Abowd, G.D., Atkeson, C.G.: Rapid prototyping of mobile context-aware applications: The cyberguide case study. In: Proceedings of the 2nd annual international conference on Mobile computing and networking, New York, United States, pp. 97–107 (1996)
[5] ISO 13407, Human-centred design processes for interactive systems. International Standard, the International Organization for Standarization (1999)
[6] Jimenez, B.: Modeling of Mobile End-User Context. M.Sc. Thesis, Helsinki University of Technology (May 2008)
[7] Eagle, N.: Machine Perception and Learning of Complex Social Systems. Doctoral dissertation, Massachusetts Institute of Technology (2005)
[8] Raento, M., Oulasvirta, A., Petit, R., Toivonen, H.: ContextPhone - A prototyping platform for context-aware mobile applications. IEEE Pervasive Computing 4(2), 51–59 (2005)
[9] Laasonen, K., Raento, M., Toivoinen, H.: Adaptative On-Device Location Recognition. In: Second International Conference on Pervasive Computing, Vienna, April 23 (2004)
[10] Kankainen, A., Tiitta, S.: Exploring everyday needs of teenagers related to context-aware mobile services. In: Proceedings of HFT 2003, Berlin, Germany, pp. 19–26 (2003)
[11] Tamminen, S., Oulasvirta, A., Toiskallio, K., Kankainen, A.: Understanding mobile contexts. In: Proceedings of Mobile HCI 2003, Udine, Italy, pp. 18–35 (2003); A revised version submitted to Personal and Ubiquitous Computing
[12] Oulasvirta, A., Kurvinen, E., Kankainen, T.: Understanding contexts by being there: case studies in bodystorming. Personal and Ubiquitous Computing 7, 125–134 (2003)
[13] Raento, M.: Exploring Privacy for Ubiquitous Computing: Tools, Methods and Experiments. Department of Computer Science, Series of publications A, Report A-2007-2 (2007)

[14] Verkasalo, H.: Handset-Based Monitoring of Mobile Customer Behaviour. Master's Thesis Series. Networking Laboratory. Department of Electrical and Telecommunications Engineering. Helsinki University of Technology, Espoo, Finland (September 2005)

[15] Verkasalo, H.: A Cross-Country Comparison of Mobile Service and Handset Usage. Licentiate's thesis, Helsinki University of Technology, Networking Laboratory, Finland (2007)

[16] Heinonen, K., Pura, M.: Classifying Mobile Services. Presented at Helsinki Mobility Roundtable, Helsinki, June 1-2 (2006)

[17] Modeling of Mobile Internet Usage and Business Project (2008), http://www.netlab.tkk.fi/tutkimus/momi/

[18] Uronen, M.: Market Segmentation Approaches in the Mobile Service Market. Master's Thesis, Networking Laboratory, Helsinki University of Technology (2008)

[19] Schmidt, A., Beigl, M., Gellersen, H.W.: There is more to Context than Location. In: Proceedings of Workshop on Interactive Applications of Mobile Computing, Rostock, Germany (November 1998)

[20] Lee, I., Kim, J., Kim, J.: Use Contexts for the Mobile Internet: A longitudinal Study Monitoring Actual Use of Mobile Internet Services. International Journal of Human-Computer interaction 18(3), 269–292 (2005)

[21] Smura, T.: Access alternatives to mobile services and content: analysis of handset-based smartphone usage data. In: ITS 17th Biennial Conference, Montreal, Canada, June 24-27 (2008)

[22] Verkasalo, H., Hämäinen, H.: Handset-Based Monitoring of Mobile Subscribers. Department of Electrical and Telecommunications Engineering. Helsinki Mobility Roundtable. Helsinki School of Economics (2006)

[23] Kivi, A.: Measuring Mobile User Behavior and Service Usage: Methods, Measurements Points, and Future Outlook. In: Proceedings of the 6th Global Mobility Roundtable, Los Angeles, California, U.S, June 1-2 (2007)

Appendix A – Distribution of Application Usage

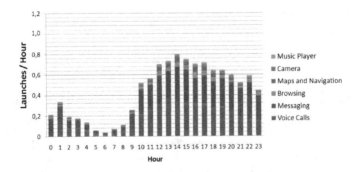

Fig. 12. Distribution of launches per hour between applications and hours of weekends

Appendix B – Propensity to Use Services

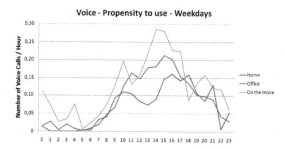

Fig. 13. Propensity to use "Voice" applications during weekdays (number of voice calls emitted/Hour)

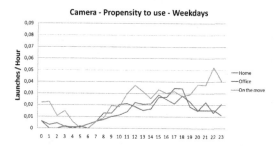

Fig. 14. Propensity to use "Camera" applications during weekdays

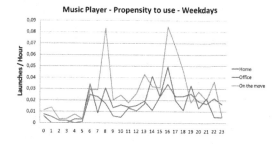

Fig. 15. Propensity to use "Music Player" applications during weekdays

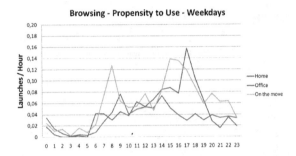

Fig. 16. Propensity to use "Browsing" applications during weekdays

Work-in-Progress and Short Papers

Improved Classification and Framework Association of Security Vulnerability, Threats and Attacks in Wireless Sensor Networks

Adnan Ashraf[1], AbdulRauf Rajput[1], Marvie Mussadiq[2], Bhawani S. Chowdhry[3], and Manzoor Hashmani[4]

[1] CREST Research Scholars, Mehran UET, Pakistan
[2] IT Consultant, Xevious Co.
[3] Fellow-Postdoc, Southampton University-UK
[4] Foreign Faculty Professor, Mehran UET
adnanlooking@ieee.org

Abstract. Security of wireless sensor network (WSN) remained an open research area throughout the current decade. New research and developments seems protecting sensor networks from various security threats but at the same time raise many questions, confusions and conflicts regarding their own viability. Such viability issues become major hindrances in security assessment of WSNs against posed security threats. This results in less reliable sensor networks and applications. In our strong opinion, there are two root-causes of this problem; 1) a comprehensive list of security threats is overlooked as researchers' work appear limited in classification of security threats and, 2) security threats are not associated with security frameworks. In this paper, we perform classification of security threats comprehensively whereas, associating these threats to a security framework; we lead in this direction. We find that specifically to assess the impact of these threats.

Keywords: WSN security, Security vulnerability, Threats and Attacks, Security Framework.

1 Introduction

The focus of this paper is the long standing open problem of developing some approach for achieving maximum security in wireless sensor networks, particularly an approach to address the fundamental security objectives that vary in applications. Such varying security objectives of applications do not allow a single security approach to best-fit another application. This is because of security objectives of an application in a sensor network could be mirrored exactly in another application depending upon the interests to be sought from that network [1] [2]. Hence, a most preferable security objective in an application can be ranked as moderated in another type of application, such as sensor-ID (source of information) in military operations and in smart-parking.

Ranking of security objectives should be carefully performed by first analyzing security threats posed to WSN and its application. In this paper, first we compile a

R. Mehmood et al. (Eds.): EuropeComm 2009, LNICST 16, pp. 269–274, 2009.

comprehensive list of security threats. Then, by classifying the security threats we associate them analytically with security assessment framework [3] [4]. We observe that such work has not been done before, in this way.

2 Related Work

Study of security vulnerability, threat and attack (VTA) aids in the development of countermeasures and security frameworks of wireless sensor network. Here we briefly review the related work, at-present issues and motivations. We observe a relatively little work in the area of classification of security threats. In the existing partial work, most of the researchers used security terms interchangeably, such as vulnerability, attacks and threats [5] [6] [7]. Using alternate terms may create problems and mislead the prospective researchers. It is not logical to use these terms interchangeably because of wide differences in these terms. In this paper, we differentiate these terms for research community for sake of research in right directions and then we comprehend a list of security threats for wireless sensor networks.

From literature, we observe that classification of WSN is based on features and mechanism that WSN exhibits today. For example, distance to base station (single or multi hops), data dependency (aggregating or non-aggregating), deployment (deterministic or dynamic), control schemes (self or non-self configurable) and application domain (features dependent) [8] [9] [10]. In a WSN, the exposure of features is application specific therefore a WSN should be selected for an application by security and reliability, instead of features, that it offers. We present here a revised classification of security VTA.

The most recent and maximum work in classification of security models of WSNs appeared by S., Kaplantzis [9] in 2006. While interchanging terms of security threats, vulnerability and attacks in WSN, the researcher has dispersed many of those in network layers [12]. Contrary to the classic work in WSN security we propose an analytical association of security threats with security framework.

3 Classification Needs of Security VTAs in WSN

It's obvious from through literature survey that WSN still experiences classical (bit modified for WSN) approaches of traditional wireless or wired networks. Probably, this is due to the likely names of attacks that are present in classical wireless networks. On the contrary, VTA (vulnerability, threat and attack) have quite different impact in the WSN due to its unique in-network communication processing. Hence, classification of VTA and development of security frameworks should be revisited to counter such security VTA.

In this paper, our approach for classification and association of security VTA is proposed to remodel application-specific WSNs that may fulfill their missions in timely manner, in hostile environments.

3.1 Security VTAs

A profound study leads to differentiate among security related terms that are being interchangeably used among researchers in published literature (discussed in section 2). In order to eliminate these ambiguities from the future literature we compile a list of vulnerabilities, threats and attacks in the light of standard definitions.

The *vulnerability* is a weak-point in the system or a network that may be exploited, whereas a *threat* is considered as an external or internal influence that may exploit the *vulnerability* (weak-point). An *attack* is the occurrence of a *threat*, causes an unwanted event to be occurred in a system such as data steal, denial of service, sniffing, spoofing, etc [11] [13][14]. An *attack* can also be termed as an *exposure* in a system.

Thinking WSN, for example, the *wireless medium* is prone to exposure or attack and it's a known vulnerability. This vulnerability may be (or may not be) exploited depending upon the nature of WSN environment. Any object blocking this communication medium from responding shall be considered as a *threat* under definition of external influence. Similarly, if any inherent feature (or circuitry) causes unwanted delay of communication signals it'll also be a *threat*.

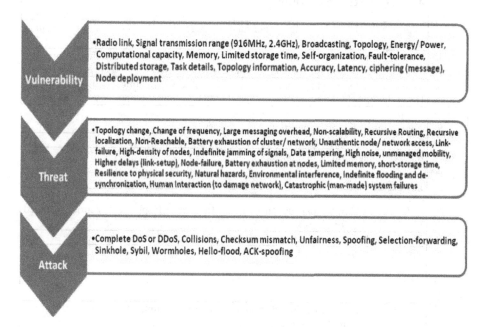

Vulnerability
- Radio link, Signal transmission range (916MHz, 2.4GHz), Broadcasting, Topology, Energy/ Power, Computational capacity, Memory, Limited storage time, Self-organization, Fault-tolerance, Distributed storage, Task details, Topology information, Accuracy, Latency, ciphering (message), Node deployment

Threat
- Topology change, Change of frequency, Large messaging overhead, Non-scalability, Recursive Routing, Recursive localization, Non-Reachable, Battery exhaustion of cluster/ network, Unauthentic node/ network access, Link-failure, High-density of nodes, Indefinite jamming of signals, Data tampering, High noise, unmanaged mobility, Higher delays (link-setup), Node-failure, Battery exhaustion at nodes, Limited memory, short-storage time, Resilience to physical security, Natural hazards, Environmental interference, Indefinite flooding and de-synchronization, Human Interaction (to damage network), Catastrophic (man-made) system failures

Attack
- Complete DoS or DDoS, Collisions, Checksum mismatch, Unfairness, Spoofing, Selection-forwarding, Sinkhole, Sybil, Wormholes, Hello-flood, ACK-spoofing

Fig. 1. A general view of vulnerability, threats and attacks in WSNs

At preliminary stages as the threat and the losses caused by such threats are unknown therefore, threats are usually considered as 'security threats'. Therefore, we comprehend a list of vulnerability, threats and attacks found in WSN in Fig 1. Concluding this section we observe that differentiating vulnerabilities, security threats and attacks resolves the terminology conflict. In the next section we classify the *security threats* while associating them to security framework.

3.2 Re-classification of Security Threats Using Security Assessment Framework

Usually, security VTAs are classified as physical-threat, accidental-error, natural, man-made, unauthorized access, malicious-user, etc. It is notable that if traditional ciphering, topology, routing and security schemes are not appropriate for WSN then how can a traditional way of security classification be appropriate for WSN? We take this opportunity first to classify the security threats using security assessment framework [3] [4] in table 1.

Table 1. Classification and Association of Security VTAs with Discrete Security Assessment Framework

N E T W O R K	*Vulnerability:* Average energy exhaustion (network), low computational capacity, limited network storage time, self-organization, fault-tolerance level, distributed storage, task details, simple ciphering, and node deployment
	Threat: Topology change, change of frequency, large messaging overhead, non-scalability, recursive routing, system failures
	Attack: Complete DoS or DDoS
L I N K	*Vulnerability:* Radio link, Signal transmission range (916MHz, 2.4GHz), Broadcasting, Topology-less infrastructure, Ad hoc Topology information
	Threat: Non-Reachable, Link-failure, High-density of nodes, Indefinite jamming of signals, Data tampering, High noise, unmanaged mobility, Higher delays (link-setup)
	Attack: Collision or checksum mismatch, Unfairness, Spoofing, Sybil, Wormholes, Hello-flood, ACK-spoofing
S I N K	*Vulnerability:* Energy exhaustion @ Sink, Task details
	Threat: Unauthorized access
	Attack: Sinkhole, de-synchronization
N O D E	*Vulnerability:* Energy exhaustion @ node, Resilience to physical security, Limited memory, short-storage time
	Threat: Node failure, Recursive localization, Indefinite flooding
	Attacks: Selective Forwarding
O T H E R S	*Vulnerability:* ---
	Threat: Natural hazards, Environmental interference, Human Interaction (to damage network), Catastrophic (man-made)
	Attack: Nil

4 Security VTAs

This paper performs a critical analysis of available literature on security classification. Criticizing the trend of interchanging terms for security VTAs, it elaborates the possible losses of this trend to research.

A comprehensive list of security VTAs is helpful to model new security protocols, frameworks, as well as to assess the existing security solutions. It allows better understanding with security issues in WSN. Customization of VTA list can also be done as per demand of an application. Similarly, any low priority constraint, threat or attack can be eliminated from the VTA list for a specific type of WSN.

Administrators of WSN will then, have a simplified management of network. Renewing policy is considered as energy hungry process in WSN. By classifying VTA, any layer of network under attack can be known and then revitalized using selective forwarding for policy renewing or countermeasures.

Distribution of security VTAs is done by assessing impact of each entry in the list and, taking into account, the infected area that could be involved in sharing losses in a WSN. Furthermore, confidentiality as task details (at node) is assumed as network asset. This ensures an uncompromised security strategy used throughout our work.

In short, we can be able to distinguish the presence of any VTA component in security layers of WSN using the assessment framework. From an application s' perspective, any vulnerability, threat or attack can be subjugated if any network layer or segment of the framework is protected by that VTA component. This is the real benefit of associating security VTA to a security framework.

5 Conclusion and Future Work

This paper differentiates among concepts of security vulnerability, threat and attack by redefining them from WSN s' perspective. On the basis of this differentiation we are able to comprehend a list of security VTAs. It helps to eliminate ambiguities regarding security literature on VTAs. Then, by examining each of VTAs we associate it with a security assessment framework for analysis. Impact of these security VTAs on a sensor network depends on various factors and is an open research issue. Also, we plan to review this approach with other security frameworks, in future to achieve good assessment in WSN applications.

References

1. Zia, T., Zomaya, A.: A security Framework for Wireless Sensor Networks. In: SAS 2006 – IEEE Sensors Application Symposium, Houston, Texas, USA, February 7-9 (2006)
2. Zou, K.C.Y.: Uncertainty-aware and Coverage-oriented Deployment for Sensor Networks. Journal of Parallel and Distributed Computing 64(7), 788–798 (2004)
3. Ashraf, A., Hashmani, M., Mussadiq, M., Chowdhry, B.S., et al.: A Pretty Safe Strategy for Analyzing Discrete Security Assessment Framework in Wireless Sensor Networks, Communications in Computer and Information Science, November 14, 2008. Book of Wireless Networks, Information Processing and Systems, vol. 20, pp. 445–448. Springer, Heidelberg (2008)
4. Ashraf, A., Hashmani, M., Mussadiq, M., Chowdhry, B.S.: Design and Analysis of the Security Assessment Framework for Achieving Discrete Security Values in Wireless Sensor Networks, Electrical and Computer Engineering, 2008. In: CCECE 2008. Canadian Conference on Electrical and Computer Engineering, May 4-7, pp. 855–860 (2008)
5. Ilyas, M., Mahgoub, I.: Handbook of Sensor Networks: Compact Wireless and Wired Sensing Systems (2004) ISBN 0-8493-1968-4, TK7872.D48.H36
6. Muraleedharan, R., Osadciw, L.A.: Jamming Attack Detection and Countermeasures. In: Wireless Sensor Network Using Ant System, Department of Electrical Engineering and Computer Science, pp. 13244–11240. Syracuse University, Syracuse

7. Crespo, R.G.: Slides on Mobile Systems Security, WSN Security Threats', Copyright Departmento de Engenharia, Electrotecnica, e de Computadores (Fall 2006)
8. Akojwar, S.G., Patrikar, R.M.: Classification Techniques with Cooperative Routing for Industrial Wireless Sensor Networks. In: Advances in Computer and Information Sciences and Engineering, pp. 503–508. Springer, Netherlands (2008)
9. Kaplantzis, S., Mani, N.: A Study on Classification Techniques for Network Intrusion Detection. In: Proceedings of the IASTED International Conference on Networks and Communication Systems, year of publication (2006)
10. Kim, Y., Jeong, S., Kim, D.: A GMM-Based Target Classification Scheme for a Node in Wireless Sensor Networks. IEICE Transactions on Communications E91-B(11), 3544–3551 (2008); doi:10.1093/ietcom/e91-b.11.3544, The Institute of Electronics, Information and Communication Engineers
11. Kim, D.S., Shazzad, K.M., Park, J.S.: A Framework of Survivability Model for Wireless Sensor Network. In: Proceedings of the First International Conference on Availability, Reliability and Security, pp. 515–522 (2006) ISBN:0-7695-2567-9
12. Kaplantzis, S., Mani, N.: Security Models of Wireless Sensor Networks, final review report for PhD (2007), http://users.monash.edu.au/~skap3/
13. Barnum, S., Gegick, M.: Defense in Depth, pp. 2005–2009. Cigital, Inc., on 2005-09-13, Copyright (2005)
14. The Living Dictionary, Series of Longman Dictionary of Contemporary English, Copyright Pearsons Education (2008)

Challenges for Mobile Social Networking Applications

Juwel Rana[1], Johan Kristiansson[2], Josef Hallberg[1], and Kåre Synnes[1]

[1] Department of Computer Science and Electrical Engineering
Luleå University of Technology, SE-971 87 Luleå
[2] Ericsson Research[*], SE-971 28 Luleå
{juwel.rana,josef.hallberg,kare.synnes}@ltu.se,
johan.j.kristiansson@ericsson.com

Abstract. This paper presents work in progress regarding utilization of social network information for mobile applications. Primarily a number of challenges are identified, such as how to mine data from multiple social networks, how to integrate and consolidate social networks, and how to manage semantic information for mobile applications. The challenges are discussed from a semantic Web perspective using a driving scenario as motivation.

The main objective is to enable mobile applications to benefit from semantic information obtained from Web services, mobile devices, or the surrounding environment. The goal is therefore to create a framework that enables integration of semantic information (location, activity, interests, etc) with social network data (from Twitter, FaceBook, LinkedIn, etc) to facilitate intelligent yet easy to use communication tools for individual persons as well as groups of persons. An ultimate goal is to make complex communication simple through utilization of semantic information and social network data for pervasive services in mobile devices.

Keywords: Mobile Social Networking, SOA.

1 Introduction

Social networks have had an almost viral growth of users during the last years, where services such as FaceBook, Twitter, LinkedIn and Delicious enable users to share personal information with family members, friends and colleagues as well as loose acquaintances and the public in general. The personal information most commonly consists of text notes/messages, photos and videos, but the personal information can also consist of social data such as contacts or list of friends. At the same time a rapid growth of mobile computing has been made possible through advanced mobile terminals connected through wireless/GSM/3G networks, which has enabled users to be ubiquitously connected and thus be 'always on'.

This rapid development in mobile computing has made social networks almost ubiquitous, where access to them can be done through a multitude of devices such as

---

[*] The work has been carried out as part of an academic research project and does not necessarily represent Ericsson views and positions.

R. Mehmood et al. (Eds.): EuropeComm 2009, LNICST 16, pp. 275–285, 2009.

a PC or a mobile phone as well as through public information displays or pervasive devices. While it is possible to access social networking services from almost anywhere, few services can today take full advantage of the mobility of the users.

Semantic information about users' location, context (such as what terminal they use) and situation (such as the current activity) can be used to filter information from social networks to support novel mobile applications. An example of such an application is to dynamically create and maintain groups (dynamic groups) based on semantic information such as using NFC-enabled mobile terminals to initiate creation of a new group or to add a member to an existing group [9]. It is also possible to automatically infer semantic information about a user into social networks (such as automated Twitter notes or LinkedIn updates).

The goal of the work is to engineer novel mobile applications through dynamic utilization of the social data available in social networks. For example, data mined from FaceBook, Twitter, LinkedIn and/or Delicious and fused can be utilized in a mobile application that presents real-time information of friends, family members and colleagues etc as a semantic contact lists or a group member list [1, 2, and 3].

This paper identifies a list of challenges for creating a platform for mobile social networking, using a top-down approach from both. The rest of the paper is structured as follows: Section 2 presents related work, Section 3 presents a motivating scenario, Section 4 introduces an architectural overview, Section 5 describes services for mobile applications, Section 6 presents challenges in mobile social networking, and finally Section 7 provides a discussion and future work.

2 Related Work

Tim-Berners Lee already in 1995 defined the Web as a collective intelligence. The viral growth of social networks today can be explained through both societal developments and technological advancements that together have enabled new types of applications where users today co-create content. 'The cloud' is the current paradigm of computing, building on this notion of co-creating both content and services [4]. Thus, Lee's vision of a collective intelligence is becoming true.

This is in particular true for social networking applications, as users feed the services with personal information and also contribute to the development of services (based on open software initiatives). Example services are:

- Wikipedia[1] harnesses collective intelligence to co-create content.
- Flickr[2] provides users with free photo sharing.
- YouTube[3] has as a service for video sharing reinvented the Web.
- Delicious[4] is an application to store, organize and share Web.
- Digg[5] enables users to share their opinion on digital contents (e.g. news, pictures, and videos) and be able to see the rank of that content.

---

[1] http://en.wikipedia.org/
[2] http://www.flickr.com/
[3] http://www.youtube.com/
[4] http://www.delicious.com/
[5] http://www.digg.com/

- LinkedIn[6] builds social networks by linking people together.
- Blogs[7] are social spaces where the users may read, write or even comment on their thoughts over the Internet to share opinions and raise open discussions.

The decentralized design techniques where end users participates in creating content provides a basic model for designing social networking applications. Creating, sharing, tagging and commenting on content while building social networks (communities) are hence central, as social needs are one reason for the viral growth of these services. However, mobile devices are now taking this even further by enabling users to be 'always on' which has many implications.

It has been shown that social context is important for designing and developing context-aware mobile applications [16], while also increasing the risk of privacy and integrity violation. In general mobile social networking applications allow users to have more social interactions and collaborations using the Web in more efficient and interesting manner [17]. For instance, the "CenceMe" system is able to collect users' present status or context information using mobile sensors and can export users' present status automatically to social networks [1]. Push-and-pull types of mobile applications are important in the context of mobile social networks [16, 1]. Pull applications may collect real-time information (e.g., micro-blogs. Status, etc) from different social networks using social API's and push applications may publish status based on sensor generated context to different mobile networks.

A dynamic group is a concept of creating and managing groups based on social data as well as semantic information [9, 15, and 3]. Related to this is a social interest discovery mechanism based on user-generated tags for discovering groups [3].

However, current API's are not enough to collect social data from social networking sites due to lack of standardization of data formats and model as well as access policies [18]. There are initiatives on open social interfaces but they have proven not to be usable in practice [19], mainly because of dependencies on social network owners (e.g. for analyzing social data) [2].

3 Motivating Scenario

Alice is a business executive at a call centre who has a large network of family members, friends and colleagues. She is very busy at work and her social life has regrettably been suffering over the last years. However, lately she has started to manage her social networks using a semantic contact application in her mobile device. It helps her by presenting status updates from the persons she is interested in (by filtering and merging information from FaceBook, Twitter, LinkedIn, etc). She also receives the latest news or interesting blogs of her friends though the application, which keeps her updated. She feels socially connected – even if busy!

Moreover, Alice uses the application for creating dynamic group that gives her a fast and easy way to communicate. This morning she plans for a lunch with her friends so she uses the application to see who are nearby and have time to chat. Four of her friends are online at the same location, so she invokes the communication tool and they decide to meet for lunch downtown.

---

[6] http://www.linkedin.com/
[7] http://www.blogger.com/home

Alice checks her calendar and todo-list, decides to take a walk downtown since the weather is lovely, and then uses the application to notify her friends that she is 'talking a walk downtown'. Her friends can then see her new status by using a similar application or by using the underlying services like Twitter or FaceBook.

A traditional contact application in a mobile phone contains contact information that most often is user-generated. However, Apple's iPhone and Google's Android platforms allow contact information to be imported from other applications. The semantic contact application described in the scenario above can automatically fetch, filter and fuse data from different data sources (social networks, news, blogs, calendars, etc), which simplifies social interaction by providing contact information updated in real-time. This means a possible shift from communication by email, phone or GSM text messages to rich communication using additional media while being able to communicate with a group as easily as an individual. Fig. 1 below depicts an Android prototype which presents a semantic contact application where information from different sources is fused and presented as semantic information about each contact in the list.

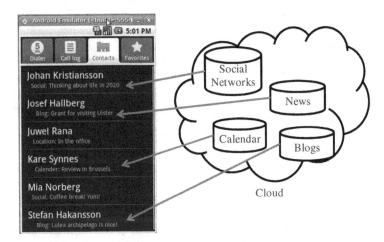

Fig. 1. Semantic Contact Application

4   Engineering a Platform for Mobile Social Networking

We investigate the feasibility of a platform for mobile social networking applications based on a Service Oriented Architecture (SOA) [6, 13]. The architecture has three main parts: the mobile client, the backend services, and the service integrator. The service integrator integrates mobile clients (e.g. mobile device software) and backend services (e.g. social data collector services or location tracking services) by providing a standard interface. In this paper we emphasize on identifying the challenges for developing a SOA-based platform for mobile social networking.

There are mainly two reasons why a SOA-based architecture is preferred for mobile social networking. The first reason is that it provides a more open and decentralized platform to adapt and integrate backend services into. The second is that the large number of social networking users and heterogeneity in applications demand sustainability, easy deployment and management as well as high integration of social applications. These criteria can be met by utilizing a SOA-based architecture.

In Fig. 2 below we can see a three layer view of the platform architecture. This view describes some of the necessary components for the platform, and is relevant in order to understand the core architecture. In the first layer we can see how the backend services collect Web data, such as social data, from different sources of the Web (e.g. Facebook, Twitter, etc.). This can be done by using social API's[8], which in turn establish connections between social networks and data collector services.

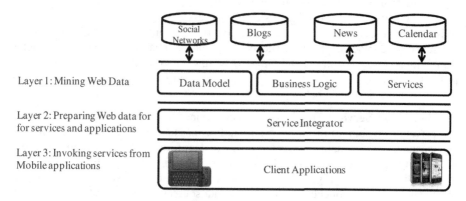

Fig. 2. Three layer view of the envision platform architecture

The service integrator is in layer 2. The role of the service integrator is to ensure interoperability of mobile clients and services. It supports interoperability by utilizing the standard specification for accessing social data [12]. Layer 3 shows how mobile clients, such as iPhone and Google Android applications, access services (e.g. social data collector services, profile builder services, etc.). Some services are associated with the mobile device software. For example, a semantic dialer application looks for unknown caller information in the social data collector service. This application also synchronizes the contact list (name, phone number, email address, status, etc) with the data from social networks via the social data collector service.

Aggregation of social data is one of the challenges in social data management. However, services which are based on reasoning techniques (e.g. profile builder services, dynamic group creator services) need a clean and complete social data set. These services provide operation for searching friends, discovering dynamic groups and so on [10]. For that purpose, the ontology based data model can be used [7, 10]. However, there are some problems in merging data, as shown in Fig. 3. By merging multi-source social data we also increase the privacy implications. A platform for aggregating and merging multi-source social data may provide a foundation for different types of services for building not only smart and flexible mobile applications but also applications such as a semantic browser. It enables mobile device software to integrate with social networks.

---

[8] http://www.programmableWeb.com/apis/directory/1?apicat=Social

5 Services for Enhancing Capacity of Mobile Applications

The semantic contact application discussed in Section 2 uses different backend services. These services enrich the capacity of mobile clients by providing real-time context-aware and social data. Therefore, the services need to use the semantic Web to ensure integrity and applicability of the data [20]. There are some problems that need to be addressed to ensure reliability of these services. One is identifying individuals from different social networks and aggregating social data for the purpose of being used in mobile applications. For example, Alice has a friend named Bob who has accounts in Facebook, Twitter and Blogger and he is using different email addresses. If Alice knows all of Bob's email addresses it is possible for her to access Bob's information from the different sources. If Alice enters the email addresses in the semantic contact application she is using the application will be able to fetch Bob's status, his blog entries, and the news he has shown interest in. For this process to work seamlessly and automatically there is a need for a number of backend services which are described below.

Profile Builder Service: The profile builder services fetch data from different public and private data sources of the Web and build consistent profile leveraging semantic Web technology. The data sources use different data formats and access policies, so it is difficult to provide a consistent data model for capturing data and building a profile on an individual basis. Fig. 3 below provides the RDF-based extended FOAF documents where data is collected from several data sources. The data refers to Bob, but the data identification keys are different. For example, in A^1 the data source is Facebook and the data owner identification key is bob@gmail.com while in A^2 the data

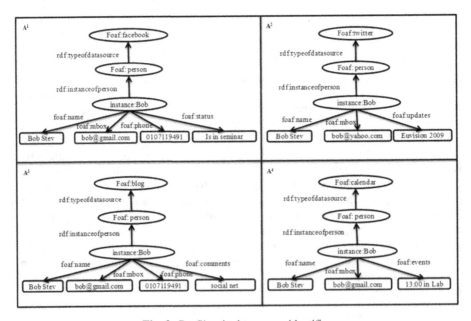

Fig. 3. Conflicts in data owner identifier

source is Twitter and the data owner identification key is bob@yahoo.com. Even if the data owner is Bob in both cases it appears as if the data owners are different because of the owner identification key.

Location Tracking Service: Location tracking services provides location information of the mobile user. Preserving privacy is one the main problem for developing such services.

Dynamic Group Creator Service: The Dynamic Group service contains all updated information of the user's contact lists and individuals. It enhances the capacity of the mobile application to perform standard query operation and build dynamic groups on the fly. This service utilizes the data collected by the data collector service and provides high value services.

Social Data Collector Service: The Social Data collector aggregates social data from different social networks.

6   Challenges

This Section describes challenges related to building a mobile social networking platform.

Interaction Design: As mentioned in the paper, semantic information obtained from the Web can be used to improve existing mobile applications, for example implementing a semantic contact application. One challenge is to investigate how to best utilize semantic information so that the application becomes easier to use, given the limited attention span of the human mind. As it also may be difficult or even impossible to develop a system with 100 percent accuracy, it is necessary to modify the application, in particular the user interface, to better deal with inaccurate or conflicting semantic information. For example, one option could be to implement a recommendation system where the user always has the final word. Another option could be to adapt the user interface (e.g. re-arrange or sort visible artifacts) to minimize user interaction. An option is also to weigh redundant information to achieve better accuracy. Optimally the user may not notice that the system sometimes fails as the application just become a bit less informative or more difficult to use in that particular case.

New Communication Services: Semantic information can be used to implement new types of communication services. For example, implementing a new Web service that forms dynamic groups of people based on location and user interest. One important research challenge is to explore how these new services should be designed and evaluate possible user benefits. This includes developing new Web frameworks and middleware as well as new user interfaces. One could for example imagine a dynamic group being visualized as third dimensional graph where the user can easily browse and navigate the currently discovered dynamic groups.

Unified Communication: When developing a new communication service it is important to get as many users as possible. When more and more communication services are deployed as Web services, it becomes possible to create mashups or aggregated Web services. As users being part of a dynamic group could be using different communication services (e.g. Twitter and Facebook) the system should automatically dispatch messages between different social networks. A challenge is therefore to make an integrated effort of consolidating social networks, or even create a virtual social network service. Although similar services (e.g. OpenSocial [19]) already exist, more advanced orchestration and Web frameworks should be developed to more easily utilize new Web APIs.

Data Mining: Data mining algorithms must be utilized in order to generate semantic information. By extracting information from social networks it is possible to automatically discover information about users. For example, automatically find phone numbers, user names and relationship between users. The information can be obtained from a wide variety of sources, including news feeds, images, videos, and text obtained from classical Web pages. However, as users may have different account or profile names, it can be difficult to map information to a one particular user. Similarly, using non unique data fields to map data can easily result in inaccurate data sets. For example, using a personal name to map data obtained from a Web page to Twitter account can easily result in inaccuracy as personal names are typically not unique.

Another problem is that the vast majority of the data on Web is not available to a crawler or even a browser, but is hidden in forms, data bases, and interactive interfaces. While many Web services now provide public APIs which makes it easier to access hidden data, they usually require some form of authentication in order to be used. This means that the data mining software must maintain credentials to different Web sites while at the same time not jeopardize the security of the users.

In addition to accessing data on the Web, data mining software should also be able to access data stored on mobile devices. For example, accessing data stored in contact list, call history, message history, and browser history etc. The call list is particularly interested as it in principle is a social network, many times reflecting the user's closest social contact or real friends [5]. One option to access local data on mobile phones it let the mobile device be accessible from the Internet (e.g. via a local Web server) so that a crawler can access the data. Another option is to let a software running on the mobile device publish relevant information to an external Web service. In both cases, it is important not to compromise the user's privacy while also preserving the battery life time of the mobile device.

Yet another enhancement could be to let the mobile devices interact with the surrounding environment. For example, detecting social interaction patterns by getting information from sensors (RFID, NFS, Bluetooth, barcodes etc.) deployed in buildings or other mobile devices. This information should be aggregated and processed with other information obtained from the Web in order to draw as good as possible.

Semantic Web and Reasoning: Once data has been fetched from the Web, it needs to be combined and refined into useful semantic information. Depending on the data received from the data mining component, the reasoning module analyses the data, draw conclusions, and store the refined data in a suitable ontology. One important research challenge is to develop suitable ontologies and rules to fuse the data into fields that fits the used ontology. Machine learning algorithms such as clustering algorithms and statistical models can be used to find useful patterns, but it could also be useful to analyze the data offline to manually find patterns, for example matching data to social sciences theories. Defining useful rules and applying machine learning algorithms to efficiently utilize vast data set containing information from the Web and sensors to improve personal communication is still a challenging research problem.

Privacy: As mentioned before, semantic information about a user must be treated carefully. The challenge is to support privacy and integrity in a simple yet powerful way. A common solution is to let the users be in control and provides some easy way for the users to share information. Typically, users will only share information if the gain is greater than possibly privacy implications. For example, people upload videos and images to YouTube and Flickr because they want other people to be able to easily access the data, or to improve their own social status. These aspects must be considered when developing new services.

7 Discussion and Future Work

This paper draws a skeleton for a mobile social networking architecture while presenting major challenges for implementing a mobile social networking platform, which in turn raises a number of research questions worthy to discuss and to study more closely in the future.

There are always inherent problems with gathering information from numerous sources, such as different social networks. Traceability of information is a logical problem about how, when and from where a particular social network is collecting social data. How can this information be trusted? How can the source of the information be relayed to the user without adding interaction overhead and confuse a user? Is it possible to fuse the information in a heterogeneous and meaningful way?

Social networks can simplify communication, not only because social networks are able to aggregate social data over the Internet, but also because of the potential influence social data can have on different applications (e.g., mobile applications or desktop applications). However, simplification often means automation and making the services more pervasive. In this lies a basic question, is it possible to find a good balance between proactivity (where the system acts in behalf of the user) and pervasiveness (where the system avoids prompting the user for a response)? Is it possible to reduce the cognitive load communication tools have on users, especially when it comes to being 'always online' and having a limited attention span?

Privacy and integrity safeguards are important, as automation of revealing personal information increases the risks of misuse of the information simply because more information will be available. It may prove vital to design the architecture from a simple yet powerful framework for privacy and integrity – otherwise users may choose not to trust the new services and thus not use them. Would dynamic groups be such a methodology for providing control of personal information? Can information be presented in less detail without loss of perceived use and without sacrificing the desired functionality of the services?

Naturally standards for social data are bound to be defined, such as OpenSocial, which are necessary in order for integration of social networks with mobile applications. Naturally also service providers will strive for the opposite in order to leverage their own services. The question here is whether it is possible to fuse information from the social networks existing today and how is that fused information perceived from perspectives of correctness, completeness and non-ambiguity? What information is possible to derive from the different social networks, as their API-based access policies are both limited and their APIs in some cases also are deprecated with no or little notification to developers?

Also, data formats and orchestration policies are not yet standardized, which means possible limitation in an open platform for social network integration with the mobile applications. Would OpenSocial currently suffice and how could it be developed to suit the needs of mobile applications? Is an extended API necessary and what parameters are of importance (flexibility, heterogeneity, etc)?

Most social networks are accesses through a Web-browser today, using Web2.0 and SOA as an enabling technologies. A mobile device has obvious limitations for presentation of graphical content, but instead are almost always carried with the user and is thus 'always on'. Would it be possible to mitigate the gap using semantic Web technology and pervasive methods based on semantic information? Less is more, as the saying, but what is lost due to the selection of information to present to the user?

Lastly, communication should be simple and intuitive. Most users use a minimum of the functionality of the mobile devices they use for communication. Can simplicity be achieved through a flexible way of creating, maintaining and using a social network for communication (e.g. utilizing dynamic groups)?

8 Conclusion

This paper presents challenges for utilizing social network information to enhance mobile applications. The three most challenging issues may be how to integrate and consolidate social networks, how to mitigate the gap between the traditional and the mobile Web through use of semantic Web technology, and how to manage semantic information for mobile applications. The challenges were discussed from a semantic Web and SOA perspective together with a driving scenario as motivation.

The main conclusion is that a mobile social networking framework would enable integration of general semantic information (location, activity, interests, etc) with social network data (from Twitter, FaceBook, LinkedIn, etc) to facilitate intelligent yet easy to use communication tools for individual persons as well as groups of persons. A goal is to make complex communication simple through utilization of pervasive technologies and semantic information from social networks. Mobile social networking would ultimately connect a person's virtual and physical world, thus enabling a wide range of novel applications that benefit from semantic information in general and social network data in particular.

References

1. Miluzzo, E., Lane, N.D., Fodor, K., Peterson, R., Lu, H., Musolesi, M., Eisenman, S.B., Zheng, X., Campbell, A.T.: Sensing meets mobile social networks: the design, implementation and evaluation of the CenceMe application. In: 6th ACM Conference on Embedded Network Sensor Systems, Raleigh, NC (2008)
2. Huberman, B.A., Romero, D.M., Wu, F.: Social networks that matter: Twitter under the microscope. In: CoRR abs/0812.1045 (2008)

3. Li, X., Guo, L., Zhao, Y.E.: Tag-based social interest discovery. In: 17th international Conference on World Wide Web, Beijing (2008)
4. Lytras, M., Damiani, E., Pablos, P.: Web 2.0: the Business Model. Springer Publishing Company, Incorporated (2008)
5. Ankolekar, A., Luon, Y., Szabo, G., Huberman, B.: Friendlee: A Mobile Application for Your Social Life. In: MobileHCI, Bonn (2009)
6. Michlmayr, A., Leitner, P., Rosenberg, F., Dustdar, S.: Publish/subscribe in the VRESCo SOA runtime. In: Second international Conference on Distributed Event-Based Systems, Rome (2008)
7. Veijalainen, J.: Developing Mobile Ontologies; Who, Why, Where, and How? In: 8th international conference on Mobile Data Management, Mannheim, pp. 398–401 (2007)
8. Web Services Description Language (WSDL) 1.1, `http://www.w3.org/TR/wsdl`
9. Hallberg, J., Norberg, M.B., Kristiansson, J., Synnes, K., Nugent, C.: Creating dynamic groups using context-awareness. In: 6th international Conference on Mobile and Ubiquitous Multimedia, Oulu, Finland (2007)
10. Christopoulou, E., Goumopoulos, C., Kameas, A.: An ontology-based context management and reasoning process for UbiComp applications. In: Joint Conference on Smart Objects and Ambient intelligence: innovative Context-Aware Services: Usages and Technologies (2005)
11. Ding, L., Zhou, L., Finin, T., Joshi, A.: How the Semantic Web is Being Used: An Analysis of FOAF Documents. In: 38th Annual Hawaii international Conference on System Sciences, vol. 04 (2005)
12. Mello, A., Rein, L.: Using Standards to Normalize Domain Specific Metadata. In: W3C Workshop on the Future of Social Networking, Barcelona (2009)
13. Borcea, C., Gupta, A., Kalra, A., Jones, Q., Iftode, L.: The MobiSoC middleware for mobile social computing: challenges, design, and early experiences. In: 1st international Conference on Mobile Wireless Middleware, Operating Systems, and Applications, Innsbruck, Austria (2008)
14. Kolan, P., Dantu, R.: Socio-technical defense against voice spamming. ACM Trans. Auton. Adapt. Syst. 2 (2007)
15. Seo, J., Croft, W.B.: Blog site search using resource selection. In: 17th ACM Conference on information and Knowledge Management, Napa Valley, California (2008)
16. Häkkilä, J., Mäntyjärvi, J.: Developing design guidelines for context-aware mobile applications. In: 3rd international Conference on Mobile Technology, Applications &Amp; Systems Bangkok (2006)
17. Zigkolis, C., Kompatsiaris, Y., Vakali, A.: Information analysis in mobile social networks for added-value services. In: The W3C Workshop on the Future of Social Networking, Barcelona (2009)
18. `http://www.programmableWeb.com/apis/directory/1?apicat=Social` (May 2009)
19. `http://www.opensocial.org/page/opensocial-foundation-faq` (May 2009)
20. Mika, P.: Social Networks and the Semantic Web (Semantic Web and Beyond). Springer, New York (2007)

Mobile Monitoring Stations and Web Visualization of Biotelemetric System - Guardian II

Ondrej Krejcar, Dalibor Janckulik, Leona Motalova, and Jan Kufel

VSB Technical University of Ostrava, Center for Applied Cybernetics,
Department of measurement and control, 17. Listopadu 15, 70833 Ostrava Poruba,
Czech Republic
Ondrej.Krejcar@remoteworld.net, Dalibor.Janckulik@hotmail.com,
Leona.Motalova@gmail.com, Jan.Kufel@awebdesign.cz

Abstract. The main area of interest of our project is to provide solution which can be used in different areas of health care and which will be available through PDAs (Personal Digital Assistants), web browsers or desktop clients. The realized system deals with an ECG sensor connected to mobile equipment, such as PDA/Embedded, based on Microsoft Windows Mobile operating system. The whole system is based on the architecture of .NET Compact Framework, and Microsoft SQL Server. Visualization possibilities of web interface and ECG data are also discussed and final suggestion is made to Microsoft Silverlight solution along with current screenshot representation of implemented solution. The project was successfully tested in real environment in cryogenic room $(-136^{0}C)$.

Keywords: PDA, Embedded Device, Biotelemetry, ECG, Silverlight, Cryogenic Room.

1 Introduction

Aim of the platform for patients' bio-parameters monitoring is to offer a solution providing services to help and make full health care more efficient without limitations for specific country. Physicians and other medical staff will not be forced to make difficult and manual work including unending paperwork, but they will be able to focus on the patients and their problems. All data will be accessible almost anytime anywhere through special applications designated for portable devices web browser or desktop clients and any made changes will be immediately at disposal to medical staff based on the security clearance. Nurses will be able to find out prescribed procedure of patient treatment which was written down by doctor during regular round. Physicians will have immediate access to the patient's newest results of accomplished examinations. In the case that the ambulance have to go to some accident, rescue team can due to portable devices send information about patient health condition directly to hospital where responsible doctors and staff will have information needed to execute immediate operation without delaying by preparation of necessary equipment. Patients who need not hospitalization will be able to be treated at home due to the

R. Mehmood et al. (Eds.): EuropeComm 2009, LNICST 16, pp. 286–293, 2009.

system capable of remote transmission of information about patient's bio-signals, so patients will be constantly under medical supervision and doctors will be able to make necessary measure if needed. All bio-signals data will be stored and automatically analyzed by neuronal network. System will evaluate presence of critical values which could be the sign of worse medical condition of a patient. In the moment of crossing the border of monitored bio-signals values inserted by doctor, system will inform responsible medical staff and provides all information which could help to determine the cause and seriousness of the problem.

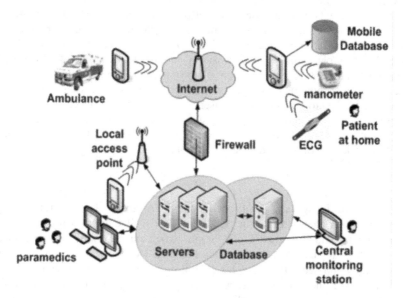

Fig. 1. Architecture of Guardian II platform

The basic idea is to create a system that controls important information about the state of a wheelchair-bound person (monitoring of ECG and pulse in early phases, then other optional values like temperature or oxidation of blood etc.), his situation in time and place (GPS) and an axis tilt of his body or wheelchair (2axis accelerometer). Values are measured with the existing equipment, which communicates with the module for processing via Bluetooth wireless communication technology. Most of the data (according to heftiness) is processed directly in PDA or Embedded equipment to a form that is acceptable for simple visualization. Two variants are possible in case of embedded equipment – with visualization and without visualization (entity with/without LCD display). Data is continually sent by means of GPRS or WiFi to a server, where it is being processed and evaluated in detail. Processing and evaluating on the server consists of - receiving data, saving data to data storage, visualization in an advanced form (possibility to recur to the older graph, zoom on a histogram (graph with historical trend), copying from the graphs, printing graphs), automatic evaluation of the critical states with the help of advanced technologies (algorithms) that use Artificial intelligence to notify the operator about the critical state and its archiving. Application in PDA, Embedded equipment is comfortable, with minimum time - the first configuration, but also configuration after downfall of application. The level of visualization will be lower. The described system can be used with small modifications for monitoring of patients in hospitals or people working in extremely hard conditions.

2 Developed Parts of Platform

Complete proposition of solution and implementation of the platform for patient's biotelemetry as it was described in previous chapter requires determination and teamwork. Every single part of the architecture has to be designed for easy application and connectivity without user extra effort, but user must be able to use given solution easily and effectively. Crucial parts of whole architecture are network servers, database servers and client applications. Due to these crucial parts the development is focused particularly on proposition and implementation of desktop client application, database structure and some other important web services.

Scenario for communication among desktop client, web services and Microsoft SQL Server is: desktop client runs on user´s computer and connects to web services on remote application server. After the desktop client is connected, web services connect to remote database server. Web services provide methods for users so users are capable to work with different data stored in database.

2.1 Mobile Parts

The main part of the system is an Embedded or PDA device. The difference in applications for measurement units is the possibility to visualize the measured data in both Real-time Graph and Historical Trend Graph, which can be omitted on an embedded device. PDA is a much better choice for Personal Healthcare, where the patient is already healthy and needs to review his condition. Embedded devices can be designed for one user, with the option to use an external display used for settings or with the possibility of usage in extreme conditions.

As measurement device is possible to connect several device with Bluetooth communication possibility. In our application we use an ECG Measurement Unit (Corbelt or BlueECG) through a virtual serial port using wireless Bluetooth technology. Measured data is stored on a SD Memory Card as a database of MS SQL Server 2005 Mobile Edition. The performance of available devices seems insufficient for sequential access; parsing of incoming packets is heavily time-consuming. Pseudo paralleling is required. A newer operating system (Windows Mobile 6) must be used to allow the processing of data from a professional EKG due to thread count limitations. The informations about user, as ID, name, surname, address and application properties are stored in the system registry (HKEY_CURRENT_USER / Software / Guardian). Working (saving, reading, finding) with registry is easier and faster as saving this informations in file. User registry values are crypted with simple algorithm (shifting char ASCII value).

Devices based on PDA type have a several limitations such as low CPU performance, low battery life or small display, which is possible to solve by embedded version of such mobile clients. We created a special windows mobile based embedded device. During the development process the several problems occurred. One of them and the most important was the need of a new operation system creation for our special architectural and device needs. We used the Microsoft PlatformBuilder for Windows CE 4.2 tools. The created operation system based on standard windows mobile has several drivers which we need to operate with communication devices and measurement devices.

2.2 Server Parts

In order to run a server, an operating system supporting IIS (Internet Information Server) is needed. IIS allow to users to connect to the web server by the HTTP protocol. The web service transfers data between the server and PDA/Embedded devices. It reads the data, sends acknowledgments, stores the data in the database and reads it from there. The service is built upon ASP.NET 2.0 technology. The SOAP protocol is used for the transport of XML data. The Wireless ECG approaches a real professional ECG with data rate as high as 800 records per second [1]. Considering 100 patients, the value gets to 288,000,000 records per hour. Even if the server accepted only 50 records per second, the sum of records for 100 patients per hour would be 18 million. That is an extreme load for both the server and the database system; hence a better way of storing data is needed. Methods that devices communicating with the web service can use include: receiving measured data, receiving patient data, deleting a patient, patient data sending. To observe measured data effectively, visualization is needed. A type of graph as used in professional solutions is an ideal solution. To achieve this in a server application, a freeware Zed Graph library can be used. For data analysis, neural nets are a convenient solution. However, there are problems in the automatic detection of critical states. Every person has a specific ECG pattern. The Neural net has to learn to distinguish critical states of each patient separately.

Important part of Guardian is central database. There are stored all data of medical staff and patients. Data of patients include different records such as diagnosis, treatment progress or data which are results of measuring by small portable devices designated to home care. These data represent the greatest problem, because amount of these data rapidly increase with increasing amount of patients. Due to this fact database servers are very loaded.

Next important parts of the platform are web services, which allow us effectively work with medical records or other data. Guardian web services are: User management, Data management, Configuration management, and User management. Each web service deals with common security module, which provides methods for one-way encryption and also implementation of methods for authorization and other security components is planned.

2.3 Visualization

We have much posibility to plotting the graphs, but in every case we can catch any disadvantage, which is caused by a lot of elements. We will try to map these solutions and find the best one for the EKG data representing.

For the main programming of the entire application it is used the ASP.NET 2.0 platform. ASP.NET is the next generation ASP, but it's not an upgraded version of ASP. It is an entirely new technology for server-side scripting. It was written from the ground up and is not backward compatible with classic ASP. It is also the major part of the Microsoft's .NET Framework.

There a lot of questions between choosing the right choice for the graphical data representing. We can use for example the Dundas Graphs, Adobe Flash or the new

Microsoft Silverlight. Dundas Graphs is a very popular choice, and we can say the best-known between commercial use. This is also the big disadvantage – we could not use it for ourselves as the open – source solution, and the customizing is disabled, too. Macromedia Flash is the best-known choice for its very good internet viewer's compatibility, but it has also many disadvantages. For example, if we have rendered .SWF file, and included into the HTML code, it is impossible for us to edit it. XAML of the Silverlight is very good solution, because it could be edited just in the notepad for example.

Microsoft Silverlight is a programmable web browser plug-in that enables features such as animation, vector graphics and audio-video playback that characterizes rich Internet applications. Silverlight provides a retained mode graphics system similar to Windows Presentation Foundation, and integrates multimedia, graphics, animations and interactivity into a single runtime environment. In Silverlight applications, user interfaces are declared in XAML and programmed using a subset of the .NET Framework. XAML can be used for marking up the vector graphics and animations. Textual content created with Silverlight is searchable and indexable by search engines as it is not compiled, but represented as text (XAML). Silverlight makes it possible to dynamically load XML content that can be manipulated through a DOM interface, a technique that is consistent with conventional Ajax techniques. With version 2.0, the programming logic can be written in any .NET language, including some derivatives of common dynamic programming languages like Iron Ruby and Iron Python.

We were focused mainly to the mapping of new possibilities about the EKG signal, next to the new technologies possibilities. As it has been appeared, there are many platforms, which we could use for the work with the EKG data and as a next step graphical solution, but we have to know, everyone has their advantages and disadvantages. We have to find the compromise, which can be easily available and we do not have to pay for it for the price of complete research of the new solution.

We mentioned about possibilities of the Dundas Graphs, Adobe Flash and in the main case Silverlight, the new platform from the Microsoft Storage, so we realized, the final solution will be best exactly with that. It is quite new technology, which come into existence with purpose of vitalize and light up the web, thanks to using their own rendering and vector graphics representing. Nowadays it is very popular between developers and even there were some problems with starting explorer compatibility, in this time it raised up and it is very good future leader on the field of vector internet graphic.

In the case of starting problems with the C# programming language it was a problem for us to find a best choice of cooperation between ASP.NET application and the Silverligh. First draft of the application program was mainly based on editing the JavaScript file and including the Silverlight files into the HTML source code. This JS file is the main file for the setting and programming the Silverlight graph behavior. It is very good to use it, because we can make our own ASP.NET project with database binding and the Silverlight is only just included component. The problems come if we want to trace the program to find some bugs. We could transfer variables between ASP and SL by the overwriting the JS file, or by the session variables. All of these solutions are just temporary, because of very slow program run and low application effectivity.

As we realized in the final part of the application, it was quite difficult to find the best choice for the application, but we would like the solution with the linear cooperation

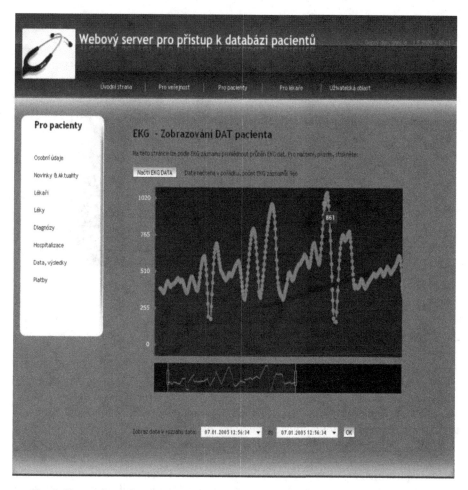

Fig. 2. User web application interface screenshot with ECG (in native Czech language)

between Visual Studio 2008 and the Silverlight Toolkit. There are so many possibilities, for example mainly saving the data right from the web-service database to the silverlight xaml.cs file. Then we have our application much faster and work is more effective. The reason is, Silverlight graph could read the source data for their graphic interpretation right from the variables, set by the Silverlight itself. We can also use very wide spread of components, for example DropDownList, Button, RichTextBox to the database components like our very good known DataGrid.

Current application interface is shown in figure [Fig. 2]. Left part consist of menu for patients with a possibilities to manage with personal data, Physicians, diagnosis, hospitalizations, data, results or payments. Upper part contains a menu for public, patients or physicians access to application. Middle part provides an access to ECG data of patient. Selection of several part of signal history is possible by mouse click or date/time setting. From the graph is possible to select several value of ECG curve and get a numerical value of these points.

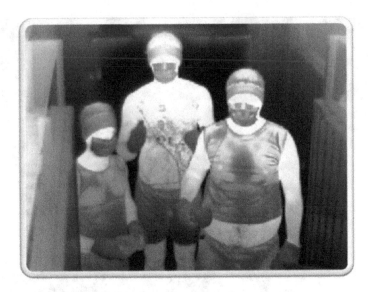

Fig. 3. Infracamera picture from Cryogenic room

3 Conclusions

The measuring device (ECG, plethysmograph) and Guardian PDA client was tested in extreme conditions in a cryogen room in Teplice (-136°C), where the final system will be installed [Fig. 3]. Implementation of the data transmission security was not solved. The whole system is classified as „work in progress" system and it is in a testing phase where we found mistakes and repaired them.

We think all the web application could be raised on the better level in the future, by the application of a few improvements. We can include to our graphical user interface some script, which could be used as the communication element between patients and doctors, for example for some messages or requests. As the final improvement in the future, the application would have some special algorithm, which could recognize any symptoms of the QRS curve, and make the job for the doctors much easier. As next improvement we would like to apply the better script for the Pan&Zoom function – it is very easy to control and we could find our place of interest very fast.

Acknowledgment. This work was supported by the Ministry of Education of the Czech Republic under Project 1M0567.

References

1. Reis, P.: Conferencia Telemedicina Onde Estamos e para onde vamos, Ericsson (2006)
2. Krejcar, O., Cernohorsky, J.: Database Prebuffering as a Way to Create a Mobile Control and Information System with Better Response Time. In: Bubak, M., van Albada, G.D., Dongarra, J., Sloot, P.M.A. (eds.) ICCS 2008, Part I. LNCS, vol. 5101, pp. 489–498. Springer, Heidelberg (2008)

3. Krejcar, O.: PDPT Framework - Building Information System with Wireless Connected Mobile Devices. In: ICINCO 2006, 3rd International Conference on Informatics in Control, Automation and Robotics, Setubal, Portugal, August 01-05, 2006, pp. 162–167 (2006)
4. Krejcar, O., Cernohorsky, J.: New Possibilities of Intelligent Crisis Management by Large Multimedia Artifacts Prebuffering. In: Ulieru, M., Palensky, P., Doursat, R. (eds.) I.T. Revolutions 2008. LNICST, vol. 11, pp. 44–59. Springer, Heidelberg (2008)
5. Arikan, E., Jenq, J.: Microsoft SQL Server interface for mobile devices. In: Proceedings of the 4th International Conference on Cybernetics and Information Technologies, Systems and Applications/5th Int. Conf. on Computing, Communications and Control Technologies, Orlando, FL, USA, July 12-15 (2007)
6. Jewett, M., Lasker, S., Swigart, S.: SQL server everywhere: Just another database? Developer focused from start to finish. DR DOBBS Journal 31(12) (2006)
7. Janckulik, D., Krejcar, O., Martinovic, J.: Personal Telemetric System – Guardian. In: Biodevices 2008, Insticc Setubal, Funchal, Portugal, pp. 170–173 (2008)
8. Krejcar, O.: Benefits of Building Information System with Wireless Connected Mobile Device - PDPT Framework. In: 1st IEEE International Conference on Portable Information Devices, PORTABLE 2007, Orlando, Florida, USA, pp. 251–254 (2007)
9. Krejcar, O., Cernohorsky, J., Janckulik, D.: Portable devices in Architecture of Personal Biotelemetric Systems. In: 4th WSEAS International Conference on Cellular and Molecular Biology, Biophysics and Bioengineering, BIO 2008, Puerto De La Cruz, Canary Islands, Spain, December 15-17, 2008, pp. 60–64 (2008)
10. Krejcar, O., Cernohorsky, J., Czekaj, P.: Secured Access to RT Database in Biotelemetric System. In: 4th WSEAS Int. Conference on Cellular and Molecular Biology, Biophysics and Bioengineering, BIO 2008, Puerto De La Cruz, Canary Islands, Spain, December 15-17, 2008, pp. 70–73 (2008)
11. Krejcar, O., Cernohorsky, J., Janckulik, D.: Database Architecture for real-time accessing of Personal Biotelemetric Systems. In: 4th WSEAS Int. Conference on Cellular and Molecular Biology, Biophysics and Bioengineering, BIO 2008, Puerto De La Cruz, Canary Islands, Spain, December 15-17, 2008, pp. 85–89 (2008)
12. Penhaker, M., Cerny, M., Martinak, L., Spisak, J., Valkova, A.: HomeCare - Smart embedded biotelemetry system. In: World Congress on Medical Physics and Biomedical Engineering, Seoul, South Korea, August 27-September 01, vol. 14, PTS 1-6, pp. 711–714 (2006)
13. Cerny, M., Penhaker, M.: Biotelemetry. In: 14th Nordic-Baltic Conference an Biomedical Engineering and Medical Physics, IFMBE Proceedings, Riga, Latvia, June 16-20, vol. 20, pp. 405–408 (2008)

Practical Issues of Wireless Mobile Devices Usage with Downlink Optimization

Ondrej Krejcar, Dalibor Janckulik, and Leona Motalova

VSB Technical University of Ostrava, Center for Applied Cybernetics,
Department of measurement and control, 17. Listopadu 15, 70833 Ostrava Poruba,
Czech Republic
Ondrej.Krejcar@remoteworld.net, Dalibor.Janckulik@vsb.cz,
Leona.Motalova@vsb.cz

Abstract. Mobile device makers produce tens of new complex mobile devices per year to put users a special mobile device with a possibility to do anything, anywhere, anytime. These devices can operate full scale applications with nearly the same comfort as their desktop equivalents only with several limitations. One of such limitation is insufficient download on wireless connectivity in case of the large multimedia files. Main area of paper is in a possibilities description of solving this problem as well as the test of several new mobile devices along with server interface tests and common software descriptions. New devices have a full scale of wireless connectivity which can be used not only to communication with outer land. Several such possibilities of use are described. Mobile users will have also an online connection to internet all time powered on. Internet is mainly the web pages but the web services use is still accelerate up. The paper deal also with a possibility of maximum user amounts to have a connection at same time to current server type. At last the new kind of database access – Linq technology is compare to ADO.NET in response time meaning.

Keywords: Mobile Device; Prebuffering; Response Time; Area Definition, Linq, ADO.NET.

1 Introduction

The usage of various mobile wireless technologies and mobile embedded devices has been increasing dramatically every year and would be growing in the following years. This will lead to the rise of new application domains in network-connected PDAs or XDAs (the "X" represents voice and information/data within one device; "Digital Assistant") that provide more or less the same functionality as their desktop application equivalents. The idea of full scale applications pursuable on mobile devices is based on current hi-tech devices with large scale display, large memory capabilities, and wide spectrum of network standards plus embedded GPS module (HTC Touch HD).

Users of these portable devices use them all time in context of their life (e.g. moving, searching, alerting, scheduling, writing, etc.). Context is relevant to the mobile user, because in a mobile environment the context is often very dynamic and the user

R. Mehmood et al. (Eds.): EuropeComm 2009, LNICST 16, pp. 294–305, 2009.

interacts differently with the applications on his mobile device when the context is different [1].

My recent research of context-aware computing has been restricted to location-aware computing for mobile applications using a WiFi network (LBS Location Based Services). The information about basic concept and technologies of user localization (such as LBS, Searching for WiFi AP) can be found in my article [2]. On localization basis, We created a special framework called PDPT (Predictive Data Push Technology) which can improve a usage of large data artifacts of mobile devices [3]. We used continual user position information to determine a predictive user position. The data artifacts linked to user predicted position are prebuffered to user mobile device. When user arrives to position which was correctly determined by PDPT Core, the data artifacts are in local memory of PDA. The time to display the artifacts from local memory is much shorter than in case of remotely requested artifact.

The idea of prebuffering may not be only one application method for user position knowledge. As well as WiFi is not only one wireless network to use for localization of user device. WiFi has advantage in speed in indoor positioning therefore the GSM/UMTS can be used in outdoor. The GPS sensor is also embedded in several types of current mobile devices, or it can be plugged by SDIO or BT interface.

We would like to describe a problem of long response in mobile device in the beginning of next chapter. Following subchapter will deal with optimal artifact size determination as well as new partial prebuffering techniques details. The position information obtaining from wireless networks (WiFi, BT, GSM, GPS) background will follow in next subchapter. The needed info about PDPT Framework design, area definition around the user and PDPT client application highlights are in the rest subchapters of chapter 2.

2   The PDPT Framework and PDPT Core

The general principle of my simple localization states that if a WiFi-enabled mobile device is close to such a stationary device – Access Point (AP) it may "ask" the provider's location position by setting up a WiFi connection. If position of the AP is known, the position of mobile device is within a range of this location provider. This range depends on type of WiFi AP. The Cisco APs are used in my test environment at Campus of Technical University of Ostrava. We performed measurements on these APs to get signal strength (SS) characteristics of all APs. The simplification of these characteristics was made to get one "super ideal characteristic" which represent a combination of characteristics of all measured APs. More details can be found in chapter 2.3 [5]. The computed equation for Super-Ideal characteristic is taken as basic equation for PDPT Core to compute the real distance from WiFi SS. This equation is in the web service code (PDPT Framework Server – Core module) to transform a Signal Strength in dB to distance from WiFi APs.

The PDA client will support the application in automatically retrieving location information from nearby location providers, and in interacting with the server. Naturally, this principle can be applied to other wireless technologies like Bluetooth, GSM or WiMAX.

To let a mobile device determine its own position is needed to have a selected adapter still powered on. This fact provides a small limitation of use of mobile devices. The complex test with several types of battery is described in my article [4] in chapter (3). The test results with a possibly to use a PDA with turned on WiFi adapter for a period of about 5 hours.

2.1 The Need of Predictive Data Push Technology

PDPT framework is based on a model of location-aware enhancement, which we have used in created system. This technique is useful in framework to increase the real dataflow from wireless access point (server side) to PDA (client side). Primary dataflow is enlarged by data prebuffering. PDPT pushes the data from SQL database to clients PDA to be helpful when user comes at final location which was expected by PDPT Core. The benefit of PDPT consists in time delay reducing needed to display desired artifacts requested by a user from PDA. This delay may vary from a few seconds to number of minutes. Theoretical background and tests were needed to determine an average artifact size for which the PDPT technique is useful. First of all the maximum response time of an application (PDPT Client) for user was needed to be specified.

Nielsen [6] specified the maximum response time for an application to 10 seconds [7]. During this time the user was focused on the application and was willing to wait for an answer. The book is over 20 years old (published in 1994). We suppose the modern user of mobile devices is more impatient so the stated value of 10 second will be shorter. This is for me even better, because my framework is more usable. We used this time period (10 second) to calculate the maximum possible data size of a file transferred from server to client (during this period). To define the amount of data is possible to download to mobile device; we executed a test of data transfer rate measurement of large data size artifacts throw the FTP protocol. we used as test devices four types of PDA (HTC Athena, HTC Universal, HTC Blueangel, HTC Roadster). Fist two devices are equipped with 802.11g standard while the rest two are only with 80211b standard of WiFi capability. These PDA devices were connected throw CISCO Wi-Fi AP. The FTP server holds 3 types of large artifacts (files) which were downloaded to internal PDA memory.

Table 1. Transmission speed on large files

data size [MB]	PDA device			
	Athena	Universal	Blueangel	Roadster
	Transfer Speed [kB{s]			
10	347	123	160	106
20	344	121	157	79
40	314	123	58	43

Unafraid the theoretical transfer rates (802.11g = 54 Mbit/s, 802.11b = 11Mbit/s) were not achieved [Tab. 1]. The maximal transfer rate of 350 kB/s has HTC Athena, but this device is not a standard PDA device. Athena is a mini-notebook with windows mobile 6 operating system. All of others devices have only a quarter amount of such speed. It is much clear that the wireless connected mobile devices have not only a limitation in wireless network module HW, but it has a problem in a slow internal bus. Finally if transfers speed wary from 40 to 160 kB/s the result file size (file which can be downloaded in a defined time of 10 seconds) wary from 400 to 1600 kB.

2.2 Determination of Optimal Artifact Size

The next step is an average artifact size definition. we use a network architecture building plan as a sample database, which contained 100 files of average size of 470 kB. The client application can download during the 10 second period from 2 to 3 artifacts. The problem is the long time delay in displaying of artifacts in some original file types. It is needed to use only basic data formats, which can be displayed by PDA natively (bmp, jpg, wav, mpg, etc.) without any additional striking time consumption.

The abysmal difference of transfer speeds from previous table [Tab. 1] vamooses, when we use for transfer smaller data files (10KB – 150KB). The testing of data transfer throw the web services was executed on all of mentioned devices. Firstly the 50 kB and then the 150 kB data file were transferred. The response time for one access and then for 100 access and finally for 500 access were measured. The test results are in [Tab. 2] and [Tab. 3].

Table 2. Response time - 50KB artifacts [ms]

Type	Number of Artifacts		
	1	100	500
Type	**Transfer Speed [kB{s]**		
Mode	101.82	5208.62	16036.61
Median	101.86	5228.54	16024.24
Average	102.00	5229.81	16022.67

The third step to determine the optimal artifact size is testing of database response for buffering. The test was executed again on all mentioned devices. The information about SQL server response of SQL Server 3.5 Compact Edition was stored.

From the executed test over the web service is evident; the artifacts of size from 50 to 150 kB are more suitable for transfer. It is because the transfer speed of them is relatively affordable in compare to transferred data amount.

Table 3. Response time - 150KB artifacts [ms]

Type	Number of Artifacts		
	1	100	500
Type	**Transfer Speed [kB{s]**		
Mode	304.82	20208.93	61029.73
Median	301.85	20227.71	61026.08
Average	302.00	20229.99	61022.86

In this case is only a higher starter costs which going to fall after first executed query. The SQL server response results are better in case of 50 to 150 kB artifacts. The artefacts transfer is not striking burdened by dependence on real speed of connection between AP and mobile device. Difference will show after a huge amount of artifacts was transferred (hundreds). The buffer stream of such size is equivalent to download of minimally 14 presentation areas. As will be shown from schema of presenting area, the most of buffered parts will not be needed. The most part of the writing time of SQL buffer from web service is due to the response from SQL server. As it is resulted in tables, writing of tens 50 kB files to the database cost about a same time as writing of one 500 kB file. With smaller files we are able to be more effective to cover buffered area.

Table 4. Response time average- SQL query - Insert of 1 artifact into SQL CE database engine [ms]

Device Type	Artifact size[kB]		
	50	150	500
HP 614c	176.2	528.3	2377.3
HTC Roadster	222.4	667.6	3004.0
HTC Advantage	226.6	679.5	3057.6
HTC Blueangel	136.4	409.0	1840.4
Samsung Omnia	185.9	557.2	2507.3

Table 5. Response time average- SQL query - Select of 1 artifact into SQL CE database engine [ms]

Device Type	Artifact size[kB]		
	50	150	500
HP 614c	83.0	95.7	118.7
HTC Roadster	91.3	103.3	128.1
HTC Advantage	79.3	91.2	113.1
HTC Blueangel	79.1	91.1	112.9
Samsung Omnia	81.1	93.1	115.5

The large artifacts are better in compare to 1Byte transferred data, but the response time is not optimal.

Such large artifact size is not only with slow transfer speed, but they also allow move with steps, which are not affordable for quicker move or more accurately presentation of position in artifact. The most of tests and problems passes from the size of artifacts. Therefore we made a change to data artifact size to maximal size of 150 kB and we change also the access to these artifacts to new way.

PDPT framework design is based on the most commonly used server-client architecture. To process data the server has online connection to the information system. Technology data are continually saved to SQL Server database.

Previous version of PDPT framework buffered the data according to the predicted position of user. In case of unexpected change of direction, the buffer in most cases cannot act on this quick change.

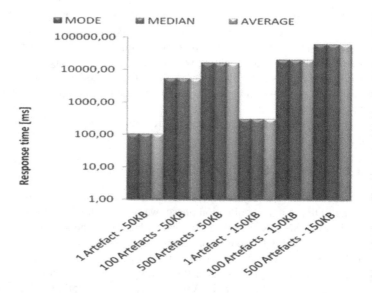

Fig. 1. Web service reaction times

The active presented area was divided to more partial artifacts [Fig. 2b]. This new modified system is now implemented to our other projects, where the position of user is needed. One of these projects is a Guardian II. This project is for hospitals areas for patients and physicians monitoring. We have implemented the new possibilities of biomedical e-health systems are discovered for increasing of interactivity. Based on position of patient, the server can select the nearest physician or nurse to act on discovered problem. By this way the response on problem can be reduced and it can help to save more human life.

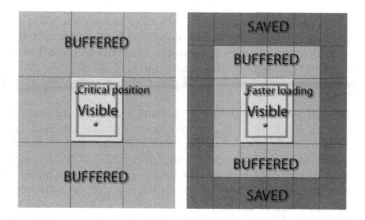

Fig. 2. a) Old application buffering (left fig.). b) New application buffering (right fig.) – visible parts merged to smaller artifacts.

Active area for move of map basis can be not only on outer margin of the whole area, but it can be on borders of several picture-boxes. By this technique is possible to move with map basis in softer grid and allow presenting the actual position of tracked object more precisely. By consequential evaluation of object moving speed, and with suitable modified map basis, we can achieve the effect of zoom of map basis. After application of such principle the system can be applicable for open space with sufficient signal for triangulation - WiFi, GSM or WiMAX. This part of framework is suitable for patient tracking in case of home care agencies. We can track the time of one attendance of nurse at the patient.

2.3 WiFi, BT, GSM and GPS Data Collection for Localization

When the use of PDPT technique is possible and it bears some advantages, the first key step of the PDPT is a data collection phase. we record information about the radio signals (WiFi, BT, GSM) as a function of a user's location. The signal information is used to construct and validate models for signal propagation.

If the mobile device knows the position of the stationary device (transmitter, BTS), it also knows that its own position is within a range of this location provider. The typical range wary from 30 to 100 m in WiFi case, respectively 50 m in BT case or 30 km for GSM. Granularity of location can be improved by triangulation of two or more visible APs (Access Points) or BTSs (Base Transceiver Stations).. The PDA client currently supports the application in automatically retrieving location information from nearby WiFi location providers, and in interacting with the PDPT server. Naturally, this principle can be applied to other wireless technologies like BT, GSM, UMTS or WiMAX. The application (locator) is implemented in C# language using the MS Visual Studio .NET with .NET Compact Framework and a special OpenNETCF library enhancement.

In previous research, we focused only to use of WiFi networks while the other wireless possibilities remained without a proper notice. Now we made an enhancement of Locator component of PDPT framework to allow operate with BT and GSM networks.

In BT network case, the position of BT APs must be known to allow the position determination. To collect BT APs position info in outdoor environment, the GPS can be used. For indoor area, the GIS (Geographic Information System) software with buildings map must be used to measure exact position of BT AP against to local environment. To manage with BT hardware of mobile device another library InTheHand 32Feet.NET is used.

GSM network is not local network but a cellular network. The problem is in position information of GSM BTSs. The operator doesn't provide any such information. One of possible solutions is based on unofficial BTSs lists which can be found on internet. The lists are typically available in HTML, TXT or CSV formats. The medium rate for BTSs with GPS position information is about 90 % of all BTSs in European countries. In case of PDPT Framework, the list must be converted to PDPT server database – GSM_BTS table.

In all three described cases of nearby BSs scanning, the data are saved to Locator Table in PDPT server DB. Data are processed from Locator Table throw the PDPT Core to Position Table. The processing techniques depend on selected wireless network. WiFi and BT network provide all visible APs nearby the user. From list of these APs is computed actual position (by triangulation).

Mobile devices with windows mobile operation system do not provide any GSM info to .NET Compact Framework. Even any special framework as in previous two cases is not known for me until now. Only possibility is in use of RIL (Radio Interface Layer) library. This library is divided into two separate components, a RIL Driver and a RIL Proxy. The RIL Driver processes radio commands and events. The RIL Proxy performs arbitration between multiple clients for access to the single RIL driver. When a module calls the RIL to get the signal strength, the function call immediately returns a response identifier. The RIL uses the function response callback to convey signal strength information to the module.

The GSM network provide only one BS info in each search cycle. This BS has the highest signal strength. The more BTSs info is collected by a several iteration cycles. During 10 cycles (per 10 seconds) the 4 BTS info is obtained on average.

The important info from BTSs is Signal Strength and Time Advance (TA). SS is refreshed every several seconds (in every scan) whereas TA is provided only during some type of communication with selected BTS (e.g. request to talk, move to another area - Location Area Code (LAC)). The list of these BTSs with info is further processed as in previous case for WiFi and BT networks. Only change is in usage of TA if it is accessible. Another possibility to get the user position in outdoor space is in GPS [8]. GPS provide a position by LONgitude and LATitude (X and Y). Only simple conversion is needed to transform a GPS coordinates to S-JTSK, which is used in PDPT Framework.

2.4 The PDPT Framework Design

The PDPT framework design is based on the server-client architecture. The PDPT framework server is created as a web service to act as a bridge between MS SQL Server (other database server eventually) and PDPT PDA Clients.

Client PDA has location sensor component, which continuously sends the information about nearby AP's intensity to the PDPT Framework Core. This component processes the user's location information and it makes a decision to which part of MS SQL Server database needs to be replicated to client's SQL Server CE database [9][10]. The PDPT Core decisions constitute the most important part of PDPT framework, because the kernel must continually compute the position of the user and track, and predict his future movement. After doing this prediction the appropriate data are prebuffered to client's database for the future possible requirements. This data represent artifacts list of PDA buffer imaginary image.

2.5 PDPT Core - Area Definition

The PDPT buffering and predictive PDPT buffering principle is not very complicated. Firstly the client must activate the PDPT on PDPT Client. This client creates a list of artifacts (PDA buffer image), which are contained in his mobile SQL Server CE database. Server create own list of artifacts (imaginary image of PDA buffer) based on area definition for actual user position and compare it with real PDA buffer image.

The area can be defined as an object where the user position is in the object centre. The PDPT Core will continue with comparing of both images. In case of some difference, the rest artifacts ale prebuffered to PDA buffer. When all artifacts for current user position are in PDA buffer, there is no difference between images. In such case the PDPT Core is going to make a predicted user position. On base of this new user position it makes a new predictive enlarged imaginary image of PDA buffer. The new cuboid has a center in direction of predicted user moving and includes a cuboid area for current user position. The PDPT Core compares the both new images (imaginary and real PDA buffer) and it will continue with buffering of artifacts until they are same. In real case of usage is better to create an algorithm to dynamic area definition to adapt a system to user needs more flexible in real time. For additional info please refer to [11].

2.6   Results – Comparisons of Two Techniques for Database Access

The PDPT framework consists of two main parts – server and client. Supposed number of users is from tens to hundreds of people with mobile device. The PDPT server has a web service interface which must be tested on adequate response time to user requests. We created special software to test these web services interfaces. The results are in table [Tab. 6].

Table 6. Median and mean response times for hundreds of users – PDPT Server web services [ms]

Users	2x4GHz + 6GB DDR2 RAM (Server)		AMD 850MHz + 512MB SD RAM (PC)	
	Median	Mean	Median	Mean
200	388	387	1413	1413
300	590	599	2099	2103
400	826	830	2851	2850
500	1061	1037	3516	3508
650	1182	1258	4574	4565
800	1662	1616	5645	5649
1000	1797	1977	7050	7046

Graph at [Fig. 3] describe the increased response time with a increased number of users. As it can be seen the values of several columns varies with small difference even for both server stations (named „Server" and „PC"). These are unfortunately only small difference. The difference between the stations increased largely from 500 simultaneous users (the difference between the stations is 2.5 s) and is growing up to 5 seconds for 1000 of users. The response time of old PC station is in this case about 7 second. This time is near the maximum response time declared by Nielsen and Hacklay [6][7]. The use of such server station is not suggested and only the new server station can manage with such amount of online users. Our created software is unfortunately possible to evaluate every web service (even the new ones) and before a real usage we can suggest a minimal server hardware configuration for adequate usage.

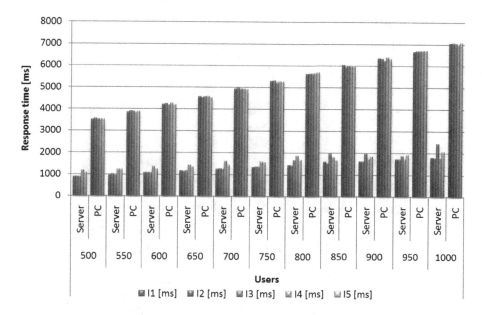

Fig. 3. Graph of response times for accessing of PDPT Server web services – 5 iteration and two server stations were tested

Table 7. Average response time – Insert of one 50KB and 150 kB artefact into SQL database through different technologies [ms]

Artifact size	50 kB		150 kB	
Device Type	Linq	ADO.NET	Linq	ADO.NET
HP 614c	229.1	202.6	686.8	607.5
HTC Roadster	289.2	255.8	867.8	767.7
HTC Advantage	294.6	260.6	883.3	781.4
HTC Blueangel	177.4	156.9	531.7	470.3
Samsung Omnia	241.6	213.7	724.3	640.8

The next step of making results is in mobile client testing. Namely the database access techniques and its response times. We made a test to accessing of SQL server buffer and the selection of better one was made. In present the testing of technologies like LINQ, ADO.NET and the direct access using SQL queries is being realized.

Preliminary test are graphed in figure [fig. 4] to provide a more visual summary. In all cases the Linq access reach higher response time value than the ADO.NET technique. The question is what the Linq technology can bring to user or developer. We evaluate several such things to find a decision which techniques is better to use. Of course the Linq is 13 % slower than the ADO.NET, but we found a several contributions in Linq to surpass this 13 %. Final decision is to use Linq access and technology in all cases which need the perfect visual response to user and access to more than one database table. These two main benefits can help to develop and use the new kind of mobile clients. PDPT Client will take advantage of these benefits in next version which is currently under the development.

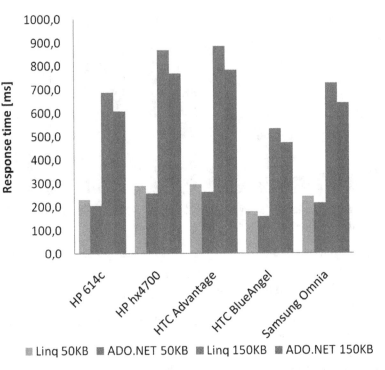

Fig. 4. Graph of average response times for inserting artifacts trough different technologies on a few devices

3 Conclusions

We are focused on the real usage of the developed PDPT Framework on a wide range of wireless connected mobile devices and its main issue at increased data transfer. For testing purpose, five mobile devices were selected with a variety of hardware and software capabilities. The high success rate found in the test data surpassed our expectations. This rate varies from 84 to 96 %. Please see the chapter 4 [5] for more info. The PDPT prebuffering techniques can improve the using of medium or large artifacts (from 50kB to 500 kB per artifact) on wireless mobile devices connected to information system. The localization part of PDPT framework is currently used in another project of biotelemetrical system for home care named Guardian II to make a patient's life safer [12]. Another utilization of PDPT consists in use of others wireless networks like BT, GSM/UMTS, WiMAX, or in GPS. This idea can be used inside the information systems like botanical or zoological gardens where the GPS navigation can be used in outdoor. Some improvements of Locator module are also described. The larger area of PDPT utilization can improve importance of PDPT Framework in wireless mobile systems.

Acknowledgment. This work was supported by the Ministry of Education of the Czech Republic under Project 1M0567.

References

1. Abowd, G., Dey, A., Brown, P., et al.: Towards a better understanding of context and context-awareness. In: Gellersen, H.-W. (ed.) HUC 1999. LNCS, vol. 1707. Springer, Heidelberg (1999)
2. Krejcar, O.: User Localization for Intelligent Crisis Management. In: AIAI 2006, 3rd IFIP Conference on Artificial Intelligence Applications and Innovation, Boston, USA, pp. 221–227 (2006)
3. Krejcar, O., Cernohorsky, J.: Database Prebuffering as a Way to Create a Mobile Control and Information System with Better Response Time. In: Bubak, M., van Albada, G.D., Dongarra, J., Sloot, P.M.A. (eds.) ICCS 2008, Part I. LNCS, vol. 5101, pp. 489–498. Springer, Heidelberg (2008)
4. Krejcar, O.: PDPT Framework - Building Information System with Wireless Connected Mobile Devices. In: ICINCO 2006, 3rd International Conference on Informatics in Control, Automation and Robotics, Setubal, Portugal, August 01-05, 2006, pp. 162–167 (2006)
5. Krejcar, O., Cernohorsky, J.: New Possibilities of Intelligent Crisis Management by Large Multimedia Artifacts Prebuffering. In: Ulieru, M., Palensky, P., Doursat, R. (eds.) I.T. Revolutions 2008. LNICST, vol. 11, pp. 44–59. Springer, Heidelberg (2008)
6. Nielsen, J.: Usability Engineering. Morgan Kaufmann, San Francisco (1994)
7. Haklay, M., Zafiri, A.: Usability engineering for GIS: learning from a screenshot. The Cartographic Journal 45(2), 87–97 (2008)
8. Evennou, F., Marx, F.: Advanced integration of WiFi and inertial navigation systems for indoor mobile positioning. Eurasip journal on applied signal processing (2006)
9. Arikan, E., Jenq, J.: Microsoft SQL Server interface for mobile devices. In: Proceedings of the 4th International Conference on Cybernetics and Information Technologies, Systems and Applications/5th Int. Conf. on Computing, Communications and Control Technologies, Orlando, FL, USA, July 12-15 (2007)
10. Jewett, M., Lasker, S., Swigart, S.: SQL server everywhere: Just another database? Developer focused from start to finish. DR DOBBS Journal 31(12) (2006)
11. Krejcar, O.: Utilization Possibilities of Area Definition in User Space for User-Centric Pervasive-Adaptive Systems. In: Hesselman, C., Giannelli, C. (eds.) Mobilware 2009 Workshops. LNICST, vol. 12, pp. 124–130. Springer, Heidelberg (2009)
12. Janckulik, D., Krejcar, O., Martinovic, J.: Personal Telemetric System – Guardian. In: Biodevices 2008, Insticc Setubal, Funchal, Portugal, pp. 170-173 (2008)

Reliable Communications Using Multi-layer Transmission

Abdel-Nasser Assimi, Charly Poulliat, and Inbar Fijalkow

ETIS, ENSEA, Université Cergy-Pontoise, CNRS
Cergy-Pontoise F-95000, France
{abdelnasser.assimi,charly.poulliat,inbar.fijalkow}@ensea.fr

Abstract. In this paper, we propose a MIMO approach for packet combining in hybrid automatic repeat request (HARQ) protocols using single-carrier multi-layer transmission over block fading channels. Based on this model, the problem of the optimization of the linear superposition coefficients is briefly addressed.

Keywords: Hybrid-ARQ, superposition coding.

1 Introduction

Multi-layer transmission is an efficient technique to improve data throughput when no channel state information (CSI) is available at the transmitter [1]. This is a promising technique for future extensions of the third generation mobile systems 3GPP-LTE (Long-Term-Evolution) standard [2]. In multi-layer transmission, multiple coded packets, each of which is referred to as a *layer*, are simultaneously transmitted using linear superposition of the modulated packets. Each layer is allocated a transmission rate and a transmitting power under the constraint of a fixed average total power per transmission. The performance of a multi-layered transmission system depends on the efficiency of the receiver in separating the different layers taking into account the effect of the channel on the transmitted signal. Reliable data communication systems usually implement HARQ protocols in order to combat against errors introduced by the communication channel. The design of HARQ protocols for multi-layer transmission must take in the account layered structure of the signal in order to help the receiver in layer separation and decoding. In this paper,[1] we address the receiver structure and the design of the HARQ protocols for better system performance.

2 Multi-layer Transmissions

We consider a multi-layered transmission where the transmitted signal $\mathbf{x}$ is formed by linear superposition of K modulated and interleaved packets $\mathbf{s}^{(k)}$,

---

[1] This work was supported by the project URC of the Pôle de compétitivité SYSTEM@TIC.

R. Mehmood et al. (Eds.): EuropeComm 2009, LNICST 16, pp. 306–309, 2009.

$$\mathbf{x} = \sum_{k=1}^{K} a^{(k)} \mathbf{s}^{(k)} \, , \tag{1}$$

with $a^{(k)} = \rho_k \exp(j \, \theta_k)$ where ρ_k is a scaling factor and θ_k is a phase-shift ($\theta_k \in [0,2\pi[$). The scaling parameters ρ_k determine the allocated power to each layer under the constraint of a unit average transmitted power, i.e. $\Sigma_k (\rho_k)^2 = 1$. Whereas, the phase-shift angles θ_k determine the shape of the combined constellation. In each layer, an information data packet $\mathbf{d}^{(k)}$, including CRC bits for error detection, is first encoded by a forward error correction code (FEC) to obtain the coded sequence $\mathbf{c}^{(k)}$ having $2N$ coded bits. Different coding rates may be used for each layer. However, we assume in this paper that the same code is used for all layers. This simplifies the system complexity by using the same encoder and decoder for all layers. The coded sequence is then interleaved using a pseudo-random interleaver $\Pi^{(k)}$ and mapped mapped to a sequence $\mathbf{s}^{(k)}$ of N complex symbols using a Gray-mapped QPSK modulation.

We consider a single-input single-output transmission system through a flat fading channel. The received signal at the instant t is given by

$$\mathbf{y}_t = \sqrt{\gamma} h_t \mathbf{x}_t + \mathbf{n}_t \, , \tag{2}$$

where $\sqrt{\gamma}$ is average transmitted power, h_t is the complex channel gain and $\mathbf{n}_t$ is the noise vector, with elements that are i.i.d. complex Gaussian random variables with zero mean and unit variance. We assume that the channel gain h remains constant during the period of one block transmission and may change from one block to another depending on the channel model. After the decoding of the received signal by the receiver, an ACK signal is returned to the transmitter for each correctly decoded layer through an error free feedback channel, whereas a NACK signal is returned for layers in error. In the case of successful decoding of all layers, the transmitter sends another block containing new K packets. Otherwise, the transmitter responds resending a block of K packets including the erroneous packets and eventually new packets on the correctly decoded layers. This is the main difference with the rateless coding [3] problem where the retransmission contains retransmitted layers only. The retransmission continues for each packet until the correct reception or a maximum number M of transmissions per packet have been reached. In the latter case, the packet in error is dropped out from the transmission buffer and an error is declared.

3 Equivalent MIMO Channel Model

At the time t, the received block contains a maximum of K layers consisting of a combination of retransmitted and new packets. Let $M_{t,k}$ be the number of transmissions of the k-th layer at the instant t. Naturally, for new transmitted layers, we have $M_{t,k} = 1$. One can see the multi-layer transmission as a multiple-input single-output (MISO) system with K transmitting antennas,

$$y_t = \sqrt{\gamma} \sum_{k=1}^{K} \tilde{h}_t^{(k)} s_t^{(k)} \, , \tag{3}$$

where $\widetilde{h}_t^{(k)} = a_t^{(k)}h_t$ is the equivalent channel for the k-th layer by considering the linear coefficients $\{a^{(k)}\}$ as part of the channel. The received block is initially stored in a buffer of size M blocks. The buffer contains the current received block and the $M-1$ previously received signal after removing the contribution of correctly decoded packets in previous transmissions. Thus, the buffered blocks contain undecoded layers only. The buffered block is referred to by the variable $\underline{y}_t$. In fact, we distinguish between three types of undecoded packets: the new packets ($M_{t,k} = 1$), the active packets which have not yet reached the maximum number of transmissions ($1 < M_{t,k} \leq M$), and the dropped packets which had been expired the maximum number of transmissions. We denote by K_n, K_a, and K_d the number of new, active and dropped packets respectively. Note that $K_n + K_a = K$. We regroup the undecoded packets in the same matrix $\mathbf{S}_t = [\mathbf{s}_1, \ldots, \mathbf{s}_{Ku}]^T$, where $K_u = K_n + K_a + K_d$. The first K_a lines include the active packets, next the K_n new packets, and then the K_d dropped packets. The equivalent MIMO model between the undecoded packets and the buffered signals can be written as

$$\underline{\mathbf{Y}}_t = \sqrt{\gamma}\mathbf{H}_t\mathbf{S}_t + \mathbf{N}_t \, , \qquad (4)$$

where $\underline{\mathbf{Y}}_t = [\underline{y}_t, \ldots, \underline{y}_{t-M+1}]^T$, $\mathbf{N}_t = [\mathbf{n}_t, \ldots, \mathbf{n}_{t-M+1}]^T$, $\mathbf{H}_t$ is the $M \times K_u$ equivalent channel response for the undecoded packets defined by their elements as

$$[\mathbf{H}]_{i,j} = \varepsilon_{i,j}\widetilde{h}_{t-i+1}^{(k_j)} \, , \qquad (5)$$

for $1 \leq i \leq M$, and $1 \leq j \leq K_u$, where k_j is the number of layer used to transmit the j-th packet. $\varepsilon_{i,j} = 1$ if an the undecoded packet $\mathbf{s}_j$ was transmitted at the time $(t - i + 1)$, and $\varepsilon_{i,j} = 0$ otherwise. Since we are interested in the decoding of active layers only, the dropped packets in our MIMO model plays the role of additional noisy transmitting antennas.

Now, having determined the equivalent MIMO channel model for multiple HARQ layered transmissions, we can apply classical methods for MIMO detection in order to separate layers as in [4]. For successive interference cancellation (SIC), the receiver performs a layer by layer detection and decoding in the descending order of the received power per layer. Under the minimum mean square error (MMSE) detection, the j-th active packet is given by

$$\hat{\mathbf{s}}_j = \mathbf{w}_j^H\underline{\mathbf{Y}}_t \, , \text{with} \quad \mathbf{w}_j^H = \sqrt{\gamma}\mathbf{h}_j^H(\mathbf{I}_M + \gamma\mathbf{H}_t\mathbf{H}_t^H)^{-1} \, , \qquad (6)$$

where $(\cdot)^H$ denotes the complex conjugate transpose and $\mathbf{h}_j$ is the j-th column of the matrix $\mathbf{H}_t$.

4 Linear Layer-Time Coding

In order to determine the best choice for the linear coefficients at the current transmission, we maximize the instantaneous channel capacity C_t assuming Gaussian source distribution $C_t = \log_2(\det[\mathbf{I}_M + \gamma\mathbf{H}_t\mathbf{H}_t^H]) = \log_2(\det[\Gamma_t])$. Applying Hadamard's inequality [5] to Γ_t, we find that the determinant of Γ_t is maximized when the lines of the channel response $\mathbf{H}_t$ are orthogonal. Since the current transmission does not contain any dropped packet, and the new transmitted packets are only contained in the current transmission, the orthogonality condition reduces to the orthogonality within the re-transmitted packets only

$$\psi_i = h_t h_{t-i}^* \sum_{j=1}^{K_a} \varepsilon_{i+1,j} a_t^{(k_j)} (a_{t-i}^{(k_j)})^* = \delta_i \ , \tag{7}$$

for $i = 0, \ldots, M-1$ This condition can not be satisfied always depending on the values of $\varepsilon_{i+1,j}$. However, minimizing the total squared correlation $\Sigma_i |\psi_i|^2$ leads to an optimal solution. In addition, the condition (7) does not specify the power repartition between the active packets and the new packets. When the channel gain is unknown to the transmitter, this problem is subject to some trade-off between the dropping rate and the data throughput in the system. For example, when the total available power is allocated to the active packets, i.e. no new packets are transmitted until the complete decoding of the active packets, this would reduce the frame error rate in the system at the expense of reduced throughput for high signal to noise ratio. This point remains subject for future works.

5 Conclusions

We presented in this paper a MIMO approach for packet combining in HARQ protocols using multi-layer transmission. This model takes into the account the colored nature of the noise for a SIC receiver and the effect of the previously dropped packets on the current decoding. Moreover, this approach allows optimizing the linear superposition coefficients for better HARQ performance.

References

1. Steiner, A., Shamai, S.: Multi-layer broadcasting hybrid-ARQ strategies for block fading channels. IEEE Trans. Wireless Commun. 7(7), 2640–2650 (2008)
2. 3GPP, Technical Specifications, 3GPP TR25.913 V7.3.0 (March 2006),
   http://www.3gpp.org/ftp/Specs/htmlinfo/25913.htm
3. Erez, U., Trott, M.D., Wornell, G.W.: Rateless Coding and Perfect Rate-Compatible Codes for Gaussian Channels. In: IEEE Int. Symp. Inf. Theory, July 9-14, pp. 528–532 (2006)
4. Chen, J., Jin, S., Wang, Y.: Reduced Complexity MMSE-SIC Detector in V-BLAST Systems. In: Proc. PIMRC 2007, September 3-7 (2007)
5. Horn, R.A., Johnson, C.: Matrix Analysis. Cambridge University Press, Cambridge (1985)

Effects of the Distinction between Long and Short Data Grants in DOCSIS Network

Joon-Young Jung[1] and Jae-Min Ahn[2]

Information and Communication Engineering Department,
Chungnam National University, Daejeon, Korea
jungjy@etri.re.kr, jmahn@cnu.ac.kr

Abstract. In this paper, we analyze the effects of the distinction between long and short data grants in the Data Over Cable Service Interface specifications (DOCSIS) protocol. According to DOCSIS specifications, the grants for a bandwidth request of a cable modem can be for either short or long data packets. The threshold value classifying a short and long data packet is a system operation parameter and is determined by a cable modem termination system (CMTS). We have tried to find the effect of the distinction at the point of efficiency and robustness. For this, we have checked the bit error rate and transmission efficiency for burst profiles defined in a commercial CMTS.

Keywords: CMTS, CM, DOCSIS, Bandwidth Allocation, Short and Long data grant.

1 Introduction

Since hybrid fiber coaxial networks provide economical access to broadband networks, many companies are exploring the support of digital interactive communications over cable television (CATV) networks [1], [2]. Data Over Cable Service Interface Specifications (DOCSIS) is a standard designed to support data communications over CATV networks. Recently, DOCSIS 3.0 was issued from Cable Television Laboratory, Inc. (CableLabs).

According to DOCSIS, the grants for a bandwidth request of a cable modem (CM) can be either for short or long data packets. The threshold value classifying a short and long data packet is a system operation parameter and is broadcasted by a cable modem termination system (CMTS). DOCSIS allows a short data grant to use forward error control (FEC) parameters that are appropriate to short packets, while a long data grant may take advantage of greater FEC coding efficiency [3]. This means that the distinction allows for the use of different levels of error correction overhead in order to provide a good balance of efficiency and robustness. However, providing such a balance is very difficult, as there are many combinations of physical parameters within the decision of system operation parameters. Therefore, using a real field system, we will check the effect of the distinction at the point of efficiency and robustness.

R. Mehmood et al. (Eds.): EuropeComm 2009, LNICST 16, pp. 310–315, 2009.

2   Robustness of DOCSIS Upstream Channel

The modulation format of a DOCSIS upstream burst can be quadrature phase shift keying (QPSK), 8 quadrature amplitude modulation (QAM), 16QAM, 32QAM, 64QAM, or 128QAM. For a general performance analysis, we assume a Gaussian channel and a matched filter reception. In this case, the bit error rate (BER) for M-QAM, where $M = 2^k$ and k is even, is

$$P_b \approx \frac{4(\sqrt{M} - 1)}{\sqrt{M}\,\log_2 M} Q\left(\sqrt{\left(\frac{3\log_2 M}{M-1}\right)\frac{E_b}{N_0}}\right),\qquad(1)$$

where E_b/N_0 is the average signal-to-noise ratio (SNR) per bit [4] and can be applied as $(5/4)(S/N)(1/log_2 M)$ in DOCSIS. When k is odd, we can use a tight upper bound,

$$P_b \le \frac{4}{\log_2 M} Q\left(\sqrt{\left(\frac{3\log_2 M}{M-1}\right)\frac{E_b}{N_0}}\right)\qquad(2)$$

for any $k \ge 1$ [5].

The DOCSIS upstream FEC is able to provide Reed-Solomon (RS) Codes over GF(256) with $T=1$ to 16, or no RS coding for each burst type. It also provides the codeword length from a minimum size of 18 bytes (16 information bytes plus two parity bytes for $T=1$ error correction) to a maximum size of 255 bytes. In a (n, k, T) RS code, when an uncorrectable error pattern occurs, if the received codeword will be not modified and output by the decoder directly, then the symbol error density at the decoder output can be expressed as

$$P_S = \sum_{i=T+1}^{n} \left(\frac{i}{n}\right)\binom{n}{i} p^i (1-p)^{n-i}\qquad(3)$$

where p is the RS symbol error probability at the decoder input.

3   Efficiency of DOCSIS Upstream Channel

To check the transmission efficiency of a DOCSIS upstream channel, we present its definition as

$$Transmission\,Efficiency = \frac{Information\,Data\,Amount}{Assigned\,Bandwidth}.\qquad(4)$$

In order to obtain the transmission efficiency of (4), it is necessary to understand the bandwidth assignment mechanism for the DOCSIS upstream channel. Factors considered for the bandwidth assignment are mini-slot size, modulation format, symbol rate, FEC overhead, preamble length, and guard time. The mini-slot size is expressed as the number of 6.25 microsecond time-ticks. The mini-slot is used as the base unit for the bandwidth assignment. The example in Table 1 relates the mini-slot to the time ticks assuming QPSK modulation [3]. The symbols/byte is a characteristic of an individual burst transmission, not of the channel. A mini-slot in this instance could represent a minimum of 16 bytes or a maximum of 48, depending on the modulation format.

Table 1. Example Relating Mini-Slot to Time Tick

Parameter	Example Value
Time Tick	6.25 microsecond
Bytes per mini-slot	16 (nominal, when using QPSK modulation)
Symbols/byte	4 (assuming QPSK)
Symbols/second	2,560,000
Mini-slots/second	40,000
Microseconds/mini-slot	25
Ticks/mini-slot	4

The FEC is divided into the fixed codeword mode and the shortened last codeword mode in DOCSIS. The total data amount, D, including the FEC overhead for each mode is calculated as follows: For the fixed mode,

$$D = \begin{cases} q \times (k + 2T) & , r = 0 \\ (q+1) \times (k + 2T) & , r \neq 0 \end{cases}, \tag{5}$$

while for the shortened last codeword mode,

$$D = \begin{cases} q \times (k + 2T) & , r = 0 \\ q \times (k + 2T) + (16 + 2T) & , 0 < r < 16 \\ q \times (k + 2T) + (r + 2T) & , r \geq 16 \end{cases}, \tag{6}$$

where q and r are respectively the quota and remainder of (m/k), and m is the total information bytes to be transmitted.

The preamble uses the QPSK constellation with preamble length 0, 2, 4,..., or 1536 bits (maximum 768 QPSK symbols). The guard time is the number of modulation intervals (e.g. symbols) measured from the end of the last symbol of one burst to the beginning of the first symbol of the preamble of an immediately following burst. Let M be the mini-slot size (i.e., time-ticks/mini-slot), T_S be the number of modulation symbols per time-tick (i.e., symbols/time-tick), S_P be the preamble length (i.e., symbols), S_G be the guard time (i.e., symbols) and B_{sym} be the number of bits per modulation symbols. Then, the required bandwidth (i.e., the number of mini-slots) for transmitting m bytes can be calculated as

$$N_{mini-slot} = \left\lfloor \left\lfloor \left(\lfloor D \times 8 / B_{sym} \rfloor + S_P + S_G \right) / T_S \right\rfloor / M \right\rfloor, \tag{7}$$

where D is the number of transmitting data bytes from (5) or (6). Therefore, the transmission efficiency of (4) can be expressed as

$$Transmission\,Efficiency = \frac{m \times 8 / B_{sym}\,(symbols)}{N_{mini-slot} \times M \times T_s\,(symbols)}.$$

(8)

4 Comparison for Short and Long Data Grant

The burst profiles of Table 2 are three default modes defined in the ARRIS CMTS, which operates in the real field. Each profile for a short and the long data grant is compared at the point of error correction performance and transmission efficiency. The transmission efficiency is evaluated by (7) and the error correction performance is evaluated by (1), (2), and (3). In these evaluations, the assumed mini-slot size is 4 time-ticks and applied modulation rate is 2.56 mega-symbols/second.

Table 2. ARRIS CMTS Burst Profiles

Mode	1		2		3	
Profile	Short	Long	Short	Long	Short	Long
Modulation Type	qpsk	qpsk	16qam	16qam	64qam	64qam
Preamble length	84	96	168	192	104	104
Diff. encoding	No	No	No	No	No	No
FEC T bytes	6	8	8	10	12	16
FEC CW Size	78	220	78	220	78	220
Scramble Seed	0x152	0x152	0x152	0x152	0x152	0x152
Max Burst Size	15	0	8	0	6	0
Guard time size	8	8	8	8	8	8
Last CW short	Yes	Yes	Yes	Yes	Yes	Yes
Scramble	Yes	Yes	Yes	Yes	Yes	Yes
Interleaver Depth	1	1	1	1	1	1
Channel type	TDMA	TDMA	TDMA	TDMA	TDMA	TDMA

Figure 1 compares the BER performances of the short and long data grant profile for each mode. Generally, the BER performance required in DOCSIS is 10E-8. In order to obtain a BER of 10E-8, the required SNR for each profile of each mode is similar. In each mode, the short profile simply has an SNR gain of about 0.3 dB at 10E-8 BER. This result shows that the performance of short and long data grants are almost the same at the point of robustness. That is, the use of a long data grant with the higher coding efficiency for a long data packet is very appropriate.

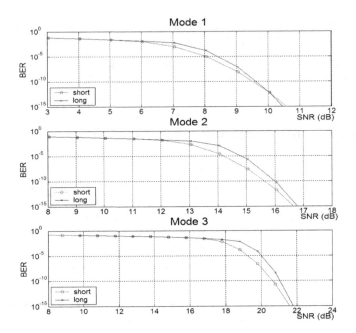

Fig. 1. BER performance comparison

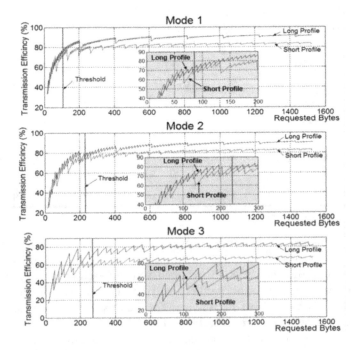

Fig. 2. Efficiency performance comparison

Figure 2 compares the transmission efficiency of short and long data grant profiles according to the number of transmitting bytes. In this comparison, when the number of transmitting bytes was small, the transmission efficiency of the short data grant profile was a little bit better. As the number of bytes increased, the transmission efficiency of the long data grant was more improved. Here, the point to pay attention to is the threshold, that is, the maximum burst mini-slot size of Table 2 classifying the short and long data grants. There exists a part in which the transmission efficiency of a long data grant is higher than that of a short one in the lower threshold. Also, the efficiency difference is very small in the lower threshold. That is, it shows that the use of a short data grant is not appropriate at the point of efficiency.

From the results of Figure 1 and 2, we have known that, without the distinction between long and short data profile, the use of one optimized profile with a high coding efficiency is effective because the advantage of using the short data grant could not be found at the point of the transmission efficiency.

5 Conclusion

From the comparisons described herein, we have found that the distinction cannot provide great effectiveness at the point of transmission efficiency. The object of the distinction is to provide a good balance of efficiency and robustness according to the packet length. But, in our analysis, the distinction provided very little benefit. Rather, it increases the complexity of the request and grant process. Therefore, we recommend that one optimized profile should be used for a data grant without a distinction between long and short. The use of one optimized profile is possible in the queue-depth based request of a DOCSIS 3.0 network.

References

1. Dai, P., Zhang, X., Wang, Q., et al.: A fast and efficient algorithm for computing bandwidth requested mini-slots over HFC. In: International Conference on WCNM 2005, September 23-26, 2005, vol. 1, pp. 419–422 (2005)
2. Kuo, W.-K., Kumar, S., Kuo, J., et al.: Improved priority access, bandwidth allocation and traffic scheduling for DOCSIS cable networks. IEEE Transactions on Broadcasting 49(4), 371–382 (2003)
3. CM-SP-MULPIv3.0-I05-070803, "DOCSIS 3.0 MAC and Upper Layer Protocols Interface Specification," Cable Television Laboratories, Inc., August 03 (2007)
4. Sklar, B.: Digital Communications: Fundamentals and Applications, 2nd edn., p. 565. Prentice Hall, Englewood Cliffs (2001)
5. Smith, D.R.: Digital Transmission Systems, 3rd edn., p. 439. Kluwer Academic Publishers (KAP), Boston (2004)

Author Index

Printed in the United States
by Baker & Taylor Publisher Services